Emergency Abdominal Surgery

CLINICAL SURGERY INTERNATIONAL

VOL 17

Emergency Abdominal Surgery

EDITED BY

R. C. N. WILLIAMSON
Professor and Director of Surgery
Royal Postgraduate Medical School
Hammersmith Hospital
London, UK

M. J. COOPER
Consultant Surgeon
Royal Devon and Exeter Hospital
Exeter, UK

CHURCHILL LIVINGSTONE
EDINBURGH LONDON MELBOURNE AND NEW YORK 1990

CHURCHILL LIVINGSTONE
Medical Division of Longman Group UK Limited

Distributed in the United States of America by Churchill
Livingstone Inc., 1560 Broadway, New York, N.Y. 10036,
and by associated companies, branches and representatives
throughout the world.

First published 1990
  Reprinted 1991

ISBN 0-443-03907-0
ISSN 0263–4422

British Library Cataloguing in Publication Data
Emergency abdominal surgery.
  1. Man. Abdomen. Acute abdomen. Surgery
  I. Williamson, Robin C. N. (Robin Charles Noel)
  II. Cooper, M. J.   III. Series
  617'.55059

Library of Congress Cataloguing in Publication Data
Emergency abdominal surgery/edited by R. C. N.
Williamson, M. J.
  Cooper.
    p. cm. — (Clinical surgery international,
  ISSN 0263–4422; vol. 17)
    1. Acute abdomen — Surgery. I. Williamson, Robin
  C. N. (Robin Charles Noel) II. Cooper, M. J. (Martin
  John)   III. Series: Clinical surgery international; v. 17.
    [DNLM: 1. Abdomen, Acute — surgery. W1 CL795U
  v. 17/WI 900 E53]
  RD540.E44 1990
  617.5'5059 — dc20
  DNLM/DLC
  for Library of Congress   89–22169
                                                  CIP

Produced by Longman Singapore Publishers (Pte) Ltd.
Printed in Singapore.

Preface

For fifty years or more emergency laparotomy has been the testing ground for the young surgeon. It is not always appropriate for out-of-hours emergencies to be delegated to juniors, since some of the conditions encountered will tax the stamina and skill of even the most experienced surgeons. Nevertheless, the discipline of reaching a diagnosis and then testing it by immediate operation will quickly refine a surgeon's powers of clinical assessment. Thus worldwide the acute abdomen offers unrivalled opportunities for surgical education, whether appendicitis, stab wounds or strangulated bowel are the commonest indication for opening the peritoneum.

In editing this book on emergency abdominal surgery we have set out to be selective rather than comprehensive, concentrating on new developments and conditions of topical interest. Thus hepatic trauma is covered but renal trauma is not; likewise peptic ulcers bleed but do not perforate. Most of the contributors are from the UK and the USA, with others from Australia and South Africa, reflecting perhaps the editors' own travel rather than any preconceived plan. We do think that we are lucky to have gathered such a strong international cast.

While it remains true that the decision to operate can be more important than the exact diagnosis, this is not always the case (for example in acute pancreatitis). In any event accurate diagnosis is not just an academic exercise: it will govern the preoperative preparation and the choice of incision, besides alerting the surgeon to the likely scope and complexity of the operation. It seems appropriate that the first chapter of this book should therefore be devoted to new methods of diagnosis applicable to the acute abdomen, including computer programmes, modern scanning techniques, laparoscopy, peritoneal lavage and fine catheter aspiration cytology.

In some parts of the world, abdominal trauma is still the commonest indication for urgent laparotomy, whether civil or military violence is to blame. Our book deals with injuries to the liver, bile ducts, pancreas, spleen, pelvis and lower urinary tract. Sepsis is the bugbear of any acute abdominal condition, and the complexities of septic shock are discussed in detail. The next ten chapters deal with most of the common gastrointestinal emergencies and some of the rarer fascinations like acute acalculous cholecystitis, colonic pseudo-obstruction and enteroliths (Chapter 13). Gynaecological emergencies are so much a part of the differential diagnosis of appendicitis that they deserve their own chapter. The book ends by considering two vascular causes of an acute abdomen, mesenteric ischaemia and ruptured aortic aneurysm.

Our goal has been to whet the appetite rather than to satiate. We have tried to include enough to stimulate abdominal surgeons at all levels of seniority, not forgetting those with impending examinations. The acute abdomen is a rigorous taskmaster, its successful management all the more satisfying.

London and Exeter, 1990   Robin Williamson
Martin Cooper

Contributors

Alan R. Berry ChM FRCS FRCSEd
Consultant Surgeon, Northampton General Hospital,
Northampton, UK

Edward L. Bradley III MD
Professor of Surgery, Emory University School of
Medicine, Atlanta, Georgia, USA

Peter L. Cass MRCOG
Lecturer and Senior Registrar, Department of
Obstetrics and Gynaecology, St Bartholomew's
Hospital, London, UK

Martin J. Cooper MS FRCS
Consultant Surgeon, Royal Devon and Exeter
Hospital, Exeter, UK

A. Cuschieri MD ChM FRCS
Professor of Surgery, Ninewells Hospital and Medical
School, Dundee, UK

Michael S. Dahn MD
Associate Professor of Surgery, Wayne State
University, Detroit, Chief, Surgical Intensive Care,
V.A. Medical Center, Allen Park, USA

Hugh Dudley CBE ChM FRCSEd FRACS
FRCS
Emeritus Professor of Surgery, London University,
London, UK

Brian F. Gilchrist MD
Department of Surgery, Oregon Health Sciences
University, Portland, Oregon, USA

D. Huber FRACS
Repatriation General Hospital, Concord, NSW,
Australia

C. D. Johnson MChir FRCS
Consultant Senior Lecturer, Department of Surgery,
Southampton General Hospital, Southampton, UK

M. R. B. Keighley MS FRCS
Professor of Surgery, The Queen Elizabeth Hospital,
Birmingham, UK

C. Kissin MRCP FRCR
Senior Registrar, Department of Radiodiagnosis,
Bristol Royal Infirmary, Bristol, UK

J. E. J. Krige FRCS FCS(SA)
Senior Lecturer, Department of Surgery, University
of Cape Town, Observatory, Cape Town, South Africa

Michael Lavelle-Jones MD FRCS FRCSEd
Lecturer in Surgery, Ninewells Hospital and Medical
School, Dundee, UK

David John Leaper MD ChM FRCS FRCSEd
Professor of Surgery, Department of Surgery,
Queen Mary Hospital, University of Hong Kong,
Hong Kong

Robert J. Lusby MD FRCS FRACS
Professor of Surgery, University of Sydney; Head,
Professorial Surgical Unit, Repatriation General
Hospital, Concord, NSW, Australia

Michael J. McMahon ChM PhD FRCS
Senior Lecturer in Surgery, University of Leeds;
Honorary Consultant Surgeon, General Infirmary,
Leeds, UK

Neil Mortensen MD FRCS
Consultant Surgeon and Clinical Lecturer in Surgery,
Department of Surgery and Gastroenterology, John
Radcliffe Hospital, Oxford, UK

Leslie W. Ottinger MD
Visiting Surgeon, Massachusetts General Hospital,
Boston, Massachusetts, USA

Simon Paterson-Brown DPhil FRCS FRCSEd
Lecturer in Surgery, Chinese University, Hong Kong

David J. Schoetz, Jr MD FACS
Chairman, Department of Colon Rectal Surgery,
Lahey Clinic Medical Center, Burlington,
Massachusetts, USA

Marcus E. Setchell FRCS FRCSEd FRCOG
Consultant Obstetrician and Gynaecologist, St
Bartholomew's and Homerton Hospitals, London, UK

Louis Solomon MD FRCS
Professor of Orthopaedic Surgery, University of
Bristol, Bristol Royal Infirmary, Bristol, UK

Michael John Stower DM FRCS
Consultant Urologist, York District Hospital, York,
UK

John Terblanche ChM FCS(SA) FRCS
FRCPS(Glasg.) FACS(Hon.)
Head of Department and Division of Surgery,
University of Cape Town Medical School,
Observatory, Cape Town, South Africa

W. E. G. Thomas BSc MS FRCS
Consultant Surgeon, Royal Hallamshire Hospital,
Sheffield, UK

Donald D. Trunkey MD
Professor and Chairman, Department of Surgery,
Oregon Health Sciences University, Portland,
Oregon, USA

J. Virjee FRCR
Consultant Radiologist, Department of
Radiodiagnosis, Bristol Royal Infirmary, Bristol, UK

Alexander J. Walt MS(Minn.) FRCS(Can.)
FRCS FACS
Professor of Surgery, Wayne State University,
Detroit, Michigan, USA

K. E. Wheatley FRCS FRCSEd
Research Fellow, The General Hospital, Birmingham,
UK

Robin C. N. Williamson MD MChir FRCS
Professor and Director of Surgery, Royal
Postgraduate Medical School, Hammersmith Hospital,
London, UK

Contents

1 *New diagnostic techniques in the acute abdomen*

This three-part Chapter reviews the use of four diagnostic techniques in the management of the acute abdomen, assessing their current value and extent of use. Two of the techniques are non-invasive, namely computer-aided diagnosis and new imaging methods (ultrasound, computerized tomography and radionuclide scanning), whereas laparoscopy and peritoneal lavage are more invasive, involving penetration of the abdominal wall and entry into the peritoneal cavity.

PART 1
Computer-aided diagnosis

D. J. LEAPER

Computer-aided diagnosis (CAD) is an exciting prospect for improving our clinical skills. Many studies have shown its value and accuracy in the field of acute abdominal pain over the last 10–15 years, yet it has become neither universally accepted nor established. Some centres, however, have found a place for CAD in patient management with an effective record, often involving junior medical staff or specially trained non-medical staff. Associated with this development has been the identification of several aspects of the clinical diagnostic process, notably why clinicians, particularly those in training, often fail to arrive at a diagnosis on which to hang a management decision. In addition, several authors have realized that by carefully documenting signs and symptoms

and following the discipline of giving a specific diagnosis to compare with a computer diagnosis, their own diagnostic record and decision making is improved.

Failure of accurate clinical diagnosis in the acute abdomen

Several studies have shown that there is a high degree of inaccuracy in the clinical diagnosis of acute abdominal pain. To some extent failure is related to the doctor's grade and experience, but several other factors are involved. It is clearly in the best interests of our patients to make the correct diagnosis and institute the correct treatment at an early stage. There is therefore the need to recognize failure and act to minimize this. An accurate diagnosis is rarely made of an acute abdomen by referring or receiving staff, often merely the diagnosis of 'acute abdomen' sufficing to admit the patient or refer them to a surgical team. There is little doubt that diagnosis at this level can be significantly improved, and this could prevent unnecessary admissions or allow referral to the most appropriate team, rather than all patients with abdominal pain being referred to the on-call surgical team. Thus pelvic inflammatory disease could be referred directly to the gynaecologists and the abdominal pain of diabetes to paediatricians or physicians. By expediting this process there is an obvious benefit to the patient plus a financial saving. In addition there is, surely, a pride in achieving a high diagnostic rate quickly without the need for prolonged or expensive investigations.

More experienced surgeons are more accurate in their diagnosis of abdominal pain. This is probably because they are able to reason heuristically and use relatively few items of information, whereas the junior surgeons in the accident and emergency department, or receiving patients on the ward, reason algorithmically. They glean all the information they can but become bogged down because they cannot utilize it effectively. This synthesis of course is what a computer can achieve easily if appropriately programmed. Nevertheless all of us are capable of poor diagnostic accuracy based on clinical assessment, presumably because we base our opinion on a wrong anecdote, cannot think in a truly probabilistic pattern or cannot handle large amounts of information.

So why has CAD not become established in the diagnosis of acute abdominal pain, with a computer terminal or access to a program available for this purpose, on surgical wards as it is for haematological and pathological results? Inevitably there must be 'physician suspicion' of computers taking over their time-honoured role. Ignorance of statistical analysis and probabilistic theory may prejudice interest, although this fear is likely to recede in the general surgical field with the continuously increasing numbers of surgeons who have written a thesis or engaged themselves in original scientific research. Another difficulty lies in the need to write down clinical information in a computer-codable form. Many would be unwilling to give their time for this, despite their acceptance of the computer in medicine. Coding can be very difficult: for example, how does one accurately and reproducibly distinguish between periodic, episodic, intermittent or colicky abdominal pain?

The realism of using a computer for diagnosis of abdominal pain is more likely to be seen by junior staff who are then able to be as effective as their seniors, particularly in out-of-hours admissions. Another way around the time factor is to use a physician's assistant, who may perhaps be resented as much as a computer presence. Although such assistants are a rarity in the UK, they can be as effective as fully trained medical staff (Lawrence et al 1987) and may allow a system to be usable in the clinic or at the bedside just like any other diagnostic aid. These assistants would be trained to translate clinical signs and symptoms into data that is acceptable to a computer, more quickly than the physician they assist. If effective, they would pay for themselves by avoiding expensive and time-wasting investigations. Clearly CAD could offer a great advantage to inexperienced staff in compromised areas: its use on submarines for diagnosing acute abdominal pain has been explored, for example (Osborne 1984).

The diagnostic process

Diagnosis, i.e. methods to achieve a management decision, is as old as medicine itself, but problems remain: we are still unable to qualify its logical steps and to facilitate the decision-making process. Many attempts have been made to dissect diagnostic pathways based on theory and on practical studies (Jaquez 1964, Lusted 1968, Gill et al 1973, Leaper et al 1973, De Dombal 1980, Wulff 1981, McCartney 1987). It is clear that senior clinicians are better diagnosticians and use few data to be effective, but how their intuition exists or works is enigmatic. It is more than just a simple pattern-matching process (De Dombal et al 1972b). There is little doubt that a computer can help to analyse much larger quantities of data, but the programming of a computer with an artificial intelligence based on experience is still a long way away. Nevertheless diagnostic dilemmas can be defined, particularly in a field such as acute abdominal pain, and signs and symptoms can be identified and recognised by computer programs. Interestingly, transcription of data to computer format and the complete filling in of proformas can improve performance. Thus the diagnostic accuracy can be improved for appendicitis (with fewer normal organs being removed) without risking an increased proportion of perforated or gangrenous appendices (De Dombal et al 1974, Adams et al 1986). The definition of terms for computer recognition is open to observer variation, but this variation lessens with practice (Gill et al 1973, Leaper et al 1973, Bjerregaard et al 1983). The importance of this definition is obvious, but it is probably changeable as disease toxonomy, let alone signs and symptoms, is arbitrary (Wulff 1981, McCartney 1987).

Methods of computer-aided diagnosis

The blunderbuss approach to CAD is to try to diagnose all diseases by simple comparison to an enormous data base (Okada et al 1977, Winter et al 1984). This approach would be impossible in practice, but a system that contained some appropriate data (rather than everything possible) or allowed some sort of dialogue, might permit diagnosis of rare disease (Pople et al 1975, Duda & Shortliffe 1983). Simple pattern matching using probabilities has been shown to be effective in abdominal pain (Graham 1977, Nixon & Rundle 1980), but more logical systems have expanded this to use simple algorithms to ask the next best question (Williams 1982), an interactive programme which guides the operator, or to employ a decision-tree pattern recognition to help with diagnosis (Kurzynski 1987).

Multiple logistic regression analysis works well with clearly defined data to help in diagnosis of pulmonary and cardiac function (Croft & Machol 1974, McCartney et al 1979, Habbema & Gelpke 1981), but it may not be so effective in the relatively imprecise field of abdominal pain (Van Way et al 1982). Cluster and connectivity analysis may allow further specificity (Atkin 1974), as they permit weighting techniques to give discrimination.

Connectivity analysis combined with 'fuzzy' logic has been used effectively in the diagnosis of acute abdominal pain. This analysis is based on a model of the vagueness of human reasoning and reflects the uncertainty of the clinical diagnostic process (Baldwin 1979, Norris et al 1985).

Knowledge-based systems, artificial intelligence or a combination of the two allow diagnosis to be modelled on human reasoning (Szolovits 1982, Spiegelhalter & Knill-Jones 1984, Reggia & Tuhrim 1985). Some workers have found this to have no great advantage over the time-honoured technique of Bayesian analysis (Fox et al 1980), which has been used extensively for CAD of acute abdominal pain and is probably the 'gold standard'.

CAD using Bayesian analysis

The 18th-century English cleric Thomas Bayes left us some of his mathematical thoughts, which were presumably formulated between his ecclesiastical chores. The principle of this type of analysis is first to set up a large data base of signs and symptoms, of preset and mutually exclusive disease processes, within a diagnostic field. This data base can be collected either retrospectively or prospectively. Acute abdominal pain is an ideal example of the sort of case to which this type of analysis can be applied and has, in fact, served as a template for research into the effectiveness of the different types of analysis. Once the probability of each sign or symptom has been determined for each disease, then new patient data can be prospectively compared with the data base and the cumulative probability of each disease can be calculated.

De Dombal's group in Leeds reported a high degree of success using Bayesian analysis of acute abdominal pain in the early 1970s (Horrocks et al 1972, De Dombal et al 1972a). In these studies they chose appendicitis, diverticulitis, perforated duodenal ulcer, non-specific abdominal pain, cholecystitis, small bowel obstruction and pancreatitis as the seven main disease categories. The overall diagnostic accuracy of the computing system (91.8%) was significantly higher than that of the most senior member of the surgical team — usually a registrar or senior registrar — who saw each case (76.9%). Many other groups have reported similar success in diagnosing abdominal pain in similar clinical circumstances (Gunn 1976) or in a different clinical environment (Wilson et al 1977, Graham & Wyllie 1979, Edwards 1986).

The difficulty with Bayesian analysis is that it gives simple probabilities only, which many clinicians may not understand when formulating a decision for management. It may be presumed to be 'right' or 'wrong', although the increased probability of a predicted disease tends to be related to increased accuracy of diagnosis. It is interesting to note that when clinicians are allowed to give their estimates of probabilities of signs or symptoms in the same categories of acute abdominal pain, they are often inaccurate. Surely, then, it is not just their inability to handle large amounts of data (which is so easily achieved by computer analysis) that makes them relatively inaccurate at prediction of disease but also the fact that they are unaware of probabilities (Leaper et al 1972)?

The data base for Bayesian analysis should be large, but it does not usually reflect changes in signs or symptoms in reaching its diagnosis, nor can it incorporate any 'weighting' of signs or symptoms easily elicited by repeated examination by the surgeon in charge. These data cannot readily by interrelated by Bayesian analysis, which makes the system rather rigid, but this does not seem to matter in practice (Seroussi 1986).

An abdominal pain data base cannot take in rare diseases, which usually have to be coded as non-specific abdominal pain. Although Meckel's diverticulitis would be diagnosed fairly accurately as appendicitis, thereby not allowing a failure in a decision to operate, salpingitis would be more likely to be diagnosed as non-specific abdominal pain and operation avoided. This category of non-specific abdominal pain is clearly unsatisfactory, particularly as follow-up of such patients can reveal important disease (Gray & Collin 1987). A second data base that only considers these more specific diagnoses may allow for greater accuracy.

The data entered into a data base might be expected to vary from area to area, but there is evidence that this is not in fact the case. The Leeds system has been shown to work on a multi-centre basis both in Finland (Ikonen et al 1983) and the UK, although it was not so accurate for diagnosis of small bowel obstruction (Adams et al 1986). It was reported as being unhelpful in a study from the United States (Van Way et al 1982), but the authors of this study used a slightly different method of analysis.

In conclusion, computer-aided diagnosis of acute abdominal pain has been proved to be effective. The use of Bayesian analysis, which is easy to operate despite certain drawbacks, is as accurate as more sophisticated, interactive, interrelated computer methods that employ artificial intelligence or 'fuzzy' logic. Why its use has not been more widespread is unclear.

REFERENCES

Adams I D, Chan M, Clifford P C et al 1986 Computer-aided diagnosis of acute abdominal pain: a multicentre study. British Medical Journal 293: 800–804

Atkin R H 1974 Mathematical structure in human affairs. Heinemann, London

Baldwin J F 1979 A new approach to approximate reasoning using a fuzzy logic. Fuzzy Sets and Systems 2: 309–325

Bjerregaard B, Brynitz S, Holst-Christensen J et al 1983 The reliability of medical history and physical examination in patients with acute abdominal pain. Methods of Information in Medicine 22: 15–18

Croft D J, Machol R E 1974 Mathematical methods in medical diagnosis. Annals of Biomedical Engineering 2: 69–89

De Dombal F T 1980 Diagnosis of acute abdominal pain. Churchill Livingstone, Edinburgh

De Dombal F T, Leaper D J, Staniland J R et al 1972a Computer-aided diagnosis of acute abdominal pain. British Medical Journal ii: 8–13

De Dombal F T, Smith R B, Modgill V K, Leaper D J 1972b Simulation of the diagnostic process: a further comparison. British Journal of Medical Education 6: 238–245

De Dombal F T, Leaper D J, Horrocks J C et al 1974 Human and computer-aided diagnosis of abdominal pain: further report with emphasis on performance of clinicians. British Medical Journal i: 376–380

Duda R O, Shortliffe E H 1983. Expert systems research. Science 220: 261–268

Edwards N H 1986 The accuracy of a Bayesian computer program for diagnosis and teaching in acute abdominal pain of childhood. Computer Programs in Biomedicine 23: 155–160

Fox J, Barber D, Bardhan K D 1980 Alternatives to Bayes? A quantitative comparison with rule-based diagnostic inference. Methods of Information in Medicine 19: 210–215

Gill P W, Leaper D J, Guillou P J et al 1973 Observer variation in clinical diagnosis — a computer-aided assessment of its magnitude and importance in 552 patients with abdominal pain. Methods of Information in Medicine 12: 108–113

Graham D F 1977 Computer-aided prediction of gangrenous and perforating appendicitis. British Medical Journal ii: 1375–1377

Graham D F, Wyllie F T 1979 Prediction of gall stone pancreatitis by computer. British Medical Journal i: 515–577

Gray D W R, Collin J 1987 Non-specific abdominal pain as a cause of acute admission to hospital. British Journal of Surgery 74: 239–242

Gunn A A 1976 The diagnosis of acute abdominal pain with computer analysis. Journal of the Royal College of Surgeons of Edinburgh 21: 170–172

Habbema J D F, Gelpke G J 1981 A computer program for selection of variables in diagnostic and prognostic problems. Computer Programs in Biomedicine 13: 251–270

Horrocks J C, McCann A P, Staniland J R et al 1972 Computer-aided diagnosis: description of an adaptable system and operational experience with 2034 cases. British Medical Journal ii: 5–9

Ikonen J K, Rokkanen P U, Gronroos P et al 1983 Presentation and diagnosis of acute abdominal pain in Finland: a computer aided study. Annales Chirurgiae et Gynaecologiae 72: 332–336

Jaquez J A 1964 The diagnostic process. Malloy, Ann Arbor

Kurzynski M W 1987 Diagnosis of acute abdominal pain using a three stage classifier. Computers in Biology and Medicine 17: 19–27

Lawrence P C, Clifford P C, Taylor I F 1987 Acute
abdominal pain: computer aided diagnosis by
non-medically qualified staff. Annals of the Royal College
of Surgeons of England 69: 231–232

Leaper D J, Horrocks J C, Staniland J R, De Dombal F T
1972 Computer-assisted diagnosis of abdominal pain using
estimates provided by clinicians. British Medical Journal
iv: 350–354

Leaper D J, Gill P W, Staniland J R et al 1973 Clinical
diagnostic process: an analysis. British Medical Journal
iii: 569–574

Lusted L B 1968 Introduction to medical decision making.
Thomas, Springfield

McCartney F J 1987 Diagnostic logic. British Medical
Journal 295: 1325–1331

McCartney F J, Rees P G, Daly K et al 1979 Angiographic
appearances of atrioventricular defects with particular
reference to distinction of ostium primum atrial septal
defect from common atrioventricular orifice. British Heart
Journal 42: 640–656

Nixon S J, Rundle J S H 1980 Computer-assisted diagnosis
of acute Crohn's disease. British Journal of Surgery
67: 352–354

Norris D, Jones R, Mathews B, Pilsworth B 1985
Developmental aspects of computer-aided diagnosis.
Bristol Medico-Chirurgical Journal 100: 101–105

Okada M, Maruyama N, Kanda T et al 1977 Medical data
base system with ability of automated diagnosis.
Computer Programs in Biomedicine 7: 163–170

Osborne S F 1984 Use of a computer-based Bayesian
method of analysis in an abdominal pain diagnostic
program. Journal of Occupational Medicine 26: 110–114

Pople H E, Myers J S, Millar R A 1975. Dialog: a model of
diagnostic logic for internal medicine. 4th International
Conference on Artificial Intelligence (quoted by Norris et
al 1985)

Reggia J A, Tuhrim S (eds) 1985 Computer assisted medical
decision making. Springer, New York

Seroussi B 1986 Computer-aided diagnosis and acute
abdominal pain when taking into account interactions.
Methods of Information in Medicine 25: 194–198

Spiegelhalter D J, Knill-Jones R P 1984 Statistical and
knowledge-based approaches to clinical decision-support
systems, with an application to gastroenterology. Journal
of the Royal Statistical Society 147: 35–77

Szolovits P 1982 Artificial intelligence in medicine.
Westview Press, Colorado

Van Way C W, III, Murphy J R, Dunn E L, Elerding S C
1982 A feasibility study of computer aided diagnosis in
appendicitis. Surgery Gynecology and Obstetrics
155: 685–688

Williams B T 1982 Clinical aids to clinical diagnosis, I–II.
CRC Press, Boca Raton

Wilson D H, Wilson P D, Walmsley R G et al 1977
Diagnosis of acute abdominal pain in the accident and
emergency department. British Journal of Surgery
64: 250–254

Winter R M, Baraitser M, Douglas J M 1984 A
computerized data base for the diagnosis of rare
dysmorphic syndromes. Journal of Medical Genetics
21: 121–123

Wulff H R 1981 Rational decision and treatment. Blackwell,
Oxford

PART 2
Methods of imaging

C. KISSIN and J. VIRJEE

Despite the rapid expansion of new diagnostic
techniques, plain radiography is still the most
commonly used imaging procedure in the evaluation of patients with acute abdominal symptoms.
The radiographs may be diagnostic in themselves
or, more frequently, they may provide information
to direct subsequent radiological evaluation. The
choice of imaging techniques available is now very
wide and includes contrast-medium examinations,
ultrasound (US), computerized tomography (CT),
nuclear medicine, angiography and magnetic
resonance imaging (MRI).

The modality that has been found to be the
most useful is ultrasound. This technique has
gained acceptance as a major diagnostic tool
largely because of the technological development
of real-time units and mechanical sector scanners.
The resultant accurate, high-resolution visualization of intra-abdominal structures has led to its
employment as the first imaging technique (after
plain films) in most abdominal emergencies, ex-
cluding those with primary bowel pathology such
as gastrointestinal bleeding, obstruction or perforation. Computerized, Doppler and endoscopic
ultrasound are also in use in some centres. Although CT has become much more widely
available over the last 10 years, it is still more expensive and time-consuming to perform than US
examination. It therefore tends to be employed
where US has failed because of bowel gas, obesity
or poor access. In addition, however, CT has particular advantages over US when an overview of
abdomen, pelvis and bony structures is required,
in assessing the extraluminal extent of gastrointestinal and vascular disease, and in enabling limited
tissue identification within a mass or collection.

The recent advances in nuclear medicine imaging involving the gastrointestinal tract have
improved the evaluation of those patients with
acute hepatobiliary pathology, acute lower
gastrointestinal bleeding and intra-abdominal
abscesses and inflammation. Contrast-media examinations of the bowel and urinary tract continue
to play an important role in the assessment of the

acute abdomen. In particular, however, the increasing awareness of pseudo-obstruction has led to an increase in the number of emergency enemas performed to identify the existence or site of an obstructing lesion, and the technique of small bowel enema examination has enabled more accurate assessment of some small bowel pathology.

The need for diagnostic angiography in the acute abdomen declined when US and CT were first introduced. It has now regained its popularity because of a wide acceptance of the value of interventional procedures and because of the development of digital subtraction techniques, which may permit the use of lower doses of contrast medium and less invasive procedures than those required for conventional arteriography. MRI is a modality which is still in its infancy in the UK. Its application to acute abdominal procedures has not yet been fully explored therefore. Indeed it is unlikely to have any real place until it is readily available in most radiology departments.

These techniques, or combinations thereof, have had an impact on the diagnosis of many conditions presenting with an acute abdomen. In particular they have a major role in the diagnosis of acute cholecystitis and pancreatitis, acute gastrointestinal haemorrhage, major trauma, aortic disease, intra-abdominal abscesses, acute appendicitis and diverticulitis.

Acute cholecystitis

Accurate diagnosis of acute cholecystitis is imperative when early cholecystectomy is to be considered, and three imaging techniques are now available. Some authors still stress the reliability of infusion cholecystography and claim a true positive rate of 88% (Dykes et al, 1984), but US and radionuclide scanning are the most popular imaging modalities at present. Cholescintigraphy is performed using one of the ^{99m}TC-labelled acetanilide iminodiacetic acid (IDA) derivatives. Non-visualization of the gallbladder with an otherwise patent biliary system implies obstruction of the cystic duct and thus acute cholecystitis (in both calculous and acalculous disease; Mauro et al 1982) (Fig. 1.1). Several similar pharmacological agents are now available (all having in common the N-

Fig. 1.1 Positive IDA scan. There is non-visualization of the gallbladder with an otherwise patent biliary system in a patient with symptoms and signs of acute cholecystitis.

substituted iminodiacetic structure), which will enable biliary visualization even with raised serum bilirubin levels. They also have a relatively low renal excretion, thus minimizing superimposition of renal activity over the gallbladder region. In the appropriate clinical setting cholescintigraphy has been reported to have over 95% sensitivity and specificity (Johnson & Coleman 1982). Following improvements in equipment and greater experience with its use, ultrasound has now been shown to have a similar predictive value. Despite the recognition of the significance of features such as uniformly decreased gallbladder wall echogenicity, the 'halo' sign (Schneider et al 1982) and the 'double wall' sign (Joseph 1983), the ultrasonographic findings most suggestive of acute cholecystitis remain the presence of gallstones, tenderness over the gallbladder and mural thickening.

Acute pancreatitis

In contrast to acute cholecystitis, the diagnosis of acute pancreatitis is essentially clinical and biochemical. Both US and CT can demonstrate the typical features of acute inflammation, but imaging techniques have a more important role in identifying complications. Contrast-enhanced CT, for

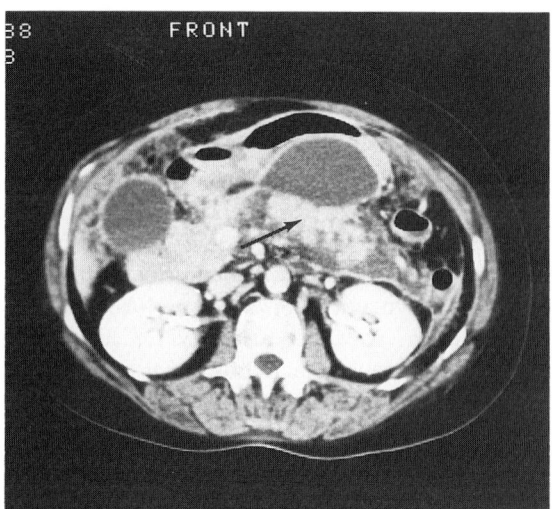

Fig. 1.2 Contrast-enhanced CT scan of the upper abdomen in a patient with severe acute pancreatitis. Viable pancreas (arrowed) takes up the intravenous contrast material as opposed to the pseudocyst that lies anteriorly and the necrotic peripancreatic fat that lies posterolaterally.

example, delineates necrotic tissue in severe necrotizing pancreatitis (Fig. 1.2), whilst US will demonstrate the presence of pseudocysts and enable their percutaneous drainage. In addition, the technique of endoscopic ultrasound is now available in some centres: the entire pancreas can be visualized by a combination of transduodenal and transgastric scanning, using a 7.5 mHz transducer incorporated into the tip of a fibroptic endoscope. The resultant high spatial resolution has been reported to demonstrate important new information about pancreatic inflammation, not obtained on previous imaging, in up to 30% of selected patients (Shorvan et al 1987).

Gastrointestinal haemorrhage

Imaging techniques play a major role in the diagnosis and management of acute gastrointestinal haemorrhage. Traditionally, endoscopy is performed as the first step in the management of upper gastrointestinal bleeding. Arteriography may then be performed if necessary, either for diagnosis or therapy. The endoscopic examination enables identification of the bleeding site and may detect features indicating the likelihood of rebleed-

ing (visible vessel, adherent clot). Endoscopic Doppler US, using a Doppler probe at the tip of the endoscope, is now being used to assess the patency of the artery beneath the bleeding point and thus predict the chances of rebleeding with greater accuracy (Beckly & Casebow 1986). Acute lower gastrointestinal bleeding does not always lend itself to endoscopy, and angiography has been considered to be the procedure of choice. However, because selective abdominal arteriography is invasive and expensive and may be difficult to perform, other less invasive diagnostic tests have been sought and radionuclide imaging studies have now gained acceptability. Two scintigraphic methods are currently in use: ^{99m}Tc sulphur colloid and ^{99m}Tc-labelled blood pool agents (red blood cells and albumin). Both are more sensitive than arteriography (Alavi & Ring 1981, McKusick et al 1981), being able to detect bleeding rates as low as 0.05–0.1 ml/min; indeed, angiography is likely to be negative if scintigraphy fails to show a bleeding focus. Sulphur colloid may be unable to identify upper GI bleeding, as hepatic and splenic activity may mask flexural bleeding sites, but labelled red cells can be used for upper and lower gastrointestinal haemorrhage and for intermittent

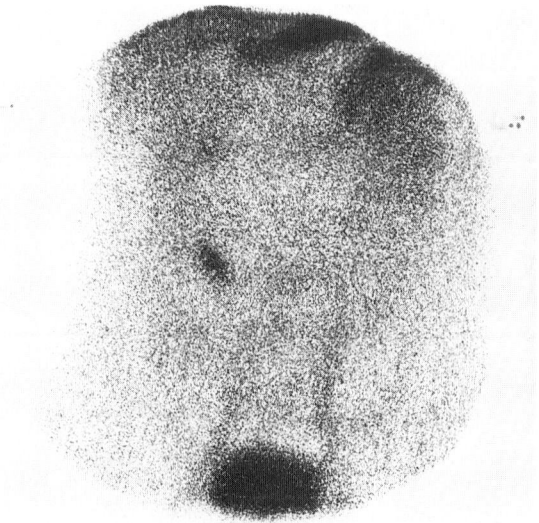

Fig. 1.3 Abnormal accumulation of ^{99m}Tc-labelled red cells indicating a bleeding site to the right of the umbilicus. Angiography was positive, and the patient (a woman of 75 years with melaena) was found to have bleeding from an inflamed jejunal diverticulum.

bleeding also. These examinations are most useful when performed before angiography either to eliminate the need for it or to guide the angiographer to the appropriate area (Fig. 1.3). Angiography itself is indicated prior to, or instead of, laparotomy, particularly where there is a history of previous surgery, suspected haemobilia or suspected small bowel bleeding, or where interventional therapy seems likely. It can identify the site and likely cause of bleeding at a rate of 0.5 ml/min and may enable non-surgical treatment by vascular infusion of constrictor drugs or by vascular embolization.

Trauma

New imaging techniques have made a large contribution to the diagnosis of visceral trauma. Abnormal fluid within the peritoneal cavity can be identified both on US and peritoneal lavage. Lavage will indicate the nature of the fluid, but US often detects the site of visceral damage, particularly in the upper abdomen. However, CT is of particular value because it is able to demonstrate the entire abdomen, pelvis, retroperitoneum and associated bony structures (Fig. 1.4) in one

examination. The expansion of angiographic catheter techniques has led to dramatic improvements in the diagnosis and therapy of major blunt pelvic trauma, in particular permitting the control of bleeding by embolization. In addition, whilst CT and US can image most retroperitoneal structures accurately, and Doppler US can be used to show renal avulsion or occlusion by detecting the absence of arterial waveforms from within the renal parenchyma (Taylor & Burns 1985), angiography remains the best modality for identifying isolated renal trauma including renal fracture and pedicular injury (Chakravarty 1986).

Aortic disease

In aortic disease US and CT have 97–100% sensitivity in the detection of aneurysmal dilatation, but angiography may still be necessary to determine if this is limited to the infrarenal portion. The diagnosis of aneurysmal rupture is usually made on clinical grounds alone and leads to immediate operation. When further evaluation is

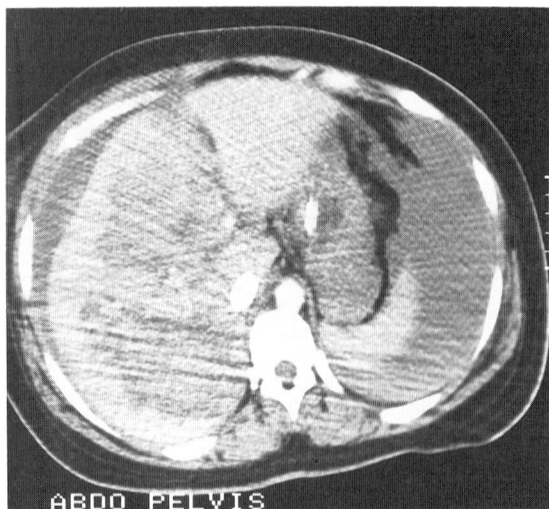

Fig. 1.4 CT scan of the upper abdomen in a 41-year-old unconscious woman after trauma. A right rib fracture was present, and there is haemorrhagic contusion of the liver with a considerable haemoperitoneum.

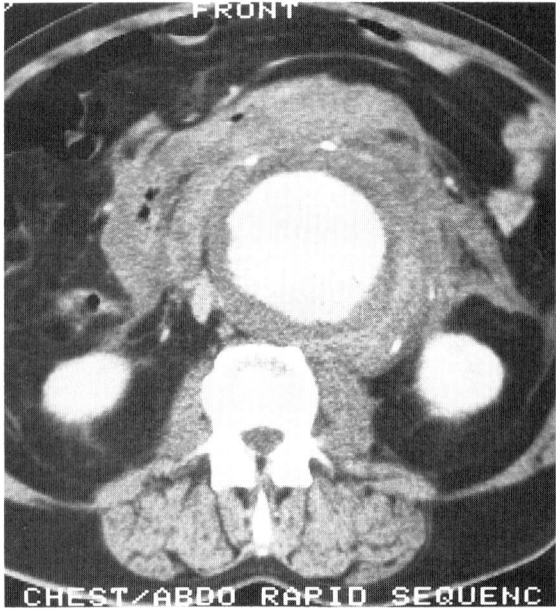

Fig. 1.5 A CT scan of the abdomen in a 70-year-old man showing marked aneurysmal dilatation of the abdominal aorta. There is a large retroperitoneal haemorrhage indicating aneurysmal rupture.

necessary, both US (provided that the accompanying ileus does not limit visualization) and CT can easily and reliably demonstrate the characteristic appearances of a dilated aorta and extensive retroperitoneal haemorrhage (Fig. 1.5). In aortic dissection real-time and Doppler US can clearly demonstrate the flap, with its characteristic undulating motion and two distinct patterns of flow in the true and false lumina, and also the extent of dissection. CT is thus often unnecessary and angiography only rarely indicated. With increasingly frequent aortic surgery, the frequency of complications presenting as an acute abdomen and the need to make accurate pre-operative diagnoses has increased. US and Doppler may demonstrate complications of aortoiliac grafts, but CT has been found to be most useful in the diagnosis of aortic graft–enteric fistulae by the identification of a periaortic mass with or without associated gas (Ackroyd et al 1985, Haaga et al 1978).

Intra-abdominal abscess

Ultrasound is usually employed as the first imaging technique in patients with suspected intra-abdominal abscesses and has an overall sensitivity of 82% (Knochel et al 1980). It may, however fail to

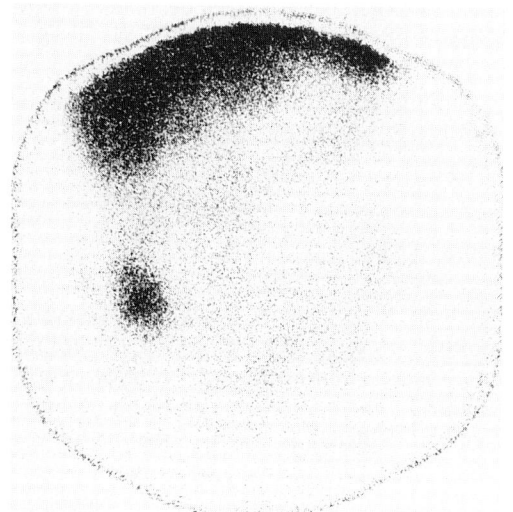

Fig. 1.6 Positive ^{111}In-labelled leucocyte scan (right iliac fossa abscess).

identify collections that are small or lie in the mid-abdomen or are obscured by bowel gas. In these situations, two radionuclide techniques are available. ^{111}In-labelled leucocyte scanning is superior to ^{67}Ga citrate owing to greater accumulation of the radionuclide in inflammatory lesions and the absence of colonic activity (Fig. 1.6), and it has a reported sensitivity of 93% in suspected intra-abdominal abscesses (Knochel et al 1980, Goldman et al 1987). However, CT has been found to be the most accurate imaging modality, with a sensitivity of 98%. All modalities have a specificity of 95% (Knochel et al 1980).

Acute appendicitis and diverticulitis

In some emergencies such as acute appendicitis and acute diverticulitis, the clinical diagnosis is obvious and appropriate treatment is implemented without radiological confirmation. In suspected acute appendicitis, however, there is still a false-positive laparotomy rate of 10–15% (Berry & Malt 1984). Attempts have therefore been made to reduce this figure and to shorten the clinical observation time in patients with atypical signs and symptoms by using accurate imaging techniques. Both sonography and scintigraphy have a high accuracy rate, but neither technique is widely utilized in the UK. The normal appendix is not visible on US scanning, but the demonstration of a non-compressible appendix with or without mural thickening, appendicoliths or localized periappendiceal fluid, has been shown to have 89% sensitivity, 95% specificity and 93% overall accuracy in the diagnosis of acute appendicitis (Puylaert 1986, Brooke Jeffrey et al 1987). In addition the ultrasound examination can identify gynaecological pathology as the cause of symptoms where appropriate. Similarly, ^{111}In-labelled leucocyte scanning is reported to have 86% sensitivity, 93% specificity, and 91% overall accuracy in the diagnosis of clinically atypical appendicitis (Navarro et al 1987).

In acute diverticulitis, when radiographic examination of the colon is indicated, the double contrast barium enema is the method traditionally used. Recently, however, CT has been advocated as an appropriate and useful imaging technique because of the superior definition of bowel wall thickness and the extent of extraluminal disease (Hulnick et al 1984; Johnson et al 1987).

New imaging techniques have thus had an appreciable impact on diagnosis in the acute abdomen. In conjunction with clinical data they enable a confident diagnosis to be made prior to, or without the need for, laparotomy in a large number of cases. The technique with the greatest impact is US, but radionuclides, CT and angiography have all made a valuable contribution.

REFERENCES

Ackroyd J, Williams T G, Lea Thomas M, Burnard K G 1985 The diagnosis of aortic graft-enteric fistulae by computed tomography. British Journal of Surgery 72: 72–73

Alavi A, Ring E J 1981 Localisation of gastrointestinal bleeding: superiority of ^{99m}Tc sulphur colloid compared with angiography. American Journal of Roentgenology 137: 741.

Beckly D E, Casebow M P 1986 Prediction of rebleeding from peptic ulcer, experience with an endoscopic Doppler device. Gut 27(1): 96–99

Berry J J R, Malt R 1984 Appendicitis near its centenary. Annals of Surgery 200: 567–575

Brooke Jeffrey R, Laing F C, Lewis F R 1987 Acute appendicitis: high resolution real-time ultrasound findings. Radiology 163: 11–14

Chakravarty M 1986 Utilisation of angiography in trauma. Radiologic Clinics of North America 24: 383–396

Dykes E H, Stewart I, Gray H et al 1984 Infusion cholecystography in the early diagnosis of acute gallbladder disease. British Journal of Surgery 71: 854–855

Goldman M, Ambrose N S, Drolc Z et al 1987 Indium-^{111} labelled leucocytes in the diagnosis of abdominal abscess. British Journal of Surgery 74: 184–186

Haaga J R, Baldwin G N, Reich N E et al 1978 CT detection of infected synthetic grafts: a preliminary report of a new sign. American Journal of Roentgenology 131: 317–319

Hulnick D H, Megibow A J, Balthazar E J et al 1984 Computed tomography in the evaluation of acute diverticulitis. Radiology 152: 491–495

Johnson D G, Coleman R E 1982 New technqiues in radionuclide imaging of the alimentary system. Radiologic Clinics of North America 20: 635–651

Johnson C D, Baker M E, Rice R P et al 1987 Diagnosis of acute colonic diverticulitis: comparison of barium enema and CT. American Journal Roentgenology 148: 541–546

Joseph A E A 1983 The gallbladder. In: Joseph A E A, Cosgrove D O, eds. Ultrasound in inflammatory disease. Churchill Livingstone, Edinburgh, pp. 161–183

Knochel J Q, Koehler P R, Lee T G et al 1980 Diagnosis of abdominal abcesses with CT, US and ^{111}In leucocyte scans. Radiology 137: 425

McKusick K A, Froelich J, Callahan R J et al 1981 Tc-99^m

red blood cells for detection of gastrointestinal bleeding: experience with 80 patients. American Journal of Roentgenology 137: 1113–1118

Mauro M A, McCartney W H, Melined J R 1982 Hepatobiliary scanning with ^{99m}Tc-PIPIDA in acute cholecystitis. Radiology 142: 193

Navarro D A, Weber P M, Kang I Y et al 1987 Indium-111 leukocyte imaging in appendicitis. American Journal of Roentgenology 148: 733–736

Puylaert J B C M 1986 Acute appendicitis: US evaluation using graded compression. Radiology 158: 355–360

Schneider M, Ribenstein W A, Auh Y H et al 1982 Ultrasonography and computed tomography in the evaluation of biliary tract disease. In: Thorbjarnason B., ed; Surgery of the biliary tract. Saunders, Philadelphia pp 19–60

Shorvan P J, Lees W R, Frost R A et al 1987 Upper gastrointestinal endoscopic ultrasonography in gastroenterology. British Journal of Radiology 60: 429–438

Taylor K J W, Burns P N 1985 Duplex doppler scanning in the pelvis and abdomen. Ultrasound in Medicine and Biology 11: 643–658

PART 3
Laparoscopy and peritoneal lavage

C. D. JOHNSON

Laparoscopy

The role of laparoscopy in the management of abdominal emergencies has been evaluated mainly in patients with abdominal trauma or acute abdominal pain. In this chapter we have considered only patients with trauma, suspected appendicitis or suspected peritonitis from causes other than appendicitis.

Trauma

In contrast to peritoneal lavage, laparoscopy has been little used in the evaluation of abdominal trauma. Yet certain advantages of laparoscopy are apparent: 1. when a haemoperitoneum is observed, the source of bleeding may be identified and subsequent operation planned appropriately; 2. the rate of bleeding and the amount of blood in the peritoneal cavity can be observed directly, enabling an early decision whether to submit the patient to laparotomy or a period of observation.

Berci and his colleagues (1983) reported an uncontrolled series in which they used a 4 mm diameter 'mini-laparoscope' to evaluate blunt abdominal trauma (97 patients) and penetrating stab wounds (9 patients). They excluded patients with gunshot wounds from their study, because there is a greater likelihood of injuries that require operation in this group. The laparoscopy was performed under local anaesthesia (with intravenous sedation when necessary) in the emergency room, intensive care unit or operating room, depending on the clinical circumstances. Patients were selected for laparoscopy if, in addition to abdominal trauma, they also had altered consciousness secondary to head injury or intoxication, or unexplained hypotension or equivocal physical signs. Fifty-seven patients (54%) had no abnormalities at laparoscopy, and all recovered uneventfully. Patients with a haemoperitoneum did not require laparotomy if the haemoperitoneum was small and no source of bleeding was found (12 patients), or if a source was found that did not require intervention, such as pelvic fractures (7 patients) or minor laceration of the liver, spleen or falciform ligament (8 patients). Patients were deemed suitable for observation in preference to laparotomy if the volume of blood was small (not filling a paracolic gutter) and did not increase, or if a moderate haemoperitoneum was found (up to 10 mm depth of blood in a paracolic gutter) and either a source was identified that was seen to have stopped bleeding, or else the blood did not reaccumulate after aspiration.

In 22 patients (21%) laparotomy was required, either because the above conditions were not met or because there was an obvious large haemoperitoneum (blood aspirated through the Verres needle prior to insufflation or loops of bowel lying in a pool of blood), or because free intestinal fluid was found within the peritoneal cavity. All but one of these patients had an injury that justified surgical intervention. These figures suggest that laparoscopy can be very helpful in the selection of patients for operation after blunt abdominal trauma or stab wounds. All the patients who required laparotomy were correctly identified, and only one (1%) unnecessary laparotomy was performed.

The results of this study appeal to the surgeon faced with abdominal trauma in that it suggests a means for more accurate assessment of intra-abdominal injuries than peritoneal lavage. Laparoscopy can be performed as speedily as lavage, and with no greater trauma to the patient, provided the narrow laparoscope is used. Confirmation of the superiority of laparoscopy in this setting is lacking, but the preliminary results of a more recent controlled trial are encouraging (Cuschieri et al 1987).

Results are available from one other large series of patients with laparoscopy for the diagnosis and management of blunt abdominal trauma, reported by Sundal and his colleagues (1982), who used laparoscopy largely to plan surgical priorities in patients with multiple trauma. Their laparoscopic findings were compatible with the surgical findings in 177 of 179 patients (99%). Sixty patients had no intra-abdominal bleeding, and all were correctly diagnosed by laparoscopy. Only two (1%) false negative laparoscopies were done. Unfortunately, insufficient details are given in this paper to judge whether laparoscopy was useful in the decision to proceed to laparotomy or to observe the patient.

Laparoscopy has also been used in the diagnosis of traumatic diaphragmatic hernia (Adamthwaite 1984). This report suggests a role for laparoscopy when this diagnosis is suspected but other investigations such as contrast radiology or CT scans are inconclusive or unavailable. The diagnosis of diaphragmatic rupture was confirmed at laparoscopy in 8 of 10 patients examined. The two patients with normal appearances at laparoscopy were managed conservatively with a successful outcome. Laparoscopy was only performed if more than 24 hours had elapsed since the injury, when intrapleural adhesions would have rendered thoracoscopy unreliable. There is a risk that laparoscopy might produce a tension pneumothorax by passage of gas through the diaphragmatic laceration, and if an intercostal drain is not already in position one should be immediately available during laparoscopy.

Appendicitis

Laparoscopy is a standard technique in gynaecology

for the diagnosis of lower abdominal and pelvic pain. General surgeons have been slow to take up this technique, but its value in the diagnosis of lower abdominal pain is becoming established. Laparoscopy can give better views of abdominal and pelvic contents than are possible through a gridiron incision. There are obvious advantages for a laparoscopy that demonstrates a normal appendix and no other condition requiring surgery. First, the patient is able to leave hospital sooner than if a normal appendix had been removed. Second, a diagnosis can often be achieved rather than presumed, without the need for a negative laparotomy, with consequent satisfaction and benefit in patient management. Minor complications after appendicectomy occur in up to 15% of cases, and major complications, though rare, may be life-threatening (Barnes et al 1962, Chang et al 1973, Lewis et al 1975, Pieper et al 1982, Dunn et al 1982).

Arguments raised against the use of laparoscopy are that if the patient does have appendicitis, then operating time has been increased by approximately 20 minutes, and also that if the appendix is removed as a diagnostic test of appendicitis, then at least the patient will never suffer appendicitis in the future. Furthermore, if the appendix is not visualized at laparoscopy, appendicectomy will still be required. These arguments appear to carry greater weight in the minds of many surgeons than the arguments in support of laparoscopic diagnosis, and the need to learn the technique, but the objective evidence favours laparoscopy as a means of reducing morbidity and hospital stay in an appreciable number of patients.

It must be conceded that in approximately one quarter of patients the appendix will not be visualized at laparoscopy. In a study where 75 patients were undergoing laparoscopy for gynaecological conditions, the appendix was not seen on 21 occasions (28%) (Paterson-Brown et al 1986a). In a further series of 81 patients with acute lower abdominal pain, the clinical diagnosis was appendicitis in 40 patients but the appendix was not visualized on nine occasions (22.5%) (Reiertsen et al 1985). Despite this handicap, laparoscopy is still able to improve diagnosis and reduce the need for surgery in patients with lower abdominal pain. Anderson and Bridgewater (1981) performed

laparoscopy in 27 patients who had presented with abdominal pain but had uncertain diagnoses. Nineteen were thought clinically to have appendicitis, but after laparoscopy only nine patients required appendicectomy. Fifteen patients had no operation after laparoscopy had shown either no abnormality or one of a variety of conditions that did not require operation.

Reiertsen and his colleagues avoided laparotomy in 16 of 40 patients thought to have appendicitis who underwent laparoscopy preoperatively. Clarke and others (1986) performed laparoscopy before operation in 46 patients with a confident diagnosis of appendicitis. Appendicectomy was avoided in 10 patients (22%).

In all these reports there is a clear preponderance of female patients, especially when laparoscopy is limited to the 'uncertain diagnosis' group. This fact is not surprising in view of the clinical difficulty of distinguishing appendicitis from disorders of the female genital tract, such as salpingitis, haemorrhage from follicular cysts and ectopic pregnancy.

Deutsch and colleagues (1982) focused on the subgroup of female patients of reproductive years, on the grounds that it is in this group that misdiagnosis and unnecessary appendicectomy is most likely. They performed laparoscopy in 36 patients in whom a diagnosis of acute appendicitis had been made. The diagnosis was revised to salpingitis or ruptured follicular cyst in one third of these cases and operation was avoided.

However, even when a more general view is taken, and patients with abdominal pain from all causes are considered, there are still demonstrable advantages to laparoscopy. Sugarbaker and co-authors (1975) compared two groups of patients with abdominal pain. In 27 with a definite clinical diagnosis requiring surgical intervention, laparotomy alone was performed and was negative in six. In 29 patients, laparoscopy was done preoperatively to establish the presence or absence of intra-abdominal disease, and 18 of these were managed without operation. One of the 11 laparotomy patients had pelvic inflammatory disease seen at laparoscopy, but operation was performed because the appendix was not visualized.

There are two points to be made concerning this

last study. For the patients with uncertain diagnoses, laparoscopy enabled a diagnosis to be made in all but one case and avoided operation in nearly two-thirds of cases. Secondly, the 'confident' diagnosis leading to laparotomy was incorrect in 22% of cases, whereas after laparoscopy the unnecessary laparotomy rate was 3%. The logical extension of these figures is to advise laparoscopy in all patients with abdominal pain, unless a confident diagnosis of a non-operative condition can be made. Universal application of laparoscopy before operation would, however, subject a considerable number of patients to a procedure that might add nothing to their management.

In a careful study, Dudley's group (Paterson-Brown et al 1986b) attempted to define the role of laparoscopy in the management of patients with abdominal pain. Of 222 consecutive patients, 42 were excluded for general contraindications to laparoscopy (see below), and 55 were not examined because of a preoperative diagnosis that was both firmly established and considered to contraindicate laparoscopy. These diagnoses were:

Intestinal obstruction
Visceral perforation
Acute pancreatitis
Abdominal trauma
Renal tract disease
Inflammatory bowel disease

They allocated the remaining patients to three groups: A, operation definitely indicated; B, operation definitely not indicated; C, decision uncertain. Group C was subdivided into those who, because of uncertainty, should have an operation ('look and see'), and those who should be observed ('wait and see'). All group C patients underwent laparoscopy. The study confirmed the previous findings of the usefulness of laparoscopy in patients in the group C category. Four 'look and see' patients and two 'wait and see' patients had their management decision altered following laparoscopy. Thus in the 31 patients in group C, six inappropriate management decisions were avoided by the use of laparoscopy. Eleven of 94 patients in groups A and B had inappropriate management, but only in group A (surgery definitely indicated) was it possible to define

clearly those who would benefit from laparoscopy. All seven of the operations which proved to be unnecessary were carried out for presumed appendicitis.

When laparoscopy is used to improve diagnosis, the more appropriate management of patients with conditions not requiring surgery significantly reduces hospital inpatient stay and hospital costs (Anderson et al 1981, Sugarbaker et al 1975). The addition of laparoscopy to a procedure such as appendicectomy has no influence on hospital stay and only marginally increases cost (Sugarbaker et al 1975). The evidence is now convincing, therefore, that the lowest error rate and the most efficient management for patients with abdominal pain will be obtained by the use of laparoscopy in those patients in whom the need for operation is uncertain and in all those in whom a diagnosis of appendicitis is made.

Diagnostic appearances at laparoscopy

Experienced surgeons should have no difficulty in recognizing the pathological conditions visible at laparoscopy. Difficulty may be encountered in visualization of the appendix, especially if it is inflamed. Adherent omentum may be gently lifted off using the laparoscope, or by using a probe or forceps inserted in the right iliac fossa. The caecum may be manipulated by rotating the pole forwards and upwards. Head-down tilt of the operating table helps this manoeuvre.

Laparoscopic signs suggestive of appendicitis when the appendix cannot be visualized:

Adherent omentum over caecum or appendix.

Inflammation of the pole of the caecum.

Any fluid in the lateral paracolic gutter or around the pole of the caecum.

Turbid fluid in the pelvis with normal pelvic organs.

The whole appendix must be seen to be normal before appendicitis can be excluded, but if another cause of pain (e.g. salpingitis) is found and none of the signs that suggest appendicitis is present, then operation is not mandatory. In all other circumstances, failure to demonstrate a normal appendix should be followed by appendicectomy.

Laparoscopic appendicectomy and laparoscopically-guided appendicectomy.

A technique has been described for intraperitoneal laparoscopic appendicectomy (Semm 1983). This procedure appears cumbersome and requires four punctures with specially designed instruments. It is in our opinion of little practical value in the management of appendicitis. However, appendicectomy through a small incision sited, under laparoscopic guidance, directly over the caecal pole is more attractive (de Kok 1977). A preliminary report of this technique recorded 15 cases and in five instances the appendix was inflamed, but no information was given about any complications after surgery (Fleming 1985).

Serious reservations will remain until larger numbers are reported, with documentation of the incidence of wound infection and intra-abdominal sepsis, as well as information about post-operative hospital stay and the rapidity of recovery to full activity. Withdrawal of an inflamed appendix through a small stab incision is likely to lead to a wound infection in a high proportion of patients, and the friable appendix could easily rupture during this manoeuvre. The technique seems particularly inappropriate for an appendix tensely distended with pus or perforated.

Laparoscopy in suspected peritonitis

There is little information on the value of laparoscopy in patients with suspected peritonitis secondary to causes other than appendicitis. Some authors have excluded patients with abdominal distension (Sugarbaker et al 1975) or with specific diagnoses that were clear-cut on clinical or radiological grounds (Paterson-Brown et al 1986b). Sundal and colleagues (1982) laparoscoped 164 patients with suspected peritonitis and achieved a 'correct diagnosis or findings compatible with the correct diagnosis' in 152 patients. Twenty-two patients with a final diagnosis of an extra-abdominal cause for their pain had a normal laparoscopy. A further 37 patients had conditions that did not require immediate surgery, in whom laparoscopy was correct or compatible with the final diagnosis in 32. It appears that in these 32 patients laparotomy was avoided. The observations of Paterson-Brown and colleagues (1986b) suggest that a more selective approach to laparoscopy, by the exclusion of patients with obvious peritonitis, perforation or obstruction, would have reduced the number of patients in whom laparoscopy contributed nothing to management but simply confirmed the decision to operate. Such a selective approach would not have reduced the usefulness of laparoscopy in the detection of patients who did not require operation.

Technical points

Laparoscopy is a simple technique to learn. Any surgeon should be able to master it quickly and perform it safely. The procedure is well described in standard textbooks, and only points of practical importance will be emphasized here.

The abdomen is distended with gas (carbon dioxide or nitrous oxide) before the introduction of the trocar; 2.5 l are usually sufficient. Over-distension should be avoided, as this carries the instruments too far away from the viscera and makes inspection and biopsy difficult. Over-distension may also increase postoperative pain by stretching the abdominal musculature and peritoneum. The pressure of gas should be observed continuously during insufflation. When the gas is flowing freely into the peritoneum the pressure will be less 10 mm Hg. Temporary obstruction of the cannula by omentum may raise this momentarily, but any prolonged rise or any rise above 25 mm Hg requires immediate cessation of insufflation. The needle tip should be freely mobile within the peritoneal cavity at all times. If flow is interrupted, the needle tip may be repositioned by movement of the hub from side to side. This manoeuvre will usually allow insufflation to continue.

The laparoscope should be warmed before use to prevent misting of the lens. A separate incision for the introduction of a probe, biopsy forceps or a sucker is nearly always useful. For this reason, the whole abdomen is prepared and exposed before insertion of the 'scope. The instrument cannula is inserted in the appropriate quadrant of the abdomen after initial inspection. All quadrants of the abdomen should be examined, and for this reason a tilting operating table is preferred, to allow exposure of the pelvis and upper abdominal organs in turn. The operator may find it convenient to stand first on one side and then on the other when examining the upper and lower abdomen.

At the end of the procedure, the gas is evacuated through the trocar as completely as possible. Rapid deflation of the abdomen should be avoided as it may precipitate cardiac arrhythmias. The incisions are closed by skin sutures or clips, although if the defect in the linea alba is accessible, it is prudent to insert a nylon stitch to close this and thereby avoid the risk of a small incisional hernia.

Contraindications to laparoscopy

Laparoscopy should not be undertaken in patients with cardiac or respiratory insufficiency in whom the abdominal distension might compromise the function of those systems. All other contraindications are relative.

A history of multiple previous abdominal operations with more than one surgical scar renders laparoscopy hazardous. The Verres needle should be introduced with care and should be aspirated before insufflation of gas. If bowel contents are aspirated the needle is withdrawn and resited. Such perforations are likely to seal without intervention if the bowel remains adherent to the abdominal wall. The Verres needle should never be introduced through a surgical scar. After successful introduction of the needle, gas is insufflated with particular attention to inflow pressure, but if difficulty is encountered in this group of patients the procedure should be abandoned. If the pneumoperitoneum is successful, the trocar is introduced at the same site as the Verres needle. Adhesions from previous surgery may limit the view obtained, but sometimes the telescope can be manipulated around them, or it may be pushed through sheets of filmy adhesions if there appears to be only gas beyond them. Dense adhesions or adhesions overlying viscera should not be approached in this way.

Obesity may render laparoscopy difficult, but it need not be a contraindication. Visualization of the viscera will be less complete and attempts to manipulate them may cause bleeding, but with care and patience useful information may be obtained to supplement the clinical findings, which, it must be remembered, may be equally difficult to interpret in obese subjects.

Intraperitoneal fluid obscures vision and should be drained before laparoscopy. The abdomen is then redistended but with an equal volume of gas. This may be much greater than the volume usually required, but it is necessary to distend the lax abdominal wall and hold it away from the bowel which floats on the surface of the remaining fluid. Residual fluid should be aspirated with a laparoscopic sucker to enable complete visualization of the parietal peritoneum and viscera. It is always necessary to close the fascial defect after laparoscopy to prevent leakage of fluid.

Complications

Laparoscopy is a safe procedure. The commonest complication is a minor wound infection at the trocar entry site, which should occur in less than 5% of cases, even when the indication for laparoscopy is an emergency presentation with abdominal pain (Sundal et al 1982, Reiertsen et al 1985, Clarke et al 1986, Paterson-Brown et al 1986a, b).

Rare major complications include perforation of bowel or retroperitoneal blood vessels and injury to the mesentery. The reported incidence of these complications is 0.006% (Chamberlain & Brown 1978). The injury should be recognized at laparoscopy. If immediate operation is undertaken to repair the injury, minimal morbidity can be anticipated. Surgical emphysema of the abdominal wall, caused by failure of the Verres needle to enter the peritoneal cavity before insufflation of gas, settles spontaneously.

Conclusion

Laparoscopy is a safe technique which can be learned quickly by general surgeons. It is useful to achieve an early diagnosis in patients with abdominal pain of uncertain origin, in those in whom the need for operation is unclear and in patients, particularly females, with a suspected diagnosis of acute appendicitis. The greater diagnostic accuracy that can be achieved with laparoscopy improves patient management and reduces hospital stay and hospital costs for those who do not require operation. Laparoscopy contributes little to the management of patients with clear-cut diagnoses other than appendicitis.

Laparoscopy may also have a place in the assessment of blunt abdominal trauma and stab wounds, but further studies are required before its general application in abdominal trauma can be recommended.

Peritoneal lavage

The usefulness of peritoneal lavage in the identification of patients who require laparotomy after closed abdominal trauma is not controversial. However the role of lavage in the management of patients with penetrating trauma is less clearly established, although it can offer useful information. Peritoneal lavage has been used in the diagnosis of suspected peritonitis by relatively few surgeons. In all three areas, peritoneal lavage should be seen as an adjunct to clinical assessment and is most useful when the clinical presentation poses unusual difficulty, for example, when consciousness is impaired or when diagnostic doubt exists.

Blunt trauma

The experience up to 1980 of peritoneal lavage in the management of blunt trauma was reviewed by Powell et al (1982). In the early use of lavage, diagnosis and management decisions depended on the depth of red coloration, as a result of blood staining, in the lavage fluid. This subjective assessment has now been superseded by the use of the red blood cell count as a quantitative measure. Red cells be found in the lavage fluid in 'negative' tops (Veith et al 1967, Barbee & Gilsdorf 1975), but most surgeons using the technique would accept a cell count of greater than 100 000 mm³ as being diagnostic of intraperitoneal injury. Other criteria of a positive lavage are fresh blood or intestinal fluid aspirated before lavage, or lavage fluid containing any one of:

Red blood cells $> 100\ 000/mm^3$

White blood cells $> 500/mm^3$

Bile

Vegetable matter

Organisms

Elevated levels of enzymes such as amylase, alkaline phosphatase (doubtful — see below)

Enzyme estimations have occasionally been reported as useful, but not all authors have found this to be so. Olsen (1973) found that fewer than 10% of patients with raised amylase levels had a significant pancreatic injury. There is experimental evidence that in lavage fluid, estimation of alkaline phosphatase is the most specific test to recognise bowel perforation soon after injury (Marx et al 1983).

The diagnostic accuracy of peritoneal lavage in blunt abdominal trauma has been shown to be in excess of 97% (Powell et al 1982). In this large collected review of over 10 000 patients, the false positive rate was 1.4% and the false negative rate was 1.3%. The value of a negative result for decision-making purposes is considerable, as it excluded, for practical purposes, significant intra-abdominal injury. If the patient's condition suggests the possibility of a false negative result, however, then repeat lavage after a delay of 6 hours or more will accurately detect major injury (Gruenberg et al 1982). Repeat lavage will also improve the accuracy of diagnosis if the red cell count is in the range 50 000–100 000/mm³, or the white cell count is 100–500/mm³ (Alyono & Perry 1982).

Indications for lavage in blunt trauma

Despite its accuracy, lavage need not be performed

in all cases of blunt abdominal trauma. If there is clear evidence of abdominal injury, from the mode of injury or the presence of external bruising, and the patient is haemodynamically unstable despite fluid replacement, then laparotomy and control of haemorrhage are required. At the other end of the scale, trauma patients without abdominal signs or symptoms do not require lavage unless one of the following complicating factors is present to make clinical evaluation difficult:

1. Coma or impaired consciousness due to injury, alcohol or drugs.
2. General anaesthetic or artificial ventilation required for non-abdominal injuries.
3. A period of unexplained hypotension.
4. Fracture of bones of trunk or femur with history or signs of abdominal injury.

Lavage is useful in patients with a history of trauma in whom signs are masked by alteration in consciousness, whether due to injury or intoxication, in patients with severe blunt trauma who are to have a general anaesthetic for treatment of non-abdominal injuries, and in those who require artificial ventilation (Reiner et al 1986, van Dongen & Boer 1985). Clearly in these circumstances accurate clinical assessment of the abdomen will not be possible. It has been suggested that, even in a patient who has normal cerebral function, if there is microscopic or gross haematuria diagnostic lavage should be performed (Trooskin et al 1985). However, it is not clear from this study how lavage contributed to the management of those patients who had no physical or radiological signs. Haematuria alone cannot be taken as an indication for lavage in our view.

Lavage in children

Lavage will safely and reliably exclude severe intra-abdominal injury after blunt trauma in children. In three series evaluating 393 children, only one false negative was reported, a case of small bowel laceration (Drew et al 1977, Dupriest et al 1982, Powell et al 1987). False positives were more troublesome, especially in the report from Powell and collegaues, who use a simple qualitat-

ive estimation of the colour of the returned lavage fluid. They suggest that caution should be used in the interpretation of a positive lavage to avoid unnecessary laparotomy. The current trend towards conservative management of splenic and hepatic injuries gives added force to this advice.

Alternatives to peritoneal lavage

Lavage is an accurate method for the assessment of blunt injury, but it is invasive and complications occur in up to 1% of patients (Powell et al 1982). Laparoscopy is safer, but it is a more complex procedure and requires special equipment. It is probably as accurate as lavage and may provide information about the site of injury that is not available with lavage (see above).

Two trials have compared computed tomography (CT) with peritoneal lavage in patients with blunt trauma (Fabian et al 1986, Pagliarello et al 1987). Both found that CT was more likely to give a false negative result. Fabian and his colleagues found a sensitivity of 60% for CT and 90% for lavage in 91 patients who had both procedures. There were no false positives with either technique. Despite the contention that CT may provide additional information, particularly when reviewed by an experienced radiologist (Fabian et al 1986, White 1986), in practice lavage is preferred because it is quicker, cheaper and more accurately defines the need for laparotomy.

Lavage in penetrating trauma

Peritoneal lavage is also useful to assess the presence of visceral injury after penetrating trauma. The criteria of a positive lavage are the same as for blunt trauma. In a series of 353 patients with penetrating trauma (Gruenberg et al 1982), the sensitivity of lavage for the detection of visceral perforation was 84% and its specificity was 98%. There was no difference in the accuracy of lavage between gunshot wounds (76 visceral injuries in 141 patients) and stab wounds (48 visceral injuries in 197 patients).

Other authors have reported similar figures (Duus et al 1986), but there are some wounds that present difficulty. Stab wounds to the chest may traverse the diaphragm and cause intra-abdominal injury. Lavage is reasonably accurate in the assessment of such patients (sensitivity 85%, specificity 97%), but isolated diaphragmatic laceration without visceral injury is a well recognized cause of a false negative result (Thal 1984). The presence of a hydrothorax or lavage fluid in the chest drain are indicators of diaphragmatic laceration.

Penetrating wounds of the colon are also identified as likely to cause false negative lavage results (Obied et al 1984). This observation may arise because there is relatively little bleeding from the injured colon and initial contamination is sealed off quickly, but the most likely cause is that some of these colonic injuries are extraperitoneal.

In conclusion, peritoneal lavage is a useful adjunct to the management of some patients with blunt or penetrating trauma, but its use must be selective. Prompt laparotomy without the results of lavage is indicated when there is unexplained hypotension and intrathoracic injuries have been excluded and when there are no complicating features such as impaired consciousness. In these cases the need for laparotomy should be judged on clinical grounds.

Lavage in peritonitis

In 1967, Veith and colleagues reported a series of 100 patients who had peritoneal lavage as a diagnostic test in acute abdominal pain. A small number of these patients had previous blunt abdominal trauma, and the authors used similar criteria for a positive lavage to those used after blunt trauma. They had one false negative and four false positives. In 11 patients it was possible to cancel a planned operation and in 12 patients an operation was performed as a result of the lavage. Evans and colleagues (1975) also found that the decision to operate or not was changed by the lavage result in over 20% of cases. Other authors (Table 1.1) have had similar experience. In a total of 344 patients in these series, the sensitivity is 93.5% and the specificity is 91.2%. Lavage appears to be useful in the diagnosis of peritonitis, therefore, but again it should only be used when there is genuine diagnostic difficulty:

Table 1.1 Accuracy of lavage results in the prediction of need for laparotomy in patients with suspected peritonitis.

Author	True positive	False positive	True negative	False negative	Total
Veith et al 1967	53	4	42	1	100
Barbee et al 1975	12	2	9	9*	32
Evans et al 1975	35	0	10	2	47
Richardson et al 1983	70	7	60	81	138
Lobbato et al 1985	14	0	13	0	27
Total	184	13	134	13	344

* This figure includes 5 patients with localized inflammation.

in patients with dementia, diminished consciousness or intoxication, or when there is doubt about the diagnosis of intra-abdominal disease, particularly in high-risk groups.

The failure of lavage to find wider acceptance in these circumstances may be related to surgeons' preferences for performing laparotomy on the basis of their clinical evaluation, even when the clinical diagnosis is not clear-cut, rather than carrying out an invasive diagnostic test which does not give information about the specific diagnosis.

Technique for lavage

The diagnostic accuracy of peritoneal lavage is not dependent on the method of introducing the catheter whether by direct percutaneous puncture or an open technique. Fears that contamination of the lavage fluid with blood from the insertion site might lead to false positive results appear groundless. In contrast, the risk of perforation of hollow viscera or retroperitoneal blood vessels is greater with the closed technique (Cochran & Sobat 1984), and it is probably more stressful for the patient. The risks are further increased in the unconscious or anaesthetised patient.

The advantages of a small peritoneal puncture, good local anaesthesia and retraction of the abdominal wall away from the bowel are confirmed by the technique of Cox and Dunham (1983). An incision is made lateral to the umbilicus, under local anaesthesia, down to and through the rectus sheath for a length of 20 mm. The rectus muscle is retracted laterally, and an artery forceps is applied to the medial edge of the sheath. The sheath and the umbilicus are lifted vertically upwards, and the trocar and catheter are passed through the posterior sheath just lateral to the umbilicus, so that the catheter passes medially, close to the abdominal wall. The trocar is withdrawn a little, and the catheter is then manipulated into the pelvis. The anterior sheath and skin are closed around the catheter, which is withdrawn at the completion of the test. This technique was used in over 700 patients with no complications, and we think it is probably the method of choice.

After insertion of the catheter, the pelvis is aspirated. The presence of blood, pus or bile indicates a positive tap. A litre of normal saline is run rapidly into the abdominal cavity; any resistance to inflow suggests misplacement of the catheter. The patient should be rolled from side to side to facilitate mixing of the fluid, and at least 200 ml of fluid should be drained by siphonage before an aliquot is examined. Use of lower volumes of return fluid is associated with more false negative results than are generally accepted (Merlotti et al 1985). Adjusting the position of the patient may be necessary to encourage fluid to drain.

In patients in whom microscopic examination of the lavage fluid is equivocal (red cell count 50 000–100 000/mm^3; WBC 100–500/mm^3) or about whom clinical diagnostic doubt still exists, the catheter should be left in place to allow a repeat lavage after an interval of six hours.

Fine catheter aspiration cytology

Stewart and his colleagues in New Zealand (1986) have developed a technique of cytological examination of peritoneal fluid. They insert a 12 or 14 gauge intravenous cannula percutaneously into the peritoneal cavity. Through this cannula they pass a fine catheter with many side holes. Aspiration through the catheter may produce fluid, which is then examined macroscopically. In all cases, after aspiration the catheter is removed and rinsed to wash off any adherent cells. The resulting suspension is filtered for cytological examination.

The most sensitive indicator of surgical pathology with this technique is the percentage of neutrophils in the peritoneal fluid sample. Stewart points out that confusion may arise with non-surgical inflammation such as pelvic inflammatory disease or pancreatitis, and that non-complicated intestinal obstruction may give a negative test. The presence of neutrophils in the aspirate indicates inflammatory pathology, as this cell type is not usually present in appreciable numbers in peritoneal fluid.

This test greatly increases the accuracy of the crucial management decision: whether or not to subject the patient to urgent laparotomy. In Stewart's pilot study, 27 patients were studied in whom the clinician had difficulty in making this decision. Two technical failures occurred, but in the remaining 25 patients a correct decision to operate or not was made in all patients after fine catheter aspiration cytology.

Recently (1988) these authors have presented the results of a further controlled study of 144 patients with acute abdominal pain. Compared with controls who had standard investigations only, patients who had fine catheter aspiration cytology were more likely to have the correct decision made about urgent laparotomy. This test deserves further evaluation in centres where cytological expertise is available for emergency examinations.

REFERENCES

Adamthwaite D N 1984 Traumatic diaphragmatic hernia: a new indication for laparoscopy. British Journal of Surgery 71: 315

Alyono D, Perry J F 1982 Significance of repeating diagnostic peritoneal lavage. Surgery 91: 656–659

Anderson J L, Bridgewater F H G 1981 Laparoscopy in the diagnosis of acute lower abdominal pain. Australian and New Zealand Journal of Surgery 51: 462–464

Barbee C L, Gilsdorf R B 1975 Diagnostic peritoneal lavage in evaluating acute abdominal pain. Annals of Surgery 181: 853–856

Barnes B A, Behringer G E, Wheelock F C, Wilkins E W 1962 Treatment of appendicitis at the Massachusetts General Hospital (1937–1959) Journal of the American Medical Association 180: 122–126

Berci G, Dunkelman D, Michel S L et al 1983 Emergency minilaparoscopy in abdominal trauma. American Journal of Surgery 146: 261–265

Chamberalain G, Brown J C 1978 The report of the working party of the confidential enquiry into gynaecological laparoscopy. London: Royal College of Obstetricians and Gynaecologists

Chang F C, Hogle H H, Welling D R 1973 The fate of the negative appendix. American Journal of Surgery 126: 752–754

Clarke P J, Hands L J, Gough M H, Kettlewell M H 1986. The use of laparoscopy in the management of right iliac fossa pain. Annals of the Royal College of Surgeons of England 68: 68–69

Cochran W, Sobat W S 1984 Open versus closed diagnostic peritoneal lavage. Annals of Surgery 200: 24–28

Cox E F, Dunham M 1983 A safe technique for diagnostic peritoneal lavage. Journal of Trauma 23: 152–154

Cuschieri A, Hennessey T P J, Stephens R, Berci G 1987 Minilaparoscopy versus peritoneal lavage in blunt abdominal trauma — preliminary results of a controlled clinical trial. British Journal of Surgery 74: 548

de Kok H J 1977 A new technique for resecting the non-inflamed, not-adhesive appendix through a mini-laparotomy with the aid of the laparoscope. Archivum Chirugicum Neerlandicum 29: 195–198

Deutsch A, Zelikovsky A, Reiss R 1982 Laparoscopy in the prevention of unnecessary appendicectomies: a prospective study. British Journal of Surgery 69: 336–337

Drew R, Perry J F, Fischer R P 1977 The expediency of peritoneal lavage for blunt abdominal trauma in children. Surgery Gynecology and Obstetrics 145: 885–888

Dunn E L, Moore E E, Elerdis S C, Murphy S R 1982 The unnecessary laparotomy for appendicitis — can it be decreased? Annals of Surgery 48: 320–323

DuPriest R W, Rodriguez A, Shatney C H 1982 Peritoneal lavage in children and adolescents with blunt abdominal trauma. The American Surgeon 48: 460–462

Duus B R, Hauch O, Damm P, Hoffman J 1986 Peritoneal lavage for the evaluation of patients with equivocal signs after abdominal trauma. Acta Chirurgica Scandinavica 152: 601–604

Evans C, Rashid A, Rosenberg I L, Pollock A V 1975 An appraisal of peritoneal lavage in the diagnosis of the acute abdomen. British Journal of Surgery 62: 119–120

Fabian T C, Mangiante E C, White T J et al 1986 A prospective study of 91 patients undergoing both computed tomography and peritoneal lavage following blunt abdominal trauma. Journal of Trauma 26: 602–608

Fleming J S 1985 Laparoscopically directed appendicectomy. Australian and New Zealand Journal of Obstetrics and Gynaecology 25: 238–239

Gruenberg J C, Brown R S, Talbert J G, Tate S S, Obied F N 1982 The diagnostic usefulness of peritoneal lavage in penetrating trauma. Annals of Surgery 48: 402–407

Lewis F R, Holcroft J W, Boey J, Dunphy J E 1975 Apendicitis. A critical review of diagnosis and treatment in 1000 cases. Archives of Surgery 110: 677–684

Lobbato V, Cioroiu M, Laraja R D et al 1985 Peritoneal lavage as an aid to diagnosis of peritonitis in debilitated and elderly patients. The American Surgeon 51: 508–510

Marx J A, Moore E E, Bar-or D 1983 Peritoneal lavage in penetrating injuries of the small bowel and colon: value of enzyme determination. Annals of Emergency Medicine 12: 68–70

Merlotti G J, Marcett E, Sheaff C M et al 1985 Use of peritoneal lavage to evaluate abdominal penetration. Journal of Trauma 25: 228–231

Obied F N, Sorensen V, Vincent G et al 1984 Inaccuracy of diagnostic peritoneal lavage in penetrating colonic trauma. Archives of Surgery 119: 906–908

Olsen W R 1973 The serum amylase in blunt abdominal trauma. Journal of Trauma 13: 200–204

Pagliarello G, Hanna S S, Gregory W D et al 1987 Abdominal pelvic computerised tomography and open peritoneal lavage in patients with blunt abdominal trauma: a prospective study. Canadian Journal of Surgery 30: 10–13

Paterson-Brown S, Olufunwa S A, Galazka N, Simmons S C 1986a Visualisation of the normal appendix at laparoscopy. Journal of the Royal College of Surgeons of Edinburgh 31: 106–107

Paterson-Brown S, Eckersley J R T, Sim A J W, Dudley H A F 1986b Laparoscopy as an adjunct to decision making in the "acute abdomen". British Journal of Surgery 73: 1022–1024

Pieper R, Kager L, Nasman P 1982 Acute appendicitis: a clinical study of 1018 cases of emergency appendicectomy. Acta Chirurgica Scandinavica 148: 51–62

Powell D C, Bivins B A, Bell R M 1982 Diagnostic peritoneal lavage. Surgery Gynecology and Obstetrics 155: 257–264

Powell R W, Green J B, Ochsner M G et al 1987 Peritoneal lavage in pediatric patients sustaining blunt abdominal trauma: a reappraisal. Journal of Trauma 27: 6–10

Reiertsen O, Rosseland A R, Hoivick B, Solheim K 1985 Laparoscopy in patients admitted for acute abdominal pain. Acta Chirurgica Scandinavica 151: 521–524

Reiner D S, Hurd R, Smith K, Kaminski D L 1986 Selective peritoneal lavage in the management of comatose blunt trauma patients. Journal of Trauma 26: 255–259

Richardson J D, Flint L M, Polk H C 1983 Peritoneal lavage: a useful diagnostic adjunct for peritonitis. Surgery 94: 826–829

Semm K 1983 Endoscopic appendicectomy. Endoscopy 15: 59–64

Stewart R J, Gupta R K, Purdie G L, Isbister W H 1986 Fine catheter aspiration cytology of peritoneal cavity improves decision-making about difficult cases of acute abdominal pain. Lancet ii: 1414–1415

Stewart R J, Gupta R K, Purdie G L, Holloway L J, Isbister W H 1988 Fine catheter aspiration cytology of peritoneal cavity for the acute abdomen: a randomised sequential clinical trial. British Journal of Surgery 75: 1229

Sugarbaker P H, Bloom B S, Sanders J H, Wilson R E 1975 Preoperative laparoscopy in diagnosis of abdominal pain. Lancet i: 442–445

Sundal E, Gyr K, Fahrlaender H 1982 Peritoneoscopy in abdominal emergencies — a valuable diagnostic tool. Endoscopy 14: 97–99

Thal E R 1984 Peritoneal lavage. Reliability of RBC count in patients with stab wounds of the chest. Archives of Surgery 119: 579–584

Trooskin S Z, Boyarsky A H, Greco R S 1985 Peritoneal lavage in patients with normal mentation and haematuria after blunt trauma. Surgery Gynecology and Obstetrics 160: 145–147

van Dongen L M, de Boer H M 1985 Peritoneal lavage in closed abdominal injury. Injury 16: 227–229

Veith F J, Webber W B, Karl R C, Deysine M 1967 Diagnostic peritoneal lavage. Annals of Surgery 166: 290–295

White T J 1986 Letter to the Editor. Journal of Trauma 26: 662–663

2 Injuries to the liver and bile ducts

J. TERBLANCHE and J. E. J. KRIGE

Liver injuries

The trauma epidemic in our modern violent society has led to a rising incidence of major liver injury. The prevalence is related to increasing civilian violence with the use of both knives and hand guns as well as the widespread misuse of high-speed motor vehicles. The problems are frequently aggravated by alcohol and drug abuse. Clinical studies have provided a better understanding of the associated problems and have resulted in improved management. Many classic beliefs have been challenged and proved to be erroneous (Walt 1978).

This chapter evaluates controversial areas of liver injury management and presents the authors' current practice, which is supported by their own experience and by recent publications, particularly from the USA (Feliciano et al 1986, Pachter et al 1986, Moore et al 1985, Meyer et al 1985).

Types of injury

Simple or complex injuries

We agree with the Houston group's view that liver injuries are best classified as either simple or complex in relation to how difficult they are to manage (Feliciano et al 1986). Of their 1000 consecutive cases of hepatic trauma seen between 1979 and 1984, 88% were simple to manage and had low morbidity and mortality rates. The Cape Town experience with 345 patients seen between 1978 and 1985 was that 80% fell into the simple category (Krige & Terblanche 1989). Others have divided liver injuries into more categories, using complex classifications. The Denver classification is probably the most widely used; this divides injuries into five classes, with classes IV and V being the equivalent of complex injuries (Moore et al 1985, Moore 1984). Although we support classification by degree of complexity, a case can be made for considering retrohepatic vena caval and hepatic vein tears as a separate sub-category of the complex group because of the extremely high mortality rate and the controversies surrounding their management.

Open or closed injuries

Liver injuries fall into two broad groups. Open injuries are either caused by stab wounds or by missile wounds. Stab wounds are usually simple, with a good prognosis. One hundred and sixty five of our 345 adult patients had stab wounds, with 98% of them being classified as simple. The only death occurred in one of the three patients whose inferior vena cava was damaged as well.

Missile wounds can be more serious. Bullet wounds are divided into low-velocity and high-velocity types. Fortunately many of the civilian injuries are due to low-velocity missiles. Seventy-four of our 345 adult patients had gunshot wounds: of these 70% were classified as simple. The mortality rate was 13.5%, with all but 2 deaths occurring in complex cases. High-velocity bullet wounds cause extensive damage and are more common in war conflict, although some civilian injuries are due to high-velocity missiles. Shrapnel wounds are often of the high-velocity type and are unfortunately beginning to increase in civilian practice due to terrorist bombs and mines.

Closed injuries occur with blunt abdominal trauma and are frequently caused by motor vehicle accidents. They tend to be more serious, although 59% of our group of 106 adult patients with blunt abdominal trauma had simple injuries (Krige & Terblanche 1989). Other causes include falling from a height, and child abuse in paediatric practice.

Mortality

Mortality is related to whether the liver injury is mild or severe and therefore whether the management is simple or complex. Overall mortality rates range between 10 and 20% and are largely dependent upon the number of complex injuries treated and the expertise of the centre (Feliciano et al 1986, Walt 1978). The Cape Town mortality in adult patients was 8.4% overall (29 of 345 patients seen over eight years) (Krige & Terblanche 1989).

The mortality rate is directly related to the number of patients presenting with massive haemorrhage, either from the liver or from the retrohepatic vena cava and hepatic veins, as well as to the extent of the liver injury. Associated non-hepatic injuries are the other important factors. Many patients with liver injuries have other lethal injuries which result in death. Associated local abdominal injuries have also been shown to increase mortality. In the Detroit series the mortality rate increased to 50% when four or more abdominal organs were involved (Walt 1978). Colon injuries are important and play a major role in the development of intra-abdominal sepsis.

The mortality audit in a unit that develops an interest and expertise in liver injuries may surprisingly not show improved survival. The reason is that if the ambulance and resuscitation facilities are improved, more fatally injured patients will arrive at the hospital or be referred to the surgical team before death and therefore be included in the mortality statistics (Walt 1978).

Pathology

Stab wounds and low-velocity missiles usually cause small defects which give rise to few problems and are simple to manage. Problems only arise if a major blood vessel or bile duct is injured. A subcapsular haematoma arises when there is a tear under Glisson's capsule without damage to the capsule itself. In the past it was feared that these would increase in size and ultimately cause delayed rupture of the liver. Although this appears to be unusual, management remains controversial. A tear or split in the liver is the typical injury with blunt trauma. This is also usually localized and minor, but can be extensive, needing complex management. Rarely, multiple tears occur in both lobes of a severely damaged liver and if extensive they can tax the ingenuity of the surgeon.

Central or contained rupture of liver with intrahepatic haematoma formation can usually be managed conservatively in a patient who is otherwise haemodynamically stable. These injuries are more common than previously realized and are increasingly being detected with modern imaging techniques. They only become important if bleeding occurs into the peritoneal cavity or into the biliary tract.

Inferior vena caval and hepatic vein injuries are fortunately uncommon but are a major cause of mortality. Modern management should improve the survival.

Diagnosis

The diagnosis will be suspected in patients with knife or gunshot wounds in the region of the liver, or with blunt trauma and evidence of injury in that area. It must be borne in mind that gunshot entry and exit wounds may be deceptively distant from the liver. The real problems of diagnosis arise in patients with altered sensorium with or without head or spinal cord injuries. The insidious onset of shock in a multiply injured or unconscious patient may easily be missed.

The aim is to diagnose continued bleeding early so that the patient can undergo emergency surgery to control haemorrhage. On the other hand those patients who are not actively bleeding can be observed, unless another organ injury requires a laparotomy. Our policy for both open and closed abdominal injuries has increasingly moved towards conservative treatment unless there is evidence of either ongoing blood loss or damaged bowel with peritoneal or retoperitoneal contamination.

The newer imaging techniques have proved particularly valuable in patients with suspected liver trauma. They should not be used in a seriously shocked patient who is obviously bleeding intra-peritoneally. Such a patient needs an immediate laparotomy, which should not be delayed while awaiting special investigations. Computerized tomography (CT) is the most widely used imaging technique and has been extensively evaluated (Meyer et al 1985). Moon & Federle (1983) have described the different types and degrees of liver injury detected by CT scanning. A CT scan clearly demonstrates parenchymal lacerations, intra-hepatic haematoma and free intraperitoneal blood. The ability to detect inhomogeneity of solid organs with CT scanning enables the attending doctor to detect that a lesion is present and also to determine its size. The same applies to free intraperitoneal fluid and blood. Currently both oral and intravenous contrast media are given to enhance the ability to localize and delineate the injury.

Ultrasound is a valuable alternative but does not give as clear a picture as a CT scan. It is useful when a CT scan is not available, or in urgent situations when the patient is in transit to the operating theatre and CT scanning is logistically impossible. Radionuclide scanning has also been utilized, but CT scanning with contrast enhancement has proved to be superior. Hepatic angiography has a limited role in the diagnosis of ongoing bleeding, but a possible therapeutic role using embolization in arterial bleeding from a segmental or subsegmental artery. A chest X-ray is essential if there is any possibility of a pneumothorax. Plain films of the abdomen are of little value. In patients with suspected renal injury or haematuria, a rapid intravenous pyelogram is essential prior to undertaking laparotomy for suspected liver injury.

We believe that the diagnosis of liver injury, as well as the decision to operate, should be made on clinical grounds. Repeated physical examination is the most important diagnostic test to decide on operative intervention in a patient in whom initial management has been conservative. Peritoneal lavage has been widely used. We believe that its use should be restricted to unconscious and/or multiply injured patients in whom the question of intra-abdominal bleeding or visceral injury arises. We do not operate on the basis of a positive tap for blood alone, but take the findings into account along with the overall clinical picture of the patient.

A potential new problem has arisen with the ready availability of non-invasive imaging. Lesions not previously detected in relatively asymptomatic patients are now being picked up by CT scanning or ultrasound (Athey 1982, Geis et al 1981). This policy has lead to unnecessary emergency surgery being undertaken on the basis of the outdated belief that all liver injuries require operative therapy. This is a false premise. Surgery should not be undertaken on the basis of imaging data alone.

Management

Principles of management

The principles of management are to stop haemorrhage, remove dead or devitalized liver tissue and to oversew or repair damaged blood vessels and bile ducts. Fortunately the majority of liver injuries are simple and can be treated without difficulty. The few complex lesions need to be diagnosed early and require major surgery by experienced hepatic surgeons if life is to be saved. Apart from death due to associated injuries, haemorrhage is the major cause of mortality. The main lifesaving aim of therapy is to stop haemorrhage. Fortunately haemorrhage can usually be stopped by packing while help is being sought or to allow the patient to be transferred to a unit where complex therapy can be undertaken.

Cape Town studies

The experience is briefly summarized to provide

the background to the policy advocated below.

Adults (1978–1985). During this 8-year period 345 adults with liver injuries were treated at Groote Schuur Hospital. Of these, 48% were stab wounds, 21% were gunshot and 31% had blunt abdominal trauma (Krige & Terblanche 1989). Ninety-seven of the 165 stab wounds were found not to be bleeding at laparotomy and no procedure was performed; 81 patients were drained, but in the other 16, not even a drain was inserted. Sixty-five patients required suture and drainage for bleeding, while 3 patients were submitted to major surgery for inferior vena cava or hepatic vein injuries. Only one patient died in the latter group.

Major complications occurred in 17% of cases, with a very low overall mortality rate (0.6%). Gunshot wounds occurred less frequently and fortunately were usually low-velocity injuries. Fifty-two of the 74 patients had simple injuries, with 29 being drained and 23 requiring suture and drainage. More major procedures, including non-anatomical debridement, lobectomy and packing, were required in the remaining patients. Three of the 4 patients with vena caval injuries due to gunshot wounds succumbed. Forty percent of these patients had major complications, and the overall mortality rate was 13.5%. Sixty-three of the 106 patients with blunt abdominal trauma had simple injuries, requiring drainage only in 29, and suture as well as drainage in 34. The complex injuries tended to be more severe with blunt trauma, and the mortality rate was higher than in the other groups. The overall mortality rate was 17%, and major complications occurred in 38% of patients.

Because we realized that a number of patients had been operated on unnecessarily, we have recently adopted a more conservative approach to stab wounds and blunt abdominal trauma when there are no clinical indications for laparotomy. This is our standard approach to other types of abdominal injury, but like others, we had previously believed that a liver injury always required a laparotomy.

Blunt abdominal trauma in children (1973–1983) Over an 11-year period at the Red Cross War Memorial Children's Hospital, Cape Town 36/216 children with abdominal trauma had liver injuries (Cywes et al 1985). In the early part of the study all patients were subjected to laparotomy after in-itial resuscitation. All but two required either simple drainage or suture and drainage. This finding led to a new policy of conservative treatment. The 23 consecutive children with blunt trauma seen after 1978 were all evaluated for conservative treatment. Only four came to laparotomy. Complications were minimal and there were no deaths. Patients were followed by serial non-invasive imaging, which demonstrated resolution and healing of the injuries after 3–6 months. We currently treat most liver injuries in children conservatively. This policy brings liver trauma management into line with both kidney and splenic trauma management in children. This approach is supported by other studies (Oldham et al 1986, Grisoni et al 1984).

Management controversies: current status

Many aspects of surgical dogma on liver injuries have been questioned recently, with a number of therapies being subjected to clinical trial. This has lead to a rethink about the management of major liver injuries, with considerable debate in the literature over the past decade. The controversies are dealt with individually below to provide the reader with background before we present our current management policy for liver injuries.

Conservatism in management This is becoming increasingly accepted for blunt liver injury in children (Oldham et al 1986, Cywes et al 1985, Grisoni et al 1984). Meyer et al (1985) proposed selective non-operative management of blunt liver injuries in adults, using CT scan as the guide. They had strict criteria for deciding on non-operative management. The Cape Town experience clearly supports a conservative approach in children as well as a less aggressive approach to liver injuries in adults, with a greater number of patients being evaluated for non-operative management. This is supported by the Johannesburg experience (Demetriades et al 1986).

A more conservative approach at operation is also evolving and has been championed by Moore et al (1985) of Denver. Even with major hepatic injuries, hepatic lobectomy is rarely indicated, with the more conservative techniques of hepatotomy and oversewing of bleeding vessels or resectional-debridement being preferred (Pachter et al 1983).

The Pringle manoeuvre and hepatic ischaemia Pringle's classic article (1908) has been misinterpreted and misquoted, perpetuating the myth that dangerous hepatic ischaemia occurs if the porta hepatis is occluded for longer than 15 minutes. This is not true: various reports have documented prolonged normothermic hepatic occlusion times using the Pringle manoeuvre without any problems. Pringle never mentioned a time limit and described porta hepatis occlusion in patients as well as experimentally in 4 rabbits, one of whom had occlusion for an hour (Pringle 1908). We have reported a patient who had 90 minutes of normothermic hepatic ischaemia and have documented prolonged hepatic ischaemia in pigs (Kahn et al 1986), while others have also emphasized the safety and efficacy of hepatic inflow occlusion under normothermic conditions (Feliciano et al 1986, Pachter et al 1983, Huguet et al 1978). The knowledge that inflow occlusion can be extended has revolutionized the management of liver injuries. For hepatic vein and vena caval injuries we advocate total hepatic isolation with porta hepatis occlusion (Pringle manoeurve) and occlusion of the vena cava above and below the liver without using a shunt. Intracaval shunts, as described by Schrock et al (1968), should be relegated to history, as the mortality rate assiociated with their use has been prohibitive (Pachter et al 1986, Feliciano et al 1981). Walt (1978) stated that 'there are possibly more authors on the subject than survivors of the procedures described'. The alternative to total hepatic isolation is the technique of Pachter et al (1986), with hepatotomy and direct exposure of the injured vessels using the Pringle manoeuvre for inflow occlusion and the finger fracture technique (Pachter et al 1983) for splitting the liver. Transthoracic aortic clamping should not be performed in liver injury because the mortality rate has again been shown to be prohibitive (Feliciano et al 1986). Temporary occlusion of the mesenteric arteries is also contraindicated.

Liver packing Packing for liver injuries fell into disrepute after World War II, where it had been widely used with surprisingly high morbidity and mortality rates. There has now been a complete reversal of this view, with the widespread ad-vocacy and correct use of packing (Feliciano et al 1986, Carmona et al 1984, Svoboda et al 1982, Feliciano et al 1981, Calne et al 1979).

For the patient who is bleeding actively at the time of the initial laparotomy, perihepatic packing with compression is essential, as it will stop most bleeding and allow the anaesthetist to catch up with blood loss and resuscitate the patient. It can be combined with porta hepatis clamping (Pringle manoeuvre) to provide greater haemostasis, but the authors usually find packing alone to be sufficient. Packs should not be inserted into a gap in a traumatized liver, as this will hold the cavity open and that can promote bleeding. They should be used as perihepatic packs to achieve compression of the liver and the bleeding vessels. If during any form of complex liver surgery, for either trauma or non-traumatic conditions, bleeding gets out of control, temporary packing should be used while the anaesthetist resuscitates the patient. Temporary packing is also advocated while awaiting more experienced surgical help or to allow transfer of the patient to a specialist centre.

At the end of a major liver resection or after dealing with severe liver trauma, packing has proved lifesaving by preventing continued bleeding, particularly in patients with coagulation defects after massive blood transfusions. Several papers confirm the success and efficacy of packing (Feliciano et al 1986, Carmona et al 1984, Svoboda et al 1982). When packs are left in the abdomen after liver surgery, the present authors remove them 24–48 h later, although others leave them in situ for 3–4 days or longer (Feliciano et al 1986).

Dry laparotomy swabs appear to be most effective for hepatic tamponade. Sufficient packs need to be inserted to ensure adequate haemostasis. The patient will usually require ventilation postoperatively because of pressure on the diaphragm. The authors' group usually insert five to eight large laparotomy swabs.

Drainage The first myth about drainage to be discarded as a result of a controlled trial was the purported necessity to drain the common bile duct after liver trauma. T-tube drainage became universally accepted as a result of misinterpretation of the paper by Merendino et al (1963). The controlled trial of Lucas and Walt (1972) showed no advantage, and since then T-tube drains have not been used in liver trauma.

Abdominal cavity drains have been presumed essential because of the likelihood of a bile leak. This dogma too has been questioned, and drains are now used selectively by many authors (Feliciano et al 1986, Mullins et al 1985). Until recently our group has used multiple open abdominal drainage, but we are now tending selectively to use closed-system irrigation drainage. Patients with liver trauma and no signs of bleeding at the time of laparotomy probably require no drainage (Feliciano et al 1986, Mullins et al 1985).

Hepatic artery ligation This is virtually never required. Operative hepatic artery ligation was popularised by Mays (1972), but its limitations have been recorded (Flint & Polk 1979) and the technique has been replaced by direct suture ligation of bleeding vessels aided by vascular inflow control using the Pringle manoeuvre.

Modern management of liver injuries

Shocked patients require urgent resuscitation. Associated injuries must be dealt with on merits, and this can be particularly important in multiple injury patients or patients with head injuries. In these patients bleeding from a liver injury can be very difficult to diagnose. Fortunately most liver injuries are relatively minor and easy to manage. The important aspect of early evaluation is to diagnose those patients who have severe liver or other intra-abdominal injuries requiring urgent laparotomy to stop haemorrhage. Patients with abdominal trauma are best explored using a midline abdominal incision. With liver trauma this must be extended as high as possible, at least up to the xiphisternum. A sternal retractor, as used for highly selective vagotomy, is helpful. The patient must be draped so that the incision can be extended to incorporate a lower median sternotomy if required (Fig. 2.1). This exposure gives the best access to the suprahepatic inferior vena cava and hepatic veins. In our experience the classical abdominothoracic extension into the left chest is very seldom required.

The extent of the intra-abdominal injuries

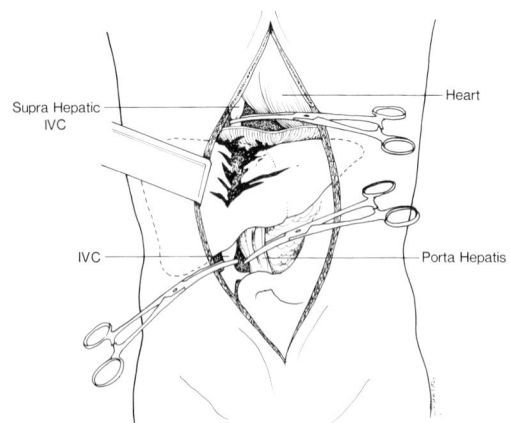

Fig. 2.1   Total hepatic isolation produced by clamping the porta hepatis (Pringle manoeuvre) and the inferior vena cava (IVC) above and below the liver. The suprahepatic IVC is exposed by splitting the lower sternum and dividing the diaphragm. A soft bowel clamp is used to occlude the porta hepatis.

should be rapidly assessed and life-threatening injuries managed first. With major liver trauma, massive bleeding may occur on opening the abdomen. This must be controlled by immediate porta hepatis compression (Fig. 2.1) and packing. If packing alone is adequate then the porta hepatis compression should be released while the patient is resuscitated. Hepatic injuries can also be controlled by packing while other injuries, such as haemorrhage from the spleen, lower abdominal vena cava or aorta, are dealt with. One of the authors had an experience of successfully packing a liver injury temporarily in a patient with high-velocity missile injuries while a potentially major intrathoracic aortic haemorrhage was dealt with, and then subsequently returning to the liver injury.

Knife wounds and minor bleeding from the liver surface will usually stop spontaneously. The management of contained subcapsular haematoma is still controversial. Many advocate that it should be left alone as it will probably not extend and cause delayed rupture. The authors prefer to open the haematoma by incising Glisson's capsule. Haemostasis is secured by diathermy to the exposed liver surface, as described later (Fig. 2.3). Deep stab wounds with extensive bleeding require hepatotomy and individual suture ligation of the bleeding vessels. The same applies to low-velocity missile injuries. Hepatic lobectomy is rarely required as a formal procedure despite recommendations for its use in the past.

In most patients with liver injuries, however caused, there will be either no bleeding from the liver, in which case nothing further need be done, or liver bleeding that is easily controlled. The patient's abdomen can then be closed with or without drainage.

Patients with major liver injuries and particularly those with hepatic vein and vena caval injuries must be identified early. Continued haemorrhage after applying porta hepatis occlusion (Pringle manoeuvre) suggests hepatic vein or vena caval injury, and once confirmed a compression perihepatic pack should be inserted: 6–8 large abdominal swabs are usually required. If the operating surgeon does not have extensive experience with liver surgery the abdomen should be closed with the packs in situ while awaiting either transfer of the patient to a specialist centre or the arrival of an experienced surgeon. Such a policy can be lifesaving and is the only acceptable procedure today for the inexperienced surgeon (Feliciano et al 1981, 1986, Carmona et al 1984, Svoboda et al 1982, Calne et al 1979).

Hepatotomy and direct vessel ligation Whenever extensive bleeding occurs during a liver split procedure or prior to the exposure of a bleeding site, it can be controlled by the Pringle manoeuvre (Pringle 1908). To achieve this the porta hepatis is exposed and encircled with a silastic snare and clamped with a soft bowel clamp to prevent damage to the vessels and bile duct (Fig. 2.1). If this procedure does not achieve complete haemostasis, then hepatic vein or vena caval injury should be suspected and dealt with as described. Hepatic inflow occlusion should be continued until haemostasis has been secured. It can be used for periods of up to an hour or longer (Kahn et al 1986, Feliciano et al 1986, Pachter et al 1983) but should preferably be used for the shortest possible time in each individual patient.

Major bleeding sites at the base of a liver tear should be exposed using the finger fracture technique (Fig. 2.2) to open through normal liver tissue, thereby extending the tear further until the bleeding site can be seen and directly ligated

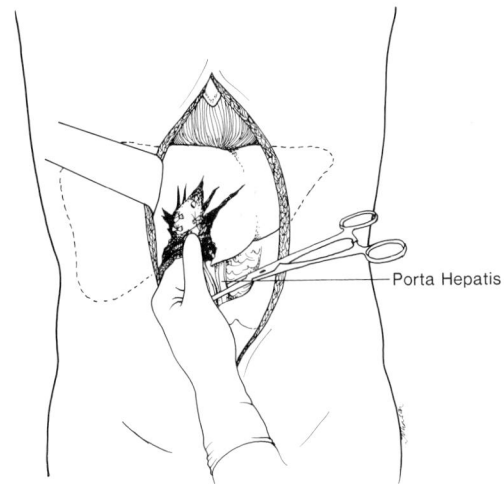

Fig. 2.2 Finger fracture technique. With the porta hepatis occluded, major bleeding sites deep in the liver tissue are exposed by separating liver tissue between the thumb and index finger and dividing vascular structures.

(Pachter et al 1983). Actively bleeding penetrating wounds should be similarly opened, extending the incision through normal liver tissue until the bleeding vessel can be seen and directly ligated. All open wounds, whether created by the initial trauma or by surgery, require careful haemostasis of the divided surfaces and inspection to find and ligate any divided bile ducts. An omental pack can be prepared and inserted into the wound as has been advocated recently (Stone & Lamb 1975, Feliciano et al 1986). The present authors have not used this technique, and have found that few patients develop bile leaks or subsequent haemorrhage if adequate attention is paid to haemostasis and ligature of small bile ducts at the time of the original procedure.

Continued oozing from the liver surface can be treated by large mattress sutures, and we use these occasionally. However, they should seldom be inserted blindly into a deep-seated bleeding liver wound. We have found high-frequency diathermy useful to stop minor oozing from the raw liver surface. The technique is shown in Fig. 2.3. A metal sucker is used and the diathermy is applied to the sucker as demonstrated. The coagulation setting on the diathermy apparatus is turned up high. Major vessels that had previously been ligated are carefully avoided. The sucker removes both blood

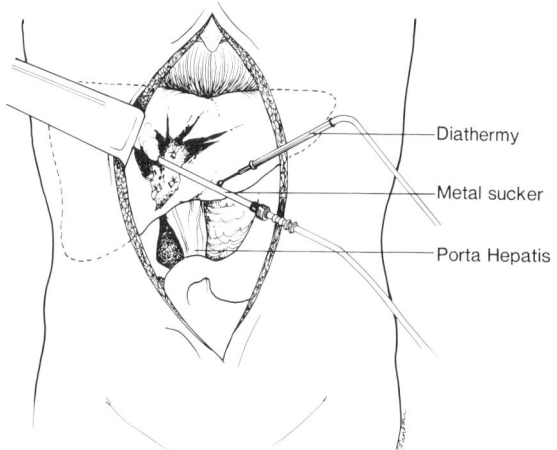

Diathermy

Metal sucker

Porta Hepatis

Fig. 2.3 Diathermy-sucker technique of achieving haemostasis. Coagulation diathermy is applied to a metal sucker. The sucker removes both blood and smoke while coagulating the raw liver surface. Previously ligated major vessels must be avoided.

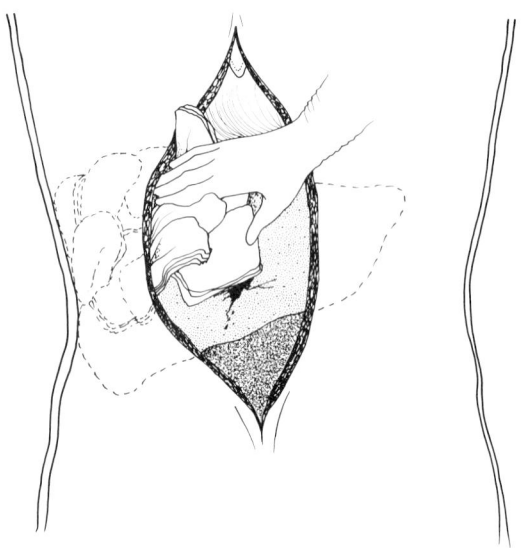

Fig. 2.4 Liver packing. Haemostasis is achieved by inserting a number of large abdominal swabs between the liver and the diaphragm or surrounding structures, thereby producing compression. Packs should not be inserted into the defects in the liver.

and smoke while coagulating the raw liver surface. Patients with major liver injuries frequently require massive blood transfusion and develop coagulopathy with extensive oozing at the end of the procedure. Under these circumstances the liver should be packed to achieve haemostasis (Feliciano et al 1986, Carmona et al 1984, Svoboda et al 1982) (Fig. 2.4). The abdomen is closed and the patient is returned to an intensive care unit. These packs are removed between 24 hours and 3–4 days later, once the haematological defects have been corrected and the patient stabilized. The pack is removed in the operating theatre under general anaesthesia. At that time bleeding will usually be no longer a problem. Any residual dead liver tissue can be removed, but further liver resection is usually unnecessary if adequate debridement was performed at the first operation. Occasionally patients with major liver injury bleed so heavily that they need to be temporally packed for 24–48 h while their haematological condition is stabilized, and then returned to theatre for the formal hepatic surgical procedures. This technique saved the life of a recent young patient who had her devitalized right liver lobe resected and a tear in the left hepatic vein and another in the vena cava repaired in a second procedure.

The edges of the liver split should be left open with drains adjacent to them, as approximation of the edges may lead to a collection of bile and blood and predispose to intrahepatic sepsis. Closed irrigation drainage is the authors' current preference, but drains may not always be required (Mullins et al 1985).

Resectional debridement All dead and devitalised liver tissue should be removed in non-anatomical planes, using the finger fracture technique (Fig. 2.2), with suture ligation of individual vessels and bile ducts as they are encountered (Pachter et al 1983). The devitalized tissue is usually clearly visible. The period of removal should also be covered by porta hepatis occlusion (Pringle manoeuvre), as this simplifies the procedure and is associated with significantly less blood loss. Formal hepatic lobectomy should only be performed when the whole of a liver lobe has been devitalized. In the authors' experience this is very rarely necessary, and then only in massive trauma in patients with associated hepatic vein injuries.

Injuries to the porta hepatis These injuries, which may involve both the blood vessels and the main bile ducts, are rare, and their management is presented below. They are complex injuries and require an experienced liver surgeon.

Hepatic vein and inferior vena caval injuries As already indicated, the inexperienced surgeon should pack the liver and either transfer the patient or await the arrival of an expert. In any event definitive surgery commences with the insertion of packs until the anaesthetist has resuscitated the patient. The liver must then be fully mobilized as for an hepatic resection. This is not a new innovation and was used by Pringle (1908) and others at the turn of the century. Extended exposure may be required, and the authors use a lower sternal split (Miller 1972) and, if necessary, a T-incision from the midline out into the right flank. Liver mobilization is performed after clamping the porta hepatis (Pringle manoeuvre). Once hepatic vein or vena caval injuries are confirmed, the area is repacked and the vena cava is exposed above the liver by opening the lower sternum and splitting the diaphragm. This gives direct access to the vena cava, which need not necessarily be encircled before applying the clamp. The vena cava below the liver is similarly exposed and clamped. This isolates the liver totally (Fig. 2.1) and allows dissection to proceed until the injured veins are visualized and repaired. Vena caval defects should be directly repaired; hepatic vein defects can be either repaired or oversewn, depending on the extent of the injury and whether the right or left lobes of the liver need to be removed as well. Total hepatic vascular isolation has enabled the authors to save the lives of patients who would otherwise have died as a result of these very complex lesions (Fig. 2.1).

An alternative rapid exposure of the suprahepatic inferior vena cava can be obtained by an 'inverted hockey stick' incision in the tendinous portion of the diaphragm overlying the liver. This is preceded by dividing the falciform ligament down to the cava. The vena cava is thus directly exposed and can be clamped above the liver within the pericardial sac (Fig. 2.5).

High-velocity missile injuries These produce extensive damage beyond the missile tract, due to shock waves. Liver injuries are frequently fatal, either in their own right or because the patient has other mortal injuries. Occasionally extensive liver resection may be required to save the life of the patient, and this is one setting in which formal liver resection may be required.

Bile duct injuries

Isolated extrahepatic bile duct or porta hepatis injuries due to external trauma are exceedingly rare (Feliciano et al 1985). Injuries to other structures in the porta hepatis are more common than isolated bile duct injuries (Sheldon et al 1985) and often preclude initial bile duct repair. Associated injury to blood vessels is the most important and is frequently life-threatening, requiring urgent treatment. Complex injuries to the extrahepatic bile ducts often require anastomosis of high bile duct to the bowel as a secondary procedure. Extrahepatic bile duct injuries are therefore dealt with briefly in this section, which is mainly devoted to iatrogenic injuries of the bile ducts; these are usually associated with cholecystectomy (Andren-Sandberg et al 1985a).

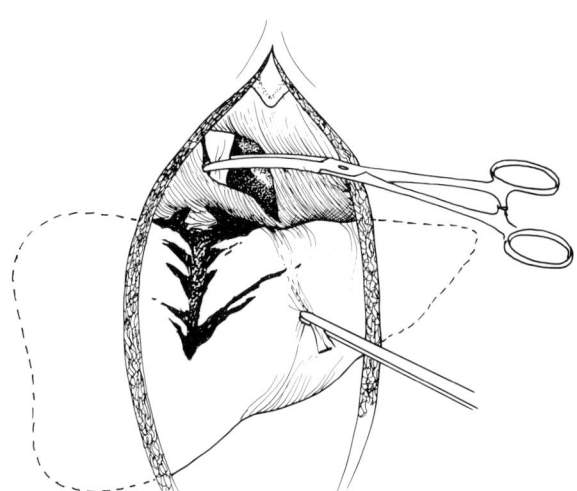

Fig. 2.5 Rapid exposure of the suprahepatic inferior vena cava in a patient with hepatic vein or vena caval injury. A 'hockey stick' incision in the diaphragm gives direct access to the suprahepatic IVC. Porta hepatis and infrahepatic IVC occlusion are also required to achieve total hepatic isolation.

External trauma to extrahepatic bile ducts

The rarity of the condition has been emphasized by Sheldon et al (1985) and Feliciano and colleagues

(1985). Less than 200 papers on this subject have appeared in the international literature. Injuries to the gallbladder, which are relatively simple to treat either by cholecystectomy or repair of the isolated damage, will not be considered.

It is of interest that bile duct injuries are seldom associated with portal vein injuries. Only 3/31 patients with porta hepatis injuries had bile duct injuries (Sheldon et al 1985). When bile duct injuries are associated with major vascular injuries, the latter take precedence in management. The priority is control of bleeding and repair of injured major vessels.

Penetrating injuries of the biliary tree are the most common, although these remain rare in relation to liver injuries (Feliciano et al 1985). Such injuries are frequently diagnosed at operation for intraperitoneal haemorrhage arising from associated vascular injuries. Blunt trauma to the extrahepatic biliary tree is distinctly rare. It is usually localized and more amenable to immediate ductal repair, but unfortunately it is commonly missed and may have serious delayed sequelae (Sheldon et al 1985). In these authors' algorithm for bile duct injury repair, direct repair is only advocated in isolated injuries or in patients in whom the associated vascular injury has been successfully dealt with. Review of these and other relatively large series (Zollinger et al 1972, Busuttil et al 1980) leads us to recommend the following policy: in porta hepatis injuries the hepatic artery should be ligated; portal vein injuries should be repaired directly. However, reports of survival after isolated portal vein ligation in porta hepatis trauma have been recorded (Petersen et al 1979). Bile duct injury, particularly high in the bile duct, should be repaired primarily with a hepaticojejunostomy (as for iatrogenic injuries) in those patients who are haemodynamically stable and where other organ injuries are controlled. Delayed repair should be undertaken in those patients with other severe injuries or who are difficult to control haemodynamically.

A recent report from Houston (Feliciano et al 1985) presented 13 cases with traumatic injury to the extrahepatic biliary system seen over a 7-year period. Only one of the patients had blunt trauma, 6 cases being stab wounds and the remaining 6 gunshot wounds. Nine patients had associated shock due to other injuries, particularly vascular injuries. Simple repair was performed in 9 patients, with 3 deaths due to other causes and only one late repair being required in the remaining 6 survivors. The other 4 had complex injuries. One died in hospital, and interestingly there were no late sequelae at long-term follow-up in the remaining 3.

We recommend that associated injuries, particularly vascular injuries, should take precedence in management. In otherwise stable patients major bile duct injuries should be repaired primarily by a hepaticojejunostomy. Small defects in the bile duct should be treated either by direct repair or initial stenting. The latter may be the only treatment required, although such patients require long-term follow-up with biochemical and ERCP confirmation that stricturing is not occurring. In patients with serious associated injuries or those who remain haemodynamically unstable for prolonged periods, stenting alone with subsequent delayed repair is probably the safest course of management.

Iatrogenic injuries to the bile ducts

Aetiology

Cholecystectomy is one of the most frequently performed operations in general surgery. Probably the most serious complication, which has a particularly high morbidity, is accidental damage to the bile duct during the operation. Fortunately this is uncommon, but the true incidence is not known because not all cases are reported. In Sweden, where about 15 000 cholecystectomies are performed annually, the health system and the Swedish Patients' Insurance Syndicate have made it possible for all 65 patients who suffered from this complication over an 8-year period to be comprehensively reviewed (Andren-Sandberg et al 1985a). In the Swedish experience, when compared with controls, injuries occurred significantly less in men than in women patients, and the patients were younger. The patients were usually otherwise fit, not obese and without evidence of suspected common bile duct stones. Most surgeons were in training, and 80% had done between 25 and 100 cholecystectomies before injuring a bile duct; they were seldom assisted by a more experienced surgeon. Inflammation and bleeding were not problems. The duct was damaged either before cholangiogram or before the films were available in the operating theatre for review in almost all cases. Most of the injuries were considered avoidable (Andren-Sanderberg et al 1985a).

In a study investigating factors responsible for bile duct injury, and also factors responsible for

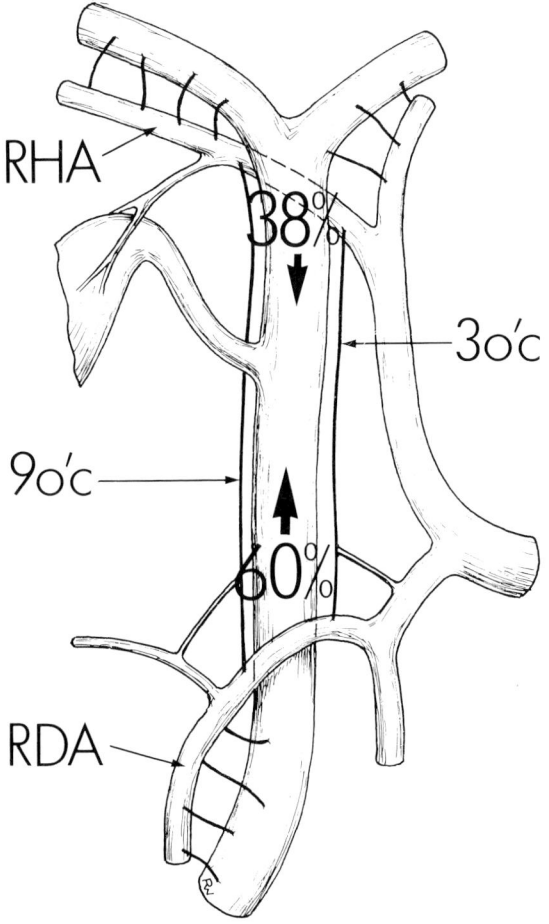

Fig. 2.6 Anterior view of the blood supply of the human bile duct. The blood supply to the bile ducts in the hilum of the liver (above) and the retropancreatic bile duct (below) from adjacent arteries is profuse. The supraduodenal bile duct blood supply is axial and tenuous, with 60% from below and 38% from above. The small main axial vessels (3 and 9 o'clock arteries) are vulnerable and easily damaged.
RHA, Right hepatic artery; RDA, retroduodenal artery.
(Reproduced with permission from Terblanche et al 1983)

leakage of the biliary anastomosis after liver transplantation or biliary tract operations, the Cape Town group, using a refined corrosion cast technique, has clearly defined the vascular supply of the human bile duct for the first time. As a result we have hypothesized on the aetiology and potential prevention of bile duct injuries (Northover & Terblanche 1978, 1979, Terblanche et al 1983). The arterial blood supply to the supraduodenal bile duct (namely, the bile duct segment between the right and left hepatic duct confluence and the first part of the duodenum) is essentially axial. The major supply (60%) comes from below, whereas the supply from above is only 38%. The main supply vessels run adjacent to the bile duct at 3 and 9 o'clock. They are very small (c. 0.3 mm in diameter), vulnerable and easily damaged (Fig. 2.6). Thus the blood supply from above to a common bile duct which is transected at a distal level is tenuous, except in the one-third of patients in whom the supraduodenal bile duct blood supply is enhanced by the newly described retroportal artery, which courses up the back of the bile duct and joins the right hepatic artery above. This has been described as the Type II pattern (Northover & Terblanche 1978) (Fig. 2.7). In contrast to the tenuous blood supply to the supraduodenal bile duct, the lower bile duct in the retropancreatic area and the higher bile ducts in the hilum of the liver have an excellent blood supply coming in laterally from adjacent arteries (Northover & Terblanche 1979) (Fig. 2.6). By amalgamating the views of previous authors (Appleby 1959, Carlson et al 1977, Douglass et al 1950), the Cape Town group has postulated that ischaemia of the supraduodenal bile duct initiates a vicious cycle where damage to the ductal mucosa allows bile to enter into the wall of the duct, thereby inducing inflammation and fibrosis, which in turn leads to further ischaemic damage to the ductal mucosa and wall with subsequent progressive stricturing.

The Cape Town group believes that this newly described anatomy helps to explain some of the previously poorly understood aspects of the aetiology of iatrogenic bile duct strictures. In addition a knowledge of the anatomy provides a better explanation for the recurrent strictures noted after repair of transected bile ducts, particularly when

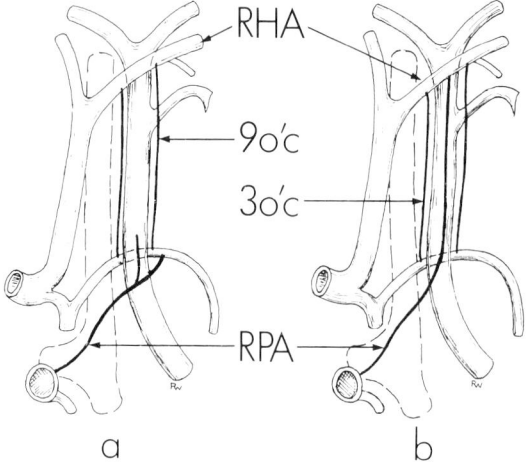

a   b

Fig. 2.7 Posterior view of the blood supply of the human bile duct, demonstrating the contribution of the retroportal artery (RPA). The RPA arises from the superior mesenteric artery (shown) or the coeliac axis. **a) Type I RPA.** In about 50% of the population it terminates by joining the retroduodenal artery, with only a small contribution to the blood supply of the supraduodenal bile duct from below **b) Type II RPA**: In one-third of the population it passes up the back of the bile duct to join the right hepatic artery (RHA) above. It is larger than the 3 and 9 o'clock arteries and, when present, can play a major role in supplying the supraduodenal bile duct from above because of its terminal connection to the right hepatic artery. (Reproduced with permission from Terblanche et al 1983)

a high anastomosis between the hepatic ducts and bowel has not been performed. Three cases illustrating this problem have been published (Terblanche et al 1983).

Clinical presentation

The detailed clinical presentations that can arise with this complication are beyond the scope of this chapter. Patients present in two main ways: Firstly with an injury that is noted at the time of the cholecystectomy, and secondly with an injury that is missed at that time and presents subsequently. When the injury is spotted at the time, the surgeon will recognize that he has mistaken the anatomy and divided the duct. The alternatives are partial division of the duct occurring during traction and attempted flush ligation of the cystic duct, and damage while attempting to control haemorrhage. The latter was formerly thought to be common,

but this is apparently no longer the case.

Patients who present late may become ill in the early postoperative period with evidence of bile leakage into the peritoneal cavity, but frequently they present even later with slowly progressive obstructive jaundice. Terblanche & Northover (1979) have postulated that initial limited damage creates a vicious cycle which can lead to increasing later damage.

Management

A high recurrent stricture rate after operative repair of iatrogenic bile duct strictures has been quoted even from specialist centres. Restricture rates of as high as 60–75% have been documented in recent literature (Pitt et al 1982, Pellegrini et al 1984, Warren & Jefferson 1973, Kune 1979). Other major series have published significantly better results. Ninety percent of the 63 patients operated on by stricture repair alone at the Hammersmith Hospital, London, had a satisfactory result with median follow-up of 3.3 years and a low operative mortality rate (Blumgart et al 1984). This group, like ourselves (Terblanche et al 1989), emphasizes high hepaticojejunostomy for repair, but concedes that longer follow-up is required to ensure that late strictures do not develop. The superiority of a high hepaticojejunal anastomosis over direct bile duct repair is supported by most of the recent major publications (Pitt et al 1982, Pellegrini et al 1984, Saber & El-Manialawi 1984, Andren-Sandberg et al 1985b).

Repair at the time of damage   Major damage should be repaired by a high hepaticojejunostomy. Minor partial incision of the duct can be treated by inserting a T-tube or a direct repair which can be stented directly at the time or subsequently, if required, at ERCP. In our view, if a clean division is to be treated by direct end-to-end duct repair, the edges should be cut back until normal tissue is reached and adequate back-bleeding should be checked prior to the direct anastomosis. The role of simple postoperative ERCP stenting for a minor leak has yet to be defined but may prove of benefit.

Delayed repair of bile duct injuries When the patient presents late, in almost all instances a high hepaticojejunostomy will be required if satisfactory results are to be achieved. The major publications supporting this view are referred to above. In those patients who present late and who have already developed associated portal hypertension, the results of surgery are very much worse (Blumgart et al 1984, Pellegrini et al 1984, Genest et al 1986).

The role of stenting after high hepaticojejunostomy remains controversial. There has been an increasing trend away from stenting if an adequate wide mucosa-to-mucosa anastomosis has been achieved, and this is the current philosophy of the present authors, although they previously used stenting (Terblanche et al 1989). We have even moved away from prolonged stenting of difficult high strictures, which was our previous policy, and currently use a jejunal access limb placed beneath the abdominal wall to provide ready access for later percutaneous dilatation should this be required (Krige et al 1987). The alternative view of prolonged stenting is supported by the group from the Lahey Clinic, who claim better results with prolonged stenting (Warren & Jefferson 1973).

Preliminary data on the use of balloon dilatation of strictured bile ducts by either the percutaneous transhepatic route or the ERCP route have been encouraging but longer follow-up is required (Mueller et al 1986, Foutch & Sivak 1985, Little et al 1986, Huibregtse et al 1986). In the authors' view, fit patients should have operative repair, but balloon dilatation should be seriously considered in poor-risk patients and patients with severe portal hypertension. As previously indicated, where adequate high bowel-to-bile duct anastomosis is not achieved, an access loop of jejunum allows for subsequent easy percutaneous dilatation (Krige et al 1987).

Cape Town data on late repair of iatrogenic bile duct strictures Eleven patients with bile duct strictures treated in our unit between 1973 and 1979 have been compared with 10 patients with repair of bile duct strictures between 1980 and 1984. The cut-off at 1979 was selected because of the recognition at that time of the importance of bile duct vascular supply in the operative repair (Northover & Terblanche 1979). The median follow-up periods for the two groups were 8 years and 4 years 4 months respectively. There were no recurrent strictures in the post-1979 patients, as opposed to 4 in the pre-1979 patients. The data could be criticized because of the sequential grouping of the patients. However both in our own experience and in other major series, two-thirds of strictures appear within 3 years of operative repair. We believe that our changed attitude towards undertaking high hepaticojejunostomy for bile duct strictures is responsible for the better results achieved in the recent series. We therefore advocate that cognizance be taken of the blood supply of the bile duct in undertaking repair of biliary strictures (Terblanche et al 1989).

REFERENCES

Andren-Sandberg A, Alinder G, Bengmark S 1985a Accidental lesions of the common bile duct at cholecystectomy. Pre- and perioperative factors of importance. Annals of Surgery 201: 328–332

Andren-Sandberg A, Johansson S, Bengmark S 1985b Accidental lesions of the common bile duct at cholecystectomy. II. Results of treatment. Annals of Surgery 201: 452–455

Appleby L 1959 Indwelling common duct tubes. Journal of International College of Surgeons 31: 631–643

Athey G W 1982 Hepatic haematoma following blunt injury: Nonoperative management. Injury 13: 302–306

Blumgart L H, Kelly C J, Benjamin I S 1984 Benign bile duct strictures following cholecystectomy: Critical factors in management. British Journal of Surgery 71: 836–843

Busuttil R W, Kitahama A, Cerise E, McFadden M, Lo R, Longmire W P 1980 Management of blunt and penetrating injuries to the porta hepatis. Annals of Surgery 191: 641–648

Calne R Y, McMaster P, Pentlow B D 1979 The treatment of major liver trauma by primary packing with transfer of the patient for definitive treatment. British Journal of Surgery 66: 338–339

Carlson E, Zukoski C F, Campbell J, Chvapil M 1977 Morphological, biophysical and biochemical consequences of ligation of the common biliary duct in the dog. American Journal of Pathology 86: 301–312

Carmona R H, Peck D Z, Lim R C Jr 1984 The role of packing and planned reoperation in severe hepatic trauma. Journal of Trauma 24: 779–784

Cywes S, Rode H, Miller A J W 1985 Blunt liver trauma in children: Nonoperative management. Journal of Pediatric Surgery 20: 14–18

Demetriades D, Rabinowitz B, Sofianos C 1986 Non-operative management of penetrating liver injuries: a prospective study. British Journal of Surgery 73: 736–737

Douglass T C, Lounsbury B F, Cutter W W, Wetzel N 1950 An experimental study of healing of the common

bile duct. Surgery Gynecology and Obstetrics
91: 301–305

Feliciano D V, Mattox K L, Jordan G L 1981
Intra-abdominal packing for control of hepatic
hemorrhage: a reappraisal. Journal of Trauma
21: 285–290

Feliciano D V, Bitondo C G, Burch J M, Mattox K L, Beall
A C, Jordan G L Jr 1985 Management of traumatic
injuries to the extrahepatic biliary ducts. American
Journal of Surgery 150: 705–709

Feliciano D V, Jordon G L, Bitondo C G, Mattox K L,
Burch J M, Cruse P A 1986 Management of 1000
consecutive cases of hepatic trauma (1979–1984). Annals
of Surgery 204: 438–445

Flint L M, Polk H C 1979 Selective hepatic artery ligation:
limitations and failures. Journal of Trauma 19: 319–323

Foutch M V, Sivak M V 1985 Therapeutic endoscopic
balloon dilatation of the extrahepatic biliary ducts.
American Journal of Gastroenterology 80: 575–580

Geis W P, Schulz K A, Giacchino J L, Freeark R J 1981
The fate of unruptured intrahepatic hematoma. Surgery
90: 689–697

Genest J F, Nanos E, Grundfest-Broniatowski S, Vogt D,
Hermann R E 1986 Benign biliary strictures: an analytic
review (1970–1984). Surgery 99: 409–413

Grisoni E R, Gauderer M L, Ferron J, Izant R J 1984
Nonoperative management of liver injuries following blunt
abdominal trauma in children. Journal of Pediatric
Surgery 19: 515–518

Huguet C, Nordlinger B, Black P, Conrad J 1978 Tolerance
of the human liver to prolonged normothermic ischemia:
A biological study of 20 patients submitted to extensive
hepatectomy. Archives of Surgery 113: 1448–1451

Huibregtse K, Katon R M, Tytgat G N J 1986 Endoscopic
treatment of post-operative biliary strictures. Endoscopy
18: 133–137

Kahn D, Hickman R, Dent D M, Terblanche J 1986 For
how long can the liver tolerate ischaemia? European
Surgical Research 18: 277–282

Krige J E J, Terblanche J 1989 Complex liver injuries.
(Submitted for publication.)

Krige J E J, Bornman P C, Harries-Jones E P, Terblanche J
1987 Modified hepaticojejunostomy for permanent biliary
access. British Journal of Surgery 74: 612–613

Kune G 1979 Bile duct injury during cholecystectomy:
causes, prevention and surgical repair in 1979. Australian
and New Zealand Journal of Surgery 49: 35–40

Little J M, Wong K P, Simmons K 1986 Percutaneous
transhepatic dilatation in the management of bile duct
strictures. Australian and New Zealand Journal of Surgery
56: 697–700

Lucas C E, Walt A J 1972 Analysis of randomized biliary
drainage for liver trauma in 189 patients. Journal of
Trauma 12: 925–930

Mays E T 1972 Lobar dearterialization for exsanguinating
wounds of the liver. Journal of Trauma 12: 397–407

Merendino K A, Dillard D H, Cammock E E 1963 The
concept of surgical biliary decompression in the
management of liver trauma. Surgery, Gynecology and
Obstetrics 117: 285–293

Meyer A A, Crass R A, Lim R C Jr, Jeffrey R B, Federle
M P, Trunkey D D 1985 Selective nonoperative
management of blunt liver injury using computed
tomography. Archives of Surgery 120: 550–554

Miller D R 1972 Median sternotomy extension of abdominal
incision for hepatic lobectomy. Annals of Surgery
175: 193–196

Moon K L, Federle M P 1983 Computed tomography in
hepatic trauma. American Journal of Roentgenology
141: 309–314

Moore E E 1984 Critical decisions in the management of
hepatic trauma. American Journal of Surgery
148: 712–716

Moore F A, Moore E E, Seagraves A 1985 Nonresectional
management of major hepatic trauma: An evolving
concept. American Journal of Surgery 150: 725–729

Mueller P R, van Sonnenberg E, Ferrucci J T, et al 1986
Biliary stricture dilatation: multicentre review of clinical
managment in 73 patients. Radiology 160: 17–22

Mullins R J, Stone H H, Dunlop W E, Strom P R 1985
Hepatic trauma: evaluation of routine drainage. Southern
Medical Journal 78: 259–261

Northover J M A, Terblanche J 1978 Bile duct blood
supply: its importance in human liver transplantation.
Transplantation 26: 67–69

Northover J M A, Terblanche J 1979 A new look at the
arterial supply of the bile duct in man and its surgical
implications. British Journal of Surgery 66: 379–384

Oldham K T, Guice K S, Ryckman F, Kaufman R A,
Martin L W, Noseworthy J 1986 Blunt liver injury in
childhood: Evolution of therapy and current perspective.
Surgery 100: 542–549

Pachter H L, Spencer F C, Hofstetter S R, Coppa G F 1983
Experience with the finger fracture technique to achieve
intra-hepatic hemostasis in 75 patients with severe injuries
of the liver. Annals of Surgery 197: 771–778

Pachter H L, Spencer F C, Hofstetter S R, Laing H C,
Coppa G F 1986 The management of juxtahepatic venous
injuries without an atriocaval shunt: Preliminary clinical
observations. Surgery 99: 569–575

Pellegrini C A, Thomas M J, Way L W 1984 Recurrent
biliary stricture. Patterns of recurrence and outcome of
surgical therapy. American Journal of Surgery
147: 175–180

Petersen S R, Sheldon G F, Lim R C Jr 1979 Management
of portal vein injuries. Journal of Trauma 19: 616–620

Pitt H A, Toshimitsu M, Parapatis S K, Tompkins R K,
Longmire W P 1982 Factors influencing outcome in
patients with post-operation biliary strictures. American
Journal of Surgery 144: 14–21

Pringle J H 1908 Notes on the arrest of hepatic hemorrhage
due to trauma. Annals of Surgery 48: 541–549

Saber K, El-Manialawi M 1984 Repair of bile duct injuries.
World Journal of Surgery 8: 82–89

Schrock T, Blaisdell F W, Mathewson C Jr 1968
Management of blunt trauma to the liver and hepatic
veins. Archives of Surgery 96: 698–704

Sheldon G F, Lim R C, Yee E S, Petersen S R 1985
Management of injuries to the porta hepatis. Annals of
Surgery 202: 539–545

Stone H H, Lamb J M 1975 Use of pedicled omentum as
an autogenous pack for control of hemorrhage in major
injuries of the liver. Annals of Surgery 141: 92–94

Svoboda J A, Peter E T, Dang C V, Parks S N, Ellyson
J H 1982 Severe liver trauma in the face of coagulopathy.
American Journal of Surgery 144: 717–721

Terblanche J, Allison H F, Northover J M A 1983 An
ischemic basis for biliary strictures. Surgery 94: 52–57

Terblanche J, Worthley C S, Spence R A J, Krige J E J 1989 High or low hepatico-jejunostomy for bile duct strictures. (Submitted for publication.)

Walt A J 1978 The mythology of hepatic trauma — or Babel revisited. American Journal of Surgery 135: 12–18

Warren K W, Jefferson M F 1973 Prevention and repair of strictures of the extrahepatic bile ducts. Surgical Clinics of North America 53: 1169–1190

Zollinger R M Jr, Keller R M, Hubay C A 1972 Traumatic rupture of the right and left hepatic ducts. Journal of Trauma 12: 563–569

3 Injuries to the spleen and pancreas

B. F. GILCHRIST and D. D. TRUNKEY

The spleen

The spleen has fascinated medicine's finest minds. The great Roman physician, Galen, viewed the spleen as 'an organ full of mystery' (Kuhn 1964), and in 1725 Sir Richard Blackmore wrote the following:

'It is impossible to inspect and contemplate this large Organ, without concluding, that it must have some important Office in the Animal Administration and that it is not a superfluous and impertinent Fungus, or an Error or Sport of Nature.' (Looareesuwan et al 1987)

Aristotle was the first to recognize that the spleen was not necessary for existence (Peck 1955). His assumption persisted through the Roman and medieval eras and was re-emphasized by Malpighi (1666). It was difficult for anyone to challenge this assumption since the function of the spleen was unknown. Early writers such as Pliny thought that the spleen controlled laughter. However, Halevi writing in the 10th century stated, 'the spleen is called laughing because of its nature to cleanse the blood and spirit from unclean obscuring matter.' (Rosner 1972) Animal experiments in the 18th century added little to knowledge of the splenic function.

The first experiments relating the spleen to infection resistance came in 1919 by Morris and Bullock who studied rat plague in splenectomized rats. They showed that the spleen is important in resisting infectious processes in rats and that its removal had a deleterious effect on resistance. Although splenectomy was compatible with survival they concluded that, 'this does not settle the problem as to whether or not a splenectomized person can weather a critical illness.' Subsequent papers challenged this very important concept and controversy continued unabated until 1952, when King and Schumacher published their classic paper on increased susceptibility to infection in infants following splenectomy.

Until recently, the spleen has been regarded as little more than a sac of blood with no essential function. As a result, general policy dictated removal should there be any evidence of injury, including minor iatrogenic tears caused by other surgical procedures. One factor that contributed to the problem was that delayed haemorrhage from the spleen was a well established surgical principle. This quiescent period is referred to as the latent period of Baudet. Although it has been referred to as a delayed rupture, we do not know of any established case in which a spleen verified as intact at laparotomy subsequently bled. A poll conducted at the Western Surgical Association could not document a case of delayed rupture (Blaisdell, 1988, personal communication). Delayed haemorrhage, in our analysis, simply implies that a spleen initially ruptured may not bleed sufficiently to produce clinical signs. However, after hours, days, or even months, a secondary haemorrhage may occur. This event can be due to further trauma to the spleen, to the expansion of a large haematoma or to continued ongoing slow haemorrhage. The highest incidence of delayed haemorrhage is within the first 24 hours. The incidence of secondary bleeding decreases geometrically with time (Olsen & Polley 1977).

Anatomy

The spleen is an elongated, ovoid body located in the left upper quadrant of the abdomen directly beneath the diaphragm, posterior and to the left of the stomach. It is protected anteriorly, laterally and posteriorly by the lower portion of the rib cage. Embryologically the spleen arises by mesenchymal differentiation along the left side of the dorsal mesogastrium in the 8 mm embryo. The size of the spleen is influenced directly by blood pressure and is also increased after meals. The average weight of the adult spleen, however, is between 75 and 100 g. There is a slight involution of this organ after the age of 60.

The hilum of the spleen is in immediate proximity to the tail of the pancreas. The anterior superior surface of the spleen is in proximity to the greater curvature of the stomach. The anterior inferior portion of the spleen has an intimate relationship to the splenic flexure of the colon. Laterally and posteriorly the spleen lies in contact with the diaphragm. Medially and posteriorly lies the left kidney. The attachments of the spleen consist of the splenophrenic ligament posteriorly (a thin leaf-like attachment which is easily disrupted by blunt dissection), the gastrosplenic ligament, in which run the short gastric vessels, and the splenocolic ligament consisting of the lateral portion of the greater omentum.

The spleen is the most vascularized organ in the body. Its blood supply includes the splenic artery, a varying number of pancreatic branches and several branches from the stomach (the vasa brevia). The splenic artery, the largest branch of the coeliac trunk, runs a highly tortuous course, particularly in older people. The main splenic artery usually divides into five or six large branches in the hilum before entering the splenic pulp (Fig. 3.1). The splenic vein is likewise formed outside the hilum. It courses along the dorsal surface of the pancreas where it joins the superior mesenteric vein to form the portal vein.

Anatomical variants in contour, fetal lobulations and shape, are common in spleens. Equally important is the incidence of accessory spleens, which may be found in up to 30% of patients. These ectopic spleens have an obviously important role

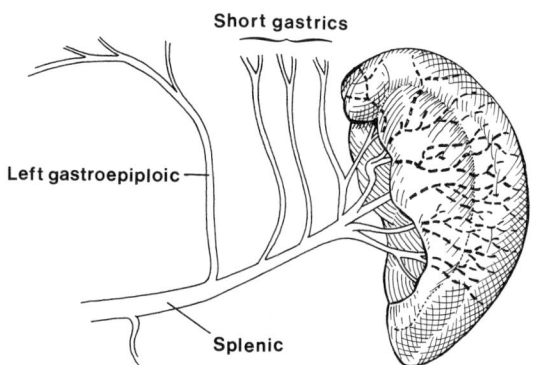

Fig. 3.1 Arterial supply of the spleen. Five to six branches take origin proximal to and in the hilum, providing segmental circulation to the spleen. The most proximal branch of the splenic artery shown here is the left gastroepiploic, followed by the short gastric arteries to the proximal portion of the greater curvature of the stomach. (Reproduced from Blaisdell & Trunkey 1982).

in function after splenectomy for trauma.

The spleen has a capsule of 1–2 mm in thickness which with the trabeculae encloses the splenic pulp. Lymphoid tissue or malpighian follicles are scattered throughout this pulp and constitute 25% of the reticuloendothelial system. The controversy as to whether the splenic circulation is closed or open is still unsettled. Nonetheless, as Peters (1983) noted, the circulation of the spleen has two functional components — the fast and the slow. The 'fast' (closed) component is routed through endothelialized vessels like other vascular beds, and is mainly nutritive. The blood of the 'slow' (open) component leaves the endothelialized vessels at the arteriolar termination and cords of Billroth. After filtering through the red pulp, where the cells are in intimate contact with immunological effector cells, the blood re-enters the circulation by passing into the splenic sinuses. The walls of these sinuses are composed of endothelial cells separated by slits measuring 1–3 μm. Cells must be deformable to negotiate this passage; those that cannot change shape are left in the cords of Billroth. The critical feature, then, of the splenic circulation is the passage of arterial blood into the venous sinuses (physiological shunt). Although the intricate dynamics of splenic circulation are still being studied today, it is definitely known that the spleen has at least five functions.

Function

Splenic function can be divided into five broad categories (Blaisdell & Trunkey 1982):

1. Filter for particulate matter, old red cells
2. Source of opsonins–tuftsin and properdin
3. Source of immunoglobulin IgM
4. Regulates T and B lymphocytes
5. Source of haematopoiesis in utero

of which four are very important to the trauma patient (Eichner 1979). The first function is that of monitoring bloodborne particulate antigens, blood cells and bacteria. The spleen is also a source of opsonins, notably tuftsin and properdin. In addition, the spleen contributes to the production of IGM antibody, which is markedly decreased after splenectomy. The spleen assists, too, in the regulation of both B and T lymphocytes. The fifth function, haematopoiesis in utero, is relatively unimportant to the trauma patient.

The spleen is the primary defence organ when the host has been invaded by bloodborne bacteria and has little or no pre-existing antibody. This capacity is due to the unique microcirculation of the splenic pulp as noted above. This circulation allows for delay, which gives splenic phagocytes time to remove even poorly opsonized bacteria. Although the liver is the most important organ for removing well opsonized bacteria, the spleen, because of its unique filter-circulation, is more effective in removing poorly opsonized bacteria.

Particulate antigens are similarly cleared by this sieving effect and in addition initiate IGM antibody response in the germinal centres. Red cells are similarly altered or eliminated as they pass through the spleen. The spleen is capable of selective removal of red cell parts: it can remove surface craters, pits from normal red cells and Howell-Jolly bodies as well as Pappenheimer siderocytes. As red cells become senescent they lose enzyme activity; the spleen, recognizing this, traps the cells and destroys them.

Asplenia leads to subnormal levels of tuftsins and properdin. Tuftsin, identified at Tufts Medical School in 1974, is a tetrapeptide that coats white cells and promotes phagocytosis of particu-

late matter, bacteria and aged blood cells. Properdin is an important component of the alternate pathway of complement activation, and subnormal levels will impair the serum opsonization of encapsulated bacteria, such as meningococci and pneumococci (Winkelstein & Lambat, 1975).

Assessment of injury

Rosoff et al (1972) have divided the clinical manifestations of traumatic rupture of the spleen into two distinct categories: the systemic symptoms of acute haemorrhage and the local symptoms of peritoneal irritation in the region of the spleen. Peritoneal haemorrhage is usually a diagnosis of exclusion, since overt signs are often absent or attenuated. Assessment of any trauma patient should include a chest X-ray, which will eliminate the hemithoraces as a significant source of blood loss. Similarly, clinical assessment of the thighs and lower legs will rule them out as a major source of haemorrhage. By exclusion the abdomen then becomes the primary cavity of suspicion for continued blood loss. This possibility is documented by repeated physical examinations, serial haematocrits, serial white counts and the use of special adjunctive procedures such as CT and ultrasound scanning (see Ch. 7). Sonography is particularly useful in detecting free fluid and may be sensitive to as little as 300 ml of blood. If the patient is unconscious, paralysed, uncooperative or otherwise lost to a proper physical examination, peritoneal lavage should be considered (see Ch. 7). Absolute signs for peritoneal exploration include involuntary guarding and unexplained shock.

Though many signs have been described and attributed to peritoneal irritation secondary to splenic rupture, very few have clinical meaning. Blood, per se, may not be irritating to the peritoneum. Clinical signs are usually secondary to diaphragmatic irritation, chest wall contusion, rib fractures or associated injuries. The Ballance sign, 'large, fixed dullness in the left flank', Kehr's sign, 'pain at the top of the left shoulder caused by irritation of the inferior surface of the left diaphragm,' and Seagesser's sign, 'pain produced in the neck by pressure over the phrenic nerve' have been only of slight help in determining splenic injury.

The enlarged, diseased spleen is easily traumatized, and rupture may result from trauma so mild that it is not remembered by the patient. The spleen is predictably prone to rupture during pregnancy, when the splenic capsule may be thinned and the spleen relatively congested. In most instances there is a history of significant trauma to the left upper quadrant or the lower rib cage. Since the hilum of the spleen is centred on the posterior axillary line, with the spleen lying between the eighth and tenth ribs, fractures of these ribs posteriorly carries a 20% chance of rupture. Therefore, assessment of the possibility of splenic rupture begins with assessment of the integrity of the chest wall. If the patient is able to take a deep breath without discomfort, the likelihood of rib fracture is slight. Conversely, if pleuritic-type pain occurs with respiration, and this is referred to the lower ribs, fracture can be assumed despite negative rib X-rays. Palpation will confirm which ribs are involved. Current adjunctive measures most useful in evaluation of splenic trauma are sonography, CT scan and arteriography. All are capable of detecting defects within the splenic parenchyma and are capable of detecting free fluid within the posterior gutters of the peritoneum.

Chest radiographs may confirm the presence of rib fractures or reveal a left pleural effusion. A flat film of the abdomen may occasionally be of value, if it shows displacement of the gastric air bubble and apparent enlargement of the spleen or a fluid collection between bowel loops. When injury is confined to the abdomen, however, we rarely utilize lavage but rely on clinical guidelines. In multiply injured patients, when monitoring blood loss is difficult, peritoneal lavage may be indicated and may lead to an earlier diagnosis of splenic injury.

A team approach is often mandatory in the patient with multiple injuries and may include decompression of space-occupying intracranial blood by neurosurgeons, while general surgeons explore the abdomen. Priorities must be established immediately. In the patients with abdominal injuries and an associated widened mediastinum, exploration of the abdomen with repair of the injuries is indicated first. Following laparotomy the patient should have an aortogram and possible thoracotomy with repair of the thoracic aorta. If the patient has associated major vascular injuries in the extremities, control of these must be obtained prior to abdominal exploration. If the patient remains unstable, exploratory laparotomy should be carried out before definitive treatment of the vascular injury.

One of the most controversial issues in regard to management of spleen injury is the so-called 'conservative' approach (Ein et al 1977). Some surgeons have advocated that children need not be operated on in the majority of instances. A careful analysis of these studies shows that the non-operated children require more blood. Those receiving more than four units of blood run a greater risk of hepatitis than of contracting postsplenectomy sepsis. Other criticisms include inappropriate deaths from splenic exsanguination. There is no question that some splenic injuries can be managed nonoperatively. However, this approach must be supported by diagnostic CT scanning to confirm that there has been minimal blood loss and no associated injuries.

Preoperative preparation

After initial assessment and resuscitation, certain preoperative adjuncts should be considered. Broad-spectrum antibiotics should be administered prior to operation when concomitant injury to the colon or small bowel is suspected. This precaution is particularly appropriate in penetrating wounds of the abdomen. If no colon or small bowel injuries are found at the time of laparotomy, the antibiotics can be discontinued. If such injuries are found, they should be continued for 24–48 h.

Operative exploration and splenic evaluation

For rapid access and wide exposure the midline incision is utilized. Our prejudice is 'that the Creator made the midline for surgeons', and we strongly recommend it here. The surgeon should always be prepared to extend the midline incision up the sternum or into the left or right chest, if necessary. The skin over the chest should always be prepared before operation along with the skin of the abdomen; the dictum we follow is that the preparation should be from 'clavicles to toes, tabletop to tabletop'.

After the initial incision has been made, the surgeon must rule out major vascular injury (Sherman 1980). First, the abdomen is entered and the patient is rapidly eviscerated. Next, blood is aspirated from all quadrants of the abdomen, with each quadrant packed to localize bleeding. The presence of clot points to the site of haemorrhage, and with splenic rupture it is usually found in the left upper quadrant surrounding the spleen. In the absence of localizing clot, the spleen should be exposed extremely gently, since the probability of injury is low and in the course of exposure, the spleen may inadvertently be traumatized.

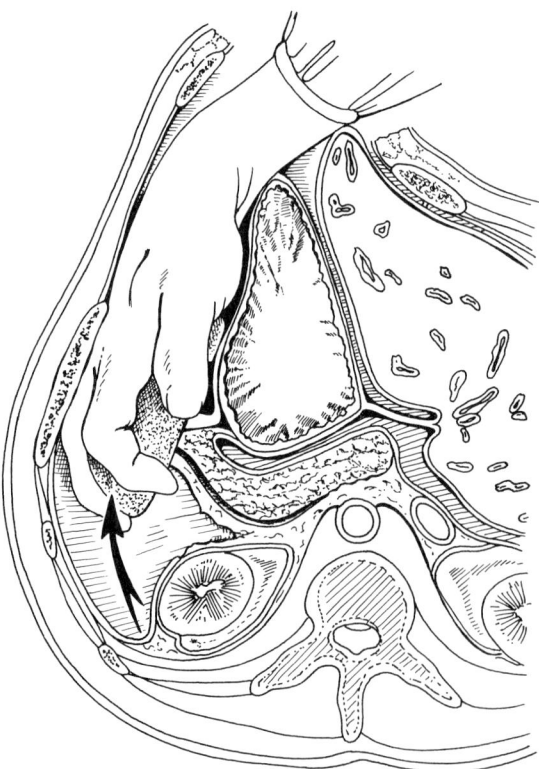

Fig. 3.2 The spleen is mobilized by traction upward and medially, developing the plane posterior to the pancreas. This is usually done most quickly by blunt digital dissection of the lateral and posterior splenic attachment. (Reproduced from Blaisdell & Trunkey 1982)

Once splenic rupture is verified by the presence of clot around the spleen, palpation of the laceration, or visualisation of ongoing haemorrhage, the spleen is mobilized by blunt dissection, severing the splenophrenic ligament posteriorly (Fig. 3.2). This manoeuvre allows for medial mobilization of the spleen. Sharp dissection of the lateral attachments of the colon facilitates the exposure. Care should be taken to avoid injury to the pancreas. Exposure and control of splenic haemorrhage is best obtained by full mobilization of the spleen into the midline. Control of the splenic blood supply should not be attempted through the lesser sac, as this may aggravate the bleeding.

Splenic injuries vary from small capsular avulsion injuries to the more extensive fragmenting types of injuries. In general, injuries to the costal surface lend themselves to repair more readily than those to the hilar area. Similarly, horizontal fractures and avulsions of the capsule are easier to control than are the larger stellate and fragmenting types of injury.

Although controversy still exists, there are certain general rules that can now be applied to splenic salvage. It is prudent to salvage all spleens when possible in both adults and (particularly) children. Factors that mitigate against splenic salvage include: uncontrolled haemorrhage from the spleen, major hilar avulsion injuries and severe associated injuries requiring considerable time to repair.

Operative treatment

In our experience, about two-thirds of injured spleens can be saved and one-third require splenectomy. The precise rules regarding splenic injury management are still undergoing evaluation. It is our position that undue enthusiasm for preserving spleens may render the patient vulnerable to more severe complications than those following splenectomy.

Once the spleen is exposed, the injury can be treated by observation, by packing with microcrystalline collagen or omentum, by suture of lacerations, by partial splenectomy, or by total splenectomy. Control of the hilar vessels can be partially obtained manually, the key being to grasp the tail of the pancreas in the thumb and the forefinger. Division of the short gastric vessels between the greater curvature of the stomach and the hilum of the spleen facilitates control of bleeding at the hilum. If there is room between the tail of the pancreas and the hilum, a soft vascular clamp (Fogarty type) can be applied to give complete haemostasis. This is best facilitated by mobilizing and separating the splenic flexure of the colon from the splenic hilum.

A small capsular tear may not require treatment. If bleeding has ceased spontaneously, it may be treated either with coagulation diathermy or with microcrystalline collagen application (Strauch 1979). Larger capsular avulsions and superficial lacerations can be treated by packing with microcrystalline collagen (Fig. 3.3). This substance is best applied with a dry sponge over the injured area, with firm pressure maintained for 5–10 min. This manoeuvre will control most superficial

bleeding satisfactorily. For deeper capsular tears, when there is associated haematoma in the splenic pulp, the haematoma should be evacuated. Larger bleeding points should be controlled by suture or by coagulation diathermy. The capsular tear must then be approximated with 5–0 or 6–0 Prolene sutures (Fig. 3.4). The sutures must be placed meticulously in a similar fashion to that utilized for a fragile vein repair. For deeper lacerations or lacerations bleeding more vigorously, mattress sutures, using a larger needle, and sutures such as polyglycolate or chromic catgut tied over Teflon bolsters may be necessary.

In some injuries, such as those involving the upper or lower pole of the spleen, segmental resection of the spleen may be possible (Buntain & Lynn 1979, Weinstein et al 1979) (Fig. 3.5). Bleeding points on the raw surface of the spleen can be controlled by suture ligature and coagulation diathermy (Fig. 3.6). Further haemostasis is obtained by microcrystalline collagen, by omental patch or by a free graft of peritoneum.

When bleeding is massive, the most conservative treatment is splenectomy (Connors 1928,

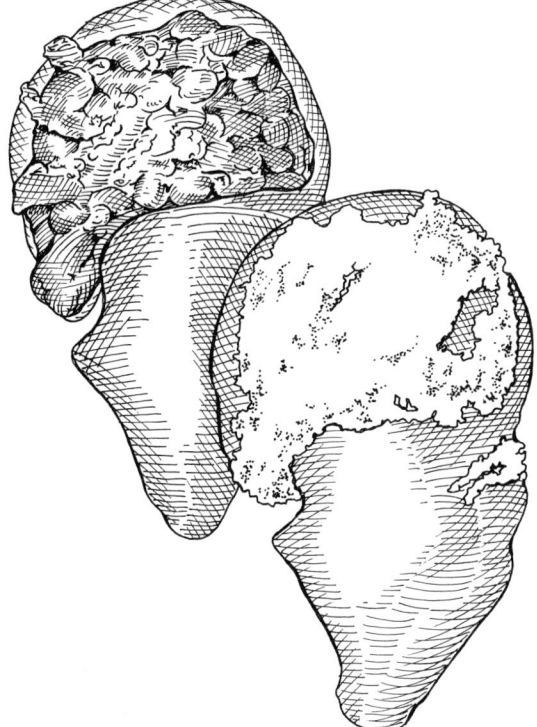

Fig. 3.3 Capsular tears or avulsions can be treated with microcrystalline collagen as shown here. (Reproduced from Blaisdell & Trunkey 1982)

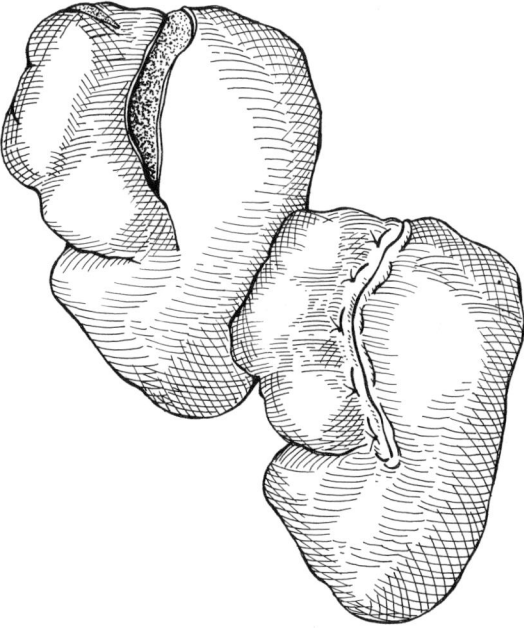

Fig. 3.4 Many lacerations of the spleen are amenable to capsular repair utilizing fine monofilament vascular suture. (Reproduced from Blaisdell & Trunkey 1982)

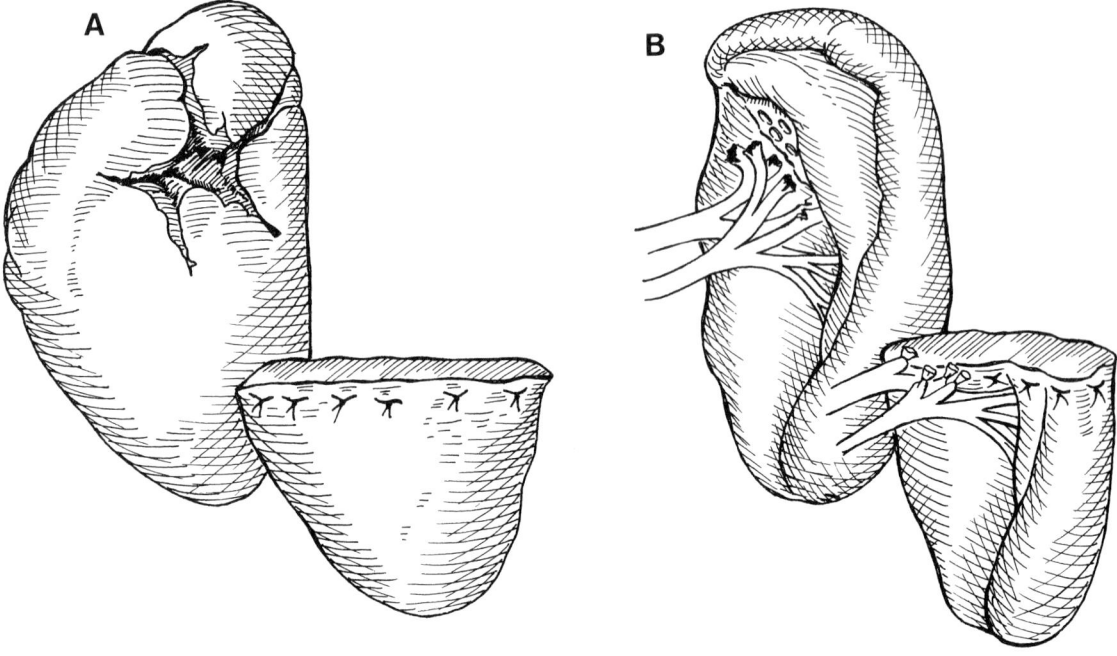

Fig. 3.5 Deeper lacerations (A) and hilar injuries (B) lend themselves to treatment by resection of the injured segment. (Reproduced from Blaisdell & Trunkey 1982)

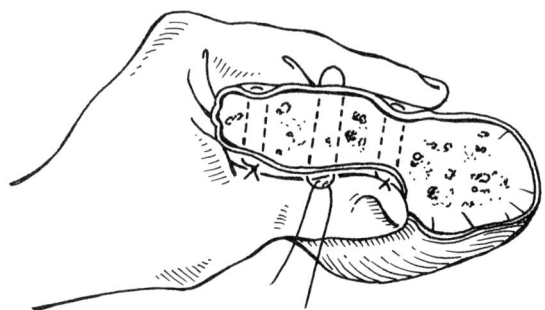

Fig. 3.6 Compression of the spleen following segmental resection provides haemostasis, facilitates identification and suturing of bleeding points and the placement of mattress sutures. (Reproduced from Blaisdell & Trunkey 1982)

Meakins 1979). Depending on the magnitude of the bleeding, the hilar vessels can be cross-clamped and divided, this immediately followed by division of the short gastric vessels. Otherwise the short gastric vessels are divided first, followed by progressive transection of the splenic hilum between multiple clamps. At the completion of splenectomy, it is necessary to recheck the security of the ligatures. This check is best accomplished by locating the tail of the pancreas by palpation and inspecting the vessels and ligatures as the vessels leave the tail of the pancreas. The greater curvature of the stomach should always be inspected, since this area is the most common source of postoperative bleeding. Frequently, one or two unligated short gastric vessels will be detected, and securing these with ligature and suture insures adequate haemostasis. Devascularization of the greater curvature of the stomach is best avoided by meticulous technique. In the absence of pancreatic or other associated injuries, the placement of drains is not necessary and may increase the incidence of infection. If there is continued blood loss in the postoperative period and the patient's spleen has been repaired, assessment of the spleen as the source of blood loss is best accomplished with CT scans and ultrasound. Arteriography may also be useful in this assessment.

Areas that remain controversial in the management of splenic trauma include splenic reimplantation, splenosis and splenic artery ligation. Reimplantation of splenic tissue has been attempted, and there is some evidence that partial splenic function may return (Fleming et al 1976). The splenic function that returns, however, is associated with its sieving of red cells. There is probably little or no return of opsonin production, but opinion on this is still divided (Constantopoulos et al 1973, Pearson et al 1978, Winkelstein & Lambert 1975). There is also evidence that diffuse peritoneal seeding of splenic tissue or splenosis does not protect the patient from overwhelming infections (Rice & James 1980).

The role of splenic artery ligation as an adjunct to splenic salvage is as yet unproven. At least one report in the literature advocates its use; however, experience at San Francisco General Hospital has not supported this procedure, since in both instances ligation of the splenic artery led to splenic necrosis (Keramidas 1979).

Postoperative care

In patients who have undergone splenectomy, the use of polyvalent pneumococcal vaccine is now an accepted treatment. However, this vaccine does not encompass all encapsulated organisms and therefore does not provide absolute protection against infection. How long prophylaxis should be continued is as yet undetermined, but most reports would indicate that susceptibility to infection and overwhelming sepsis lasts for many years. Therefore in young susceptible patients prophylactic, limited-spectrum antibiotics such as oral penicillin have been advocated by some. Nevertheless, the patient should be advised to start oral antibiotics such as ampicillin at the first signs of any upper respiratory illness and to see a physician immediately.

Asplenia increases the risks of other postoperative complications, including wound infection, subphrenic abscess, and thromboembolic phenomena. The use of prophylactic antibiotics is probably not warranted in simple noncontaminated injuries, but they probably should be utilized for at least 24–48 h following contaminated and complex injuries. Anticoagulation may be of value in selected instances when the injury has been limited to the spleen, but it is often contraindicated in more complex trauma cases because of the immediate complications of bleeding. When utilized, low-dose heparin is probably not adequate and larger doses are required, for example 75–150 units/kg by initial bolus followed by 15–20 u/kg per hour by continuous intravenous infusion.

In those patients in whom splenic salvage has been accomplished, bed rest and inactivity may be a useful adjunct for up to three weeks after the operation. This precaution may reduce the chances of postoperative haemorrhage and haematoma formation.

Postoperative complications

Although the injury may appear relatively trivial, the complications of splenic injury may be lethal (Table 3.1). The most likely initial complication is bleeding. Bleeding is either from the short gastric vessels or from the hilar vessels in the tail of the pancreas. If the patient manifests more than a unit or two of blood loss in the first 24 h, reoperation is indicated to control the bleeding point and to evacuate blood and haematoma. We believe in an aggressive approach to postoperative bleeding in order to prevent subsequent complications, including subphrenic abscess and pulmonary complications related to irritation of the diaphragm.

Trauma to the pancreas from the original injury or during splenectomy may result in postoperative pancreatitis. This condition is manifested by increased fluid requirement, by the presence of an ileus and/or a distended tender abdomen. The

Table 3.1 Complications of splenectomy (Blaisdell and Trunkey 1982)

1. Persistent intraperitoneal bleeding
2. Postoperative pancreatitis
3. Devascularization of the stomach
    Gastric fistula
    Subphrenic abscess
    Peritonitis
4. Thromboembolic complications
    Thrombosis suprarenal veins
    Thrombosis of deep veins
    Pulmonary embolism
5. Infection
    Acute postoperative
    Catastrophic late

serum amylase may or may not be elevated. If the surgeon is certain that a primary pancreatic ductal division has not been missed, the treatment is conservative, utilizing nasogastric suction, intravenous fluids and observation.

In rare instances, devascularization of the greater curvature of the stomach due to division of the gastroepiploic and short splenic vessels may result in a gastric leak or fistula. This complication is usually manifested three or four days following injury by the development of fever, abdominal tenderness and elevation of the white cell count. Reoperation is indicated if this injury is suspected. Attempts at direct suture of the stomach will usually be unsuccessful, and the acceptance of a fistula is usually necessary. Good posterior drainage should be instituted and combined with nasogastric drainage and total parenteral hyper-alimentation.

Thromboembolic complications have been a much feared complication of splenectomy. The exact incidence is disputed and difficult to determine. However, in the series at San Francisco General Hospital it was found that the incidence of thromboembolic complications approached 5% (Steele & Lim 1975). Thromboembolism is manifest by thrombophlebitis in veins receiving intravenous infusions, clotting in leg veins or pulmonary manifestations of embolism. Tragic deaths in young patients have occasionally resulted from thromboembolism. In theory, this complication could be prevented by prophylactic anticoagulation, but anticoagulation of the injured postoperative surgical patient is usually contraindicated for at least 24 h. Mild forms of prophylaxis that we employ consist of antiplatelet-aggregating agents, such as enteric-coated aspirin, low molecular weight dextran or, in high risk patients, heparin anticoagulation.

Another complication is infection, either acute infection complicating the immediate postoperative period, or late devastating infections by encapsulated organisms, such as pneumococcus and meningococcus (Singer 1973). The risk of the latter is greater in infants and children but has been documented in young adults. The advent of pneumococcal vaccine appears to prevent many pneumococcal complications but is of no use against other encapsulated organisms.

The pancreas

The pancreas lies in a relative anatomical fortress, well guarded both anteriorly and posteriorly. Anteriorly the pancreas has a position behind all of the intraperitoneal organs, and posteriorly it is protected by the large, thick paraspinal muscles and vertebral column. The pancreas is a very difficult organ to injure alone. To injure the pancreas, either a very forceful blunt injury must occur or a weapon must penetrate very deeply. Pancreatic injuries are most often associated with multiple injuries, a fact that gives some insight into the high mortality rates that occur.

A thorough understanding and appreciation of pancreatic anatomy and relationships are paramount for the trauma surgeon. The anatomy is exquisite in detail and inherently complex. Major vascular conduits, biliary ducts, bowel and the pancreatic parenchyma are all a part of the equation when pancreatic injury occurs.

Anatomy

The pancreas is 120–150 mm in length and extends almost transversely across the posterior abdominal wall, posterior to the stomach. The area it covers spans the duodenum to the spleen. The *head* is the broad, right-hand extremity which connects to the main part of the organ, the *body*. The connection between the head and the body is via the *neck*, an important surgical landmark. The leftward extremity of the pancreas, which passes slightly upwards is called the *tail*. The topographical areas that the pancreas traverses are the epigastrium and the left hypochondrial regions (Clemente 1985).

The positions of the different parts of the pancreas in relation to other organs are of both anatomical and surgical importance. The *head* is situated within the curve of the duodenum. In fact, sometimes a small part of the head of the pancreas is actually embedded in the wall of the descending part of the duodenum. From the lower and left parts of the head issues an elongation, the *uncinate process*. This process projects upwards and to the left behind the superior mesenteric vessels. From the anterosuperior aspect of the head of the pancreas, the neck juts forward, upwards, and towards the left, to be continued into the body of the pancreas. The boundary between the head and neck, on the right side, is a groove for the gastroduodenal artery. On the left side, and behind, a deep notch intervenes between the head and the neck, and in it the superior mesenteric and splenic vessels unite to form the portal vein. Below and to the right of the neck the anterior surface of the head is in contact with the transverse colon, with only areolar tissue intervening. The lower surface is covered with peritoneum, which is continuous with the inferior layer of the transverse mesocolon. The uncinate process is covered anteriorly by the superior mesenteric vessels.

The posterior surface of the head of the pancreas is related to the inferior vena cava, which runs upwards behind it and covers nearly the whole of this aspect. In addition, it is related to the terminal parts of the renal veins and the right crus of the diaphragm. The uncinate process passes in front of the aorta. The bile duct lies either in a groove on the upper and lateral parts of the posterior surface of the head of the pancreas or in a canal within its substance.

The neck, approximately 20 mm long, extends forwards, upwards and to the left from the head, and merges imperceptibly into the body. Its anterior surface is covered with peritoneum and adjoins the pylorus, with part of the omental bursa intervening. The gastroduodenal and the anterior superior pancreaticoduodenal arteries descend in front of the gland at the right side of the junction of the neck with the head. Its posterior surface is in relation with the superior mesenteric vein and the beginning of the portal vein.

The tail is narrow and generally lies in contact with the inferior part of the gastric surface of the spleen. It is contained within two layers of lienorenal ligament, together with splenic vessels to which it is clearly related.

The main pancreatic duct traverses the pancreas from left to right, lying nearer its posterior than its anterior surface. It receives the ducts of the various lobules composing the gland. These minor ducts join the main duct almost at right angles, producing what Gray's *Anatomy* describes as a 'herringbone pattern' (Clemente 1985). Considerably augmented in size, the main duct reaches the neck of the pancreas. Turning downwards, backwards and to the right, it comes into relation with the bile duct, which lies to its right side. Together the two ducts pass obliquely into the wall of the descending part of the duodenum and there unite to form a short dilated hepatopancreatic ampulla. The constricted distal end of this ampulla opens on the summit of the major duodenal papilla. As a rule, the two ducts do not unite until they approach very close to the opening on the major duodenal papilla. Sometimes the pancreatic duct and the bile duct open separately into the duodenum. Frequently, there is an additional duct which receives the ducts from the lower part of the head and is known as the accessory pancreatic duct. It runs upward in front of the main pancreatic duct, to which it is connected by a communicating duct, and opens into the duodenum about 20 mm above and slightly ventral to the major duodenal papilla.

Incidence

Although pancreatic injuries are seen with greater frequency today, pancreatic trauma is still uncommon. It occurs in about 2% of all abdominal injuries. Nearly one-fourth of pancreatic injuries are caused by blunt trauma and three-fourths by penetrating trauma. There has been a relative increase in frequency in pancreatic trauma in the last 30 years, as violence in western civilization has increased and more injurious weapons are used. Additionally, the steady increase in the number of automobiles and automobile accidents have

Table 3.2 Associated organ injuries in 1031 patients with pancreatic wounds. (Reproduced, with permission, from Mattox et al 1988)

Organ Injured	Total	
	No.	%
Liver	483	46.8
Stomach	436	42.3
Major arteries and veins	426	41.3
Spleen	289	28.0
Kidney	241	23.4
Duodenum	199	19.3
Colon	175	17.0
Small bowel	151	14.6
Common bile duct	35	3.4
Gallbladder	15	1.4

increased the incidence. The organ most frequently injured in association with pancreatic trauma is the liver, followed closely by the stomach (Table 3.2). Mattox and colleagues (1988) have shown that 45% of patients with pancreatic wounds have associated injuries of major arteries or veins.

Diagnosis

Diagnostic peritoneal lavage

To make the diagnosis of pancreatic injury, the diagnosis must first be entertained. We have followed the dictum that any patient sustaining a stab wound of the upper abdomen or sustaining blunt trauma to the upper abdomen has a pancreatic injury until proven otherwise. Our sequence of diagnosis, however, depends on the type of weapon used in penetrating the abdomen. When the weapon is a knife and the wound appears superficial, the stab wound is explored under local anaesthesia. If the peritoneum has not been violated and there are no signs of obvious intraperitoneal injury, we utilize peritoneal lavage. If the patient has been shot in the upper abdomen, unless there is proof that the wound was tangential, the patient undergoes exploratory celiotomy. Those who have suffered from blunt trauma to the upper abdomen are evaluated by clinical and laboratory modalities (Friend et al 1985). Obviously, if peritonitis or intraperitoneal haemorrhage are discernible, we go directly to the operating room. If not, we advocate the liberal use of contrast-enhanced computed tomography. Although peritoneal lavage can be useful in this setting, the CT scan is the test that gives us the most information and allows us to make a precise diagnosis.

CT scan

Computerized tomography is uniquely suited for evaluation of pancreatic trauma. However, in selected cases CT diagnosis may be quite difficult (Federle et al 1981). In certain cases of pancreatic laceration or fracture, there are few changes in density, and as such these cannot be well defined

by CT. This is, of course, in contradistinction to lesions of the liver and kidney. Additionally, areas of pancreatic injury may be difficult to distinguish on scans due to motion or streak artefacts in the region of the pancreas. Gastric decompression, patient sedation and the use of very dilute oral Gastrografin may aid in obviating these artefacts. Faster scanning may also reduce artefact.

The timing of CT scanning in pancreatic trauma may also be very important. False negative scans have been found if performed within 12 h of the trauma. However, thickening of the anterior renal fascia may be a very subtle early sign indicating pancreatic injury. Although this lining may be related to past or current inflammatory lesions in the anterior pararenal spaces, in the trauma setting the signs should alert the radiologist and surgeon to possible parenchymal pancreatic injuries.

Amylase

The use of amylase in pancreatic trauma has been subject to intense scrutiny and controversy (Bouwman et al 1984). Many traumatized patients have elevations of serum amylase, which often lead to a diagnosis of pancreatitis or pancreatic injury. However, in the presence of multiple injuries the picture is obscured, as serum amylase is derived from both pancreatic and salivary glands. Greenlee and colleagues (1984) have shown that fractionation of the amylase may aid in making a precise diagnosis of pancreatic injury; however, Bouwman and his colleagues drew opposite conclusions. The paramount point is that elevation of total serum amylase in the injured patient does not of itself indicate pancreatic injury. Therefore, measurement of amylase and amylase fractions is still controversial and imprecise in determining pancreatic injuries.

Serum amylase levels are not helpful in those patients who have sustained penetrating injury to the pancreas. The amylase is not elevated in 75% of penetrating pancreatic injuries. This fact is in contradistinction to the 80% elevation in patients sustaining blunt trauma to the pancreas (Berne et al 1968). The caveat that must be kept in mind is that any perforation of the duodenum or upper gastrointestinal tract may also produce an elevated serum amylase concentration. This elevation occurs as a result of spillage of intraluminal amylase into the peritoneal cavity, where it is quickly absorbed.

ERCP

Some of the trauma literature indicates the effectiveness of endoscopic retrograde cholangiopancreatography (ERCP) in the diagnosis of pancreatic injury (Bozymski et al 1981). We have not used ERCP as a preoperative diagnostic procedure because the time and effort involved do not seem to warrant its use. It has also been pointed out that ERCP can exacerbate damage already done. ERCP should be held in abeyance for those operative settings in which clear delineation of ductal structures is not evident. ERCP can then be carried out while the patient is in the operating room under anaesthesia.

The fact remains that the specific diagnosis of pancreatic injury is most often made in the operating room. Patients who are operated upon for upper abdominal trauma must undergo very careful exploration of the pancreas, including opening of the lesser sac through the gastrocolic omentum to inspect the entire anterior surface. To explore the posterior aspect of the pancreas, a Kocher manoeuvre should be employed. There are some who feel that the peritoneum along the entirety of the inferior border of the pancreas should be incised to allow elevation of the body and tail of the pancreas and to look at the posterior surface of the tail. Failure to do a complete evaluation of the pancreas has led to disastrous results, all of which can be obviated by a compulsive, circumspect inspection.

Combined duodenal injury

One cannot discuss pancreatic injuries without some mention of duodenal trauma as well. Injury that involves both the pancreas and the duodenum is clearly more severe than single organ injury (Berne et al 1968). Such an injury demands thorough evaluation of the retroperitoneum and cognizance of those relationships emphasized in the anatomy overview. Morbidity and mortality in these injuries is directly proportional to the extent and location of the injury and of other associated injuries. It has been shown, however, that the types of surgical repair used can have a profound effect on long-term sequelae (Campbell & Kennedy 1980). There is not, however, a unanimity of opinion on the treatment of individual injuries to these organs, as the breadth of injuries is such that a unified approach is simply not possible. Some consensus in therapy is offered by Jordan & Reber (1986), however.

A methodical and conservative approach is advised, and close inspection of the entire pancreas is the first step in operative evaluation. Contusions or lacerations that do not involve a main duct, be it Wirsung's canal or Santorini's duct, can be well handled by either open penrose drainage or closed sump suction. We favour the latter.

Ductal transections which are some distance away from the head are usually handled by resection. Resection of the pancreas in these cases usually necessitates the taking of the spleen. As already mentioned, however, the spleen should be saved in children whenever possible. There is one qualification to this specific operative therapy of resection: if such a resection necessitates the removal of 80% of the pancreas, then a Roux-en-Y ought to be fashioned to the pancreatic body in lieu of its removal. The Roux-en-Y lowers the incidence of post-traumatic endocrine insufficiency (Lucas 1977).

Evaluation of the pancreatic duct is a major concern in these cases, and there are a number of options available, some of which are more practicable than others. Some authors advocate operative pancreatography via the duodenum or through the distal duct after resection. This manoeuvre will generally give a clear delineation of the anatomy, but most experienced trauma surgeons rely most often on local inspection and exploration to determine if a major duct has been injured (Linos et al 1983) (Fig. 3.7). As noted by Feliciano and colleagues (1984), this procedure eliminates performing a duodenotomy in the presence of a pancreatic injury. Should a duct injury be missed and a fistula result, it is now infrequent that reoperation will need to be undertaken, as many fistulae will close on their own.

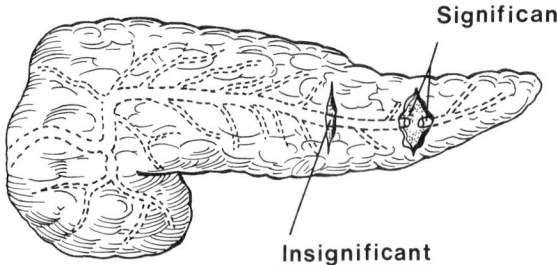

Significant

Insignificant

Fig. 3.7 Demonstration of significant (disruption of pancreatic duct) vs. proximal insignificant injury (in which duct is intact). (Reproduced from Blaisdell & Trunkey 1982)

Wöltering (personal communication 1988) has shown a 78% decrease in pancreatic output within 24 hours with the use of the somatostatin analogue, Sandostatin® (Sandoz Co. East Hanover, N J)

Pancreaticoduodenectomy is reserved for those who have a ductal disruption in the head of the pancreas with associated devitalizing injuries to the duodenum, common bile duct, or significant injury to the ampulla of Vater; or to control an exsanguinating bleed emanating from the pancreatic head (Henarejos et al 1983). Pancreaticoduodenectomy has also been used to gain control of haemorrhage from the retropancreatic portal vein. This extensive exercise in surgical anatomy is indicated for only 2–3% of most patients with pancreatic injuries. Most trauma surgeons note its 20–30% mortality rate and argue that it should be used rarely (Gustafsson et al 1983). We feel that it should be used when its indications warrant it.

Repair of duodenal perforation or blowout is well managed with a two-layered closure. Those duodenal injuries that are more extensive need to be handled in an aggressive surgical manner, as numerous studies have shown an appreciable morbidity rate if a fistula develops (Lal et al 1978). Aggressive surgical approaches include duodenal diverticulization as described by Berne et al (1968). This procedure necessitates antrectomy with a gastrojejunostomy and a tube duodenostomy (Fig. 3.8). This diverticulization diverts the gastrointestinal stream away from the repaired site, and a tube duodenostomy vents the area of repair. This is a technique used by many, but critics point out that such a procedure necessitates resection of

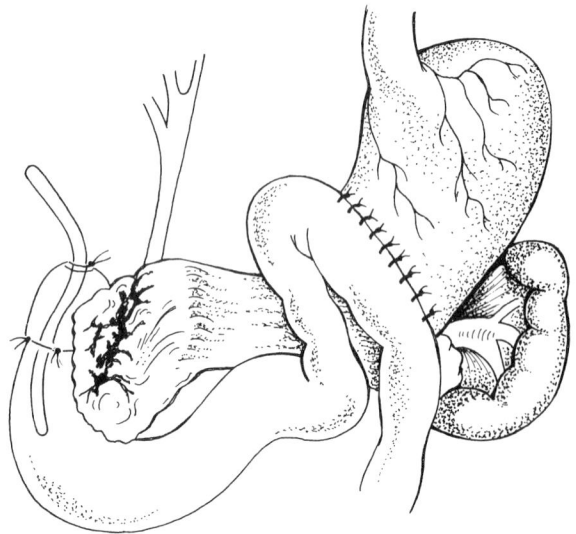

Fig.3.8 Duodenal diverticulization procedure. This is suitable for patients with severe injury to the head of the pancreas with or without duodenal injury but with an intact pancreatic ductal system. (Reproduced with permission, from Lucas 1977)

healthy tissue (antrum) and creation of a second hole in the injured duodenum.

Pyloric exclusion is another method of diverting the gastrointestinal stream from a repaired area. Here no normal tissue is resected and the diversion is temporary. It has been shown that 90–95% of the patients who undergo pyloric exclusion have a patent pylorus 2–3 weeks after the procedure. Critics point out that the ulcerogenic potential of this operation is high when truncal vagotomy is not performed. Stone and co-workers (1962) have developed a third major technique for diversion and decompression. They routinely use gastrostomy and retrograde jejunostomy in association with a feeding jejunostomy and have been very successful, however, others have not been so successful with this technique. Many criticize it because of the need to create both gastrostomy and jejunostomy incisions in a patient who already has serious duodenal injury.

In conclusion, combined pancreaticoduodenal injuries are most commonly caused by penetrating wounds. Usually the patient will also have other intra-abdominal injuries. The mortality rate of these combined injuries is, of course, higher than for either organ alone. Almost 50% of all deaths occur in the perioperative period. Sepsis and multiple organ failure account for more than 80% of late deaths.

Injury to the pancreas alone

Injuries to the pancreas-alone are treated according to the type of injury sustained. Table 3.3

Table 3.3 Recommended treatment of pancreatic wounds according to type of injuries (Mattox et al 1988)

Type of Wound	Treatment
Haematoma	Drainage
Superficial laceration	Drainage
Contusion, tissue viable	Drainage
Deep laceration	Repair of laceration and drainage
Severe contusion of tail of pancreas with injury to spleen or splenic vessels	Splenectomy and distal pancreatectomy
Total transection of pancreas, no other injuries	Closure of proximal transected end and Roux-en-Y jejunostomy to distal end
Total transection with damage to splenic vessels or spleen	Distal pancreatectomy and splenectomy
Total transection in association with multiple organ injuries, particularly with severe haemorrhage	Distal pancreatectomy
Deep laceration of the pancreas with transection of the pancreatic duct but intact posterior capsule	Only pancreatojejunostomy
Combined pancreatoduodenal injuries	Independent repair of each organ separately and drainage
Simple stab wound or low calibre bullet wound, injuring head of pancrease and duodenum	
More severe wounds of pancreas and duodenum requiring complicated duodenal repair or the possibility of stricture formation	Repair and closure of the pylorus and gastrojejunostomy
Total destruction of duodenum and head of pancreas	Whipple operation
Total destruction of the pancreas	Total pancreatectomy

outlines the general consensus on how these types of wounds should be treated. The central thesis is that conservation of pancreatic tissue is paramount. Resection of pancreatic tissue should be done only when the extent of damage is so great that primary repair is not feasible. The need for resection is self-evident in the combined pancreatic and duodenal injuries as outlined.

Those patients who have suffered only minor contusions or lacerations of the pancreatic parenchyma need only drainage of the wound. Larger lacerations, of course, necessitate repair by simple suture. Catgut suture in this setting should never be used, as pancreatic secretions will dissolve this material. If a major pancreatic duct is transected, the pancreas distal to the transection should be resected. This manoeuvre often necessitates the removal of the spleen owing to the anatomical constraints involved.

Total transection of the pancreas through the neck will also necessitate resection. Here the distal pancreas is removed and the proximal aspect of the pancreas is closed with nonabsorbable suture or staples. The reason why resection is carried out in this setting instead of attempts at reanastomosing the duct is because other associated injuries are usually involved. These injuries necessitate expeditious treatment of the pancreas, and resection aids in exposing the other injuries.

If the pancreas is transected at the neck and no other serious injuries have occurred, anastomosis of the duct and the pancreatic substance is an option. This is a difficult technical exercise, and even with stenting of the duct the patency rate is not high. The toughest therapeutic decision operatively to be made is when the pancreatic head is injured alone. If major ductal injury has occurred, pancreaticoduodenectomy and sometimes total pancreatectomy are indicated. If it can be seen that there is no ductal injury, the treatment is simply drainage of the area as one would do with injuries to the body or tail of the pancreas.

Mortality

The overall mortality rate for pancreatic wounds is between 15 and 25% today (Levison et al 1984).

The highest rates are found in those patients who have had to have large resections of pancreatic tissue. The major causes of death are haemorrhage and shock. Thus most patients die within 24–48 h.

Those who live beyond 48 h and who ultimately succumb are invariably seen to have either intra-abdominal sepsis or adult respiratory distress syndrome (ARDS).

REFERENCES

Berne C J, Donovan A J, Hagen W E 1968 Combined duodenal-pancreatic trauma. Archives of Surgery 96: 712–719

Blaisdell F W, Trunkey D D 1982 Trauma management, vol 1. Thieme-Stratton, New York

Bouwman D L, Weaver D W, Walt A J 1984 Serum amylase and its isoenzymes: a clarification of their implications in trauma. Journal of Trauma 24: 573

Bozymski E M, Orlando R C, Holt J W, III 1981 Traumatic disruption of the pancreatic duct demonstrated by endoscopic retrograde pancreatography. Journal of Trauma 21: 244

Buntain W L, Lynn H P 1979 Splenorrhaphy: changing concepts for the traumatized spleen. Surgery 86: 748

Campbell R, Kennedy T 1980 The management of pancreatic and pancreaticoduodenal injuries. British Journal of Surgery 67: 845–850

Clemente C D 1985 Gray's Anatomy, 30th American edn

Connors J F 1928 Splenectomy for trauma. Annals of Surgery 88: 388

Constantopoulos A, Najjar V A, Wish J B, Necheles T H, Stolbach L L 1973 Defective phagocytosis due to tuftsin deficiency in splenectomized subjects. American Journal of Diseases of Children 125: 663–665

Eichner E R 1979 Splenic function: normal, too much, and too little. American Journal of Medicine 66: 311

Ein S H, Shandling B, Simpson J S, Stephens C A, Bandi S K, Biggar W D, Freedman M H 1977 The morbidity and mortality of splenectomy in children. Annals of Surgery 185: 307–310

Federle M P, Goldberg H I, Kaiser J A, Moss A A, Jeffrey R B, Jr, Mall J C 1981 Evaluation of abdominal trauma by computed tomography. Radiology 138: 637–644

Feliciano D V, Bitondo C G, Steed G N et al 1984 Five hundred open taps or lavages in patients with abdominal stab wounds. American Journal of Surgery 148: 772–777

Fleming R C, Dickson R E, Harrison E G 1976 Splenosis: autotransplantation of splenic tissues. American Journal of Medicine 61: 414

Friend P J, Jamieson N V, MacFarland R 1985 Blunt pancreatic injury: two case reports and a review of the literature. Injury 16: 391

Gopal V, Bisno A L 1977 Fulminant pneumococcal infections in "normal" asplenic hosts. Archives of Internal Medicine 137: 1576

Greenlee T, Murphy K, Ram M D 1984 Amylase isoenzymes in the evaluation of trauma patients. Annals of Surgery 50: 637

Gustafsson L, Falk A, Darle N, Gamklou R 1983 Surgical management of pancreatic injuries. Acta Chirurgica Scandinavica 149: 629–631

Henarejos A, Cohen D M, Moossa A R 1983 Management of pancreatic trauma. Annals of the Royal College of Surgeons of England 65: 297

Jordan G L Jr, Reber H A (eds) 1986 Surgical diseases of the pancreas. Lee & Febiger, Philadelphia, p 875

Keramidas D C 1979 The ligation of the splenic artery in the treatment of traumatic rupture of the spleen. Surgery 85: 530

King H, Schumacher H B Jr 1952 Splenic studies. I. Susceptibility to infection after splenectomy performed in infancy. Annals of Surgery 136: 239

Kuhn C G (ed) 1964 Galen (Concerning the uses of the parts of the human body) Book 5, chap. 15. In: Complete works of Claudius Galen Vol 3. Olms, Hildesheim, p 316

Lal S K, Gross E, Holbrook I B, Irving M H 1978 Metabolic problems in the management of a traumatic pancreatic fistula. Injury 9: 323

Levison M A, Petersen S R, Sheldon G F, Trunkey D D 1984 Duodenal trauma: experience of a trauma center. Journal of Trauma 24: 475–480

Linos D A, King R M, Much P, Farnell M B 1983 Blunt pancreatic trauma. Minnesota Medicine 68: 153–160

Looareesuwan S, Ho M, Wattanagoon Y et al 1987 Dynamic alteration in splenic function during acute falciparum malaria. New England Journal of Medicine 317: 675–679

Lucas C E 1977 Diagnosis and treatment of pancreatic and duodenal injury. Surgical Clinics of North America 57: 49

Malpighi M 1666 De Liene. In: Malpighi M, De viscerum structura excertitatio anatomica. Golonga, J Monitus, pp 101–150

Mattox K L, Moore E E, Feliciano D V 1988. In: Appleton and Lange (eds) Trauma. Norwalk C T, San Mateo C A, pp 479, 481, 483

Meakins J L 1979 Splenectomy for rupture of the spleen: a reappraisal. Canadian Medical Association Journal 121: 11–12

Morris D H, Bullock F D 1919 The importance of the spleen in resistance to infection. Annals of Surgery 70: 513

Olsen W R, Polley T Z 1977 A second look at delayed splenic rupture. Archives of Surgery 112: 442

Pearson H A, Johnston D, Smith K A, Touloukian R J 1978 The born-again spleen: return of splenic function after splenectomy for trauma. New England Journal of Medicine 298: 1389–1392

Peck A L (trans) 1955 Aristotle: Parts of animals, Book III, chap 12. Harvard University Press, Cambridge MA

Peters A M 1983 Splenic blood flow and blood cell kinetics. Clinical Hematology 12: 421–447

Rice H M, James P D 1980 Ectopic splenic tissue failed to prevent fatal pneumococcal septicaemia after splenectomy for trauma. Lancet 565: (1) 8168

Rosner F 1972 The spleen in the Talmud and other early Jewish writing. Bulletin of the History of Medicine 46: 82–85

Rosoff L, Cohen J L, Telfer N, Halpern M 1972 Injuries of the spleen. Surgical Clinics of North America 52: 667–697

Sherman R 1980 Perspectives in management of trauma to the spleen. Journal of Trauma 20: 1

Singer D B 1973 Postsplenectomy sepsis. Perspectives in
Pediatric Pathology 1: 285–311

Steele M, Lim R C 1975 Advances in management of
splenic injuries. American Journal of Surgery
130: 159

Stone H H, Stowers K B, Shippey S H 1962 Injuries to the
pancreas. Archives of Surgery 85: 525–530

Strauch G O 1979 Preservation of splenic function in adults
and children with injured spleens. American Journal of
Surgery 137: 478

Weinstein M E, Govin G G, Rice C L, Virgilio R W 1979.
Splenorrhaphy for splenic trauma. Journal of Trauma
19: 692–697

Winkelstein J A, Lambert G H 1975 Pneumococcal serum
opsonizing activity in splenectomized children. Journal of
Pediatrics 87: 430

4

Fracture of the pelvic ring

L. SOLOMON and M. J. STOWER

Fractures of the pelvis account for less than 5% of all skeletal injuries, but they are particularly important because of the associated soft tissue injuries which are a major cause of morbidity and mortality. Like other serious injuries, they demand a combined approach by experts in various fields.

About two-thirds of all pelvic fractures occur in road accidents involving pedestrians; over 10% of these patients will have associated visceral injuries, and in this group the mortality rate is probably in excess of 10% (Levine & Crampton 1963, Peltier 1965, Froman & Stein 1967, Eid 1981).

Anatomy

The pelvic ring is made up of the two innominate bones and the sacrum, articulating in front at the symphysis pubis (the anterior or pubic bridge) and posteriorly at the sacroiliac joints (the posterior or sacroiliac bridge). This basin-like structure transmits weight from the trunk to the lower limbs and provides protection for the pelvic viscera: the large vessels and nerves, bowel, bladder and genitourinary organs.

The stability of the pelvic ring depends upon the rigidity of the bony parts and the integrity of the strong ligaments that bind the three segments together at the symphysis pubis and the sacroiliac joints. The strongest and most important of the tethering ligaments are the sacroiliac and iliolumbar ligaments; as long as they are intact, weightbearing is unimpaired. This is an important factor in differentiating between 'stable' and 'unstable' injuries of the pelvic ring.

The major branches of the common iliac arteries arise within the pelvis between the level of the sacroiliac joint and the greater sciatic notch. With their accompanying veins they are particularly vulnerable in fractures through the posterior part of the pelvic ring. The nerves of the lumbar and sacral plexuses, likewise, are at risk with posterior pelvic injuries.

The bladder lies behind the symphysis pubis. The trigone is held in position by the lateral ligaments of the bladder and, in the male, by the prostate. The prostate lies between the bladder and the pelvic floor. It is held laterally by the medial fibres of the levator ani, whilst anteriorly it is firmly attached to the pubic bones by the puboprostatic ligament. In the female the trigone is attached also to the cervix and the anterior vaginal fornix. The urethra is held by both the pelvic floor muscles and the pubourethral ligament. Consequently in females the urethra is much more mobile and less prone to injury.

In severe pelvic injuries the membranous urethra is damaged when the prostate is forced backwards whilst the urethra remains static. When the puboprostatic ligament is torn, the prostate and base of the bladder can become grossly dislocated from the membranous urethra.

The pelvic colon, with its mesentery, is a mobile structure and therefore not readily injured. However, the rectum and anal canal are more firmly tethered to the urogenital structures and the muscular floor of the pelvis and are therefore vulnerable in pelvic fractures.

Classification of pelvic ring fractures

For practical purposes pelvic fractures can be divided into three types: 1. Isolated fractures that do not disrupt the pelvic ring; 2. Fractures that disrupt the pelvic ring; 3. Acetabular fractures, which are really a special class of ring fracture. While it is possible for almost any fracture to be associated with damage to the intrapelvic structures, only pelvic ring fractures carry a high risk of serious visceral injury. In this chapter we shall deal only with injuries that disrupt the pelvic ring.

Most fractures of the pelvic ring are, in reality, double breaks. Often the second break is not visible on a radiograph, either because it is only very slightly displaced or because it is immediately reduced. Certainly if the visible fracture is displaced, or if the pelvis looks asymmetrical, one must assume that there is a second point of disruption (Fig. 4.1). This can be important in planning treatment. In 1859 Malgaigne drew attention to those cases in which fracture of the superior and inferior pubic rami anteriorly was as-sociated with fracture or dislocation in the vicinity of the sacroiliac joint (Fig. 4.2); these double breaks of the ring are still referred to as 'Malgaigne fractures', although the term now carries less distinctive connotations than it did in the past. What is more important is whether the fracture is stable or unstable, and this depends almost entirely on whether the bony and ligamentous bridge across the sacroiliac region has remained intact or come apart (Bucholz 1981).

The following simple classification, based mainly on the radiographic appearances, has practical implications for treatment and prognosis.

Type I — Undisplaced single break This presents as either fracture of the pubic rami on one side or moderate separation of the symphysis pubis. There may be partial disruption of the sacroiliac ligaments, but this is usually overlooked. The fracture is stable and is seldom associated with visceral injury.

Type II — Displaced single break Here, too, the break is usually through the ipsilateral pubic rami or the symphysis pubis, but displacement is more

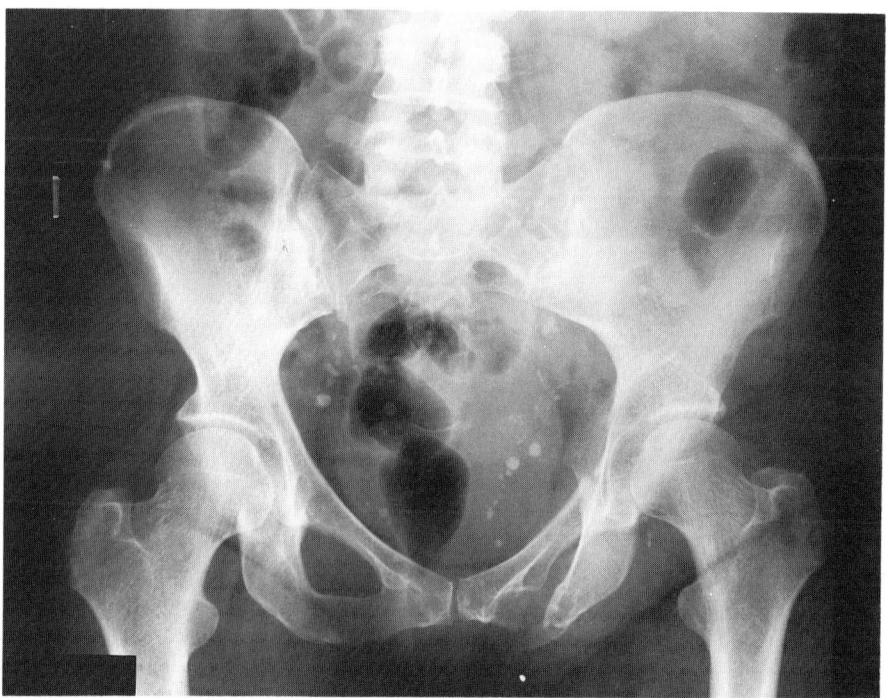

Fig. 4.1 Radiograph of the pelvis showing fractures of the inferior and superior pubic rami on the left side. Although there is no obvious asymmetry of the pelvic ring, there is a strong suspicion of disruption of the right sacroiliac joint.

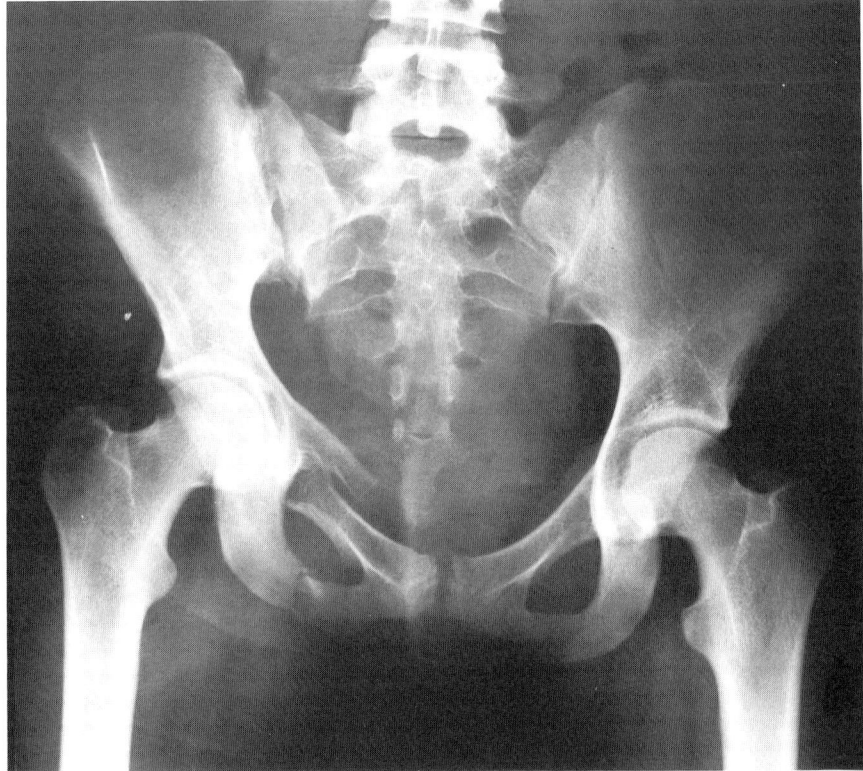

Fig. 4.2   Radiograph showing fractures of the superior and inferior pubic rami on the right, disruption of the ipsilateral sacroiliac joint and vertical displacement of the right side of the pelvis (the Malgaigne fracture).

marked. It is assumed that the sacroiliac ligaments are torn, but the posterior break may not be obvious on X-ray. There may be associated visceral injury.

Type III — Double break, with or without displacement. These are further subdivided into:

A. Bilateral fractures of both pubic rami or fractures of the pubic rami and separation of the symphysis — often associated with injury to the bladder or urethra.
B. Fractures or dislocation of the pubic bridge and obvious fracture or disruption of the sacroiliac bridge. If the sacroiliac break is much displaced the pelvis will be unstable.
C. Anterior and posterior breaks with vertical displacement of the innominate bone (Fig. 4.2). These are shear injuries, usually due to a fall from a height. The sacroiliac

bridge is completely disrupted and the pelvis is unstable. There is a high incidence of visceral injury and retroperitoneal haemorrhage.

Clinical features

Fracture of the pelvis should be suspected in every patient with serious abdominal or lower limb injuries. There may be a history of a road accident or a fall from a height or crush injury. Often the patient complains of pain, and there may be swelling or bruising of the lower abdomen, the thighs, the perineum, the scrotum or the vulva. All these areas should be rapidly inspected, looking for evidence of extravasation of urine. However, the first priority, always, is to assess the patient's general condition and to look for signs of blood loss. It may be necessary to start resuscitation before the examination is completed.

The abdomen should be carefully palpated. Signs of irritation suggest the possibility of intraperitoneal bleeding. The pelvic ring can be gently compressed from side to side and back to front. Tenderness over the sacroiliac region is particularly important and may signify disruption of the posterior bridge.

A rectal examination is then carried out in every case. The coccyx and sacrum can be felt and tested for tenderness. If the prostate can be felt, which is often difficult due to pain and swelling, its abnormal position may indicate a urethral injury.

Enquire when the patient passed urine and look for bleeding at the external meatus. An inability to void and blood at the external meatus are the classical features of a ruptured urethra. However, the absence of blood at the meatus does not exclude a urethral injury, because the external sphincter may be in spasm, halting the passage of blood from the site of injury. Thus every patient who has a pelvic fracture must be considered to be at risk.

The patient can be encouraged to void; if he is able to do so, either the urethra is intact or there is only minimal damage which will not be made worse by the passage of urine. No attempt should be made to pass a catheter as this could convert a partial to a complete tear of the urethra. If a urethral injury is suspected, this can be diagnosed more accurately and more safely by retrograde urethrography.

A ruptured bladder should be suspected in patients who do not void or in those in whom a bladder is not palpable after adequate fluid replacement. This palpation is often difficult because of abdominal wall haematoma. The physical findings initially can be minimal, with normal bowel sounds, as extravasation of sterile urine produces little peritoneal irritation. Only a very small proportion of patients with a ruptured bladder are hypotensive, so if the patient is hypotensive another cause must be sought.

Neurological examination is important; there may be damage to the lumbar or sacral plexus.

If the patient is unconscious, the same routine is followed. However, early X-ray examination is essential in these cases.

Radiography

X-ray of the pelvis

Once you have assured yourself that the patient's life is not in danger, a plain anteroposterior radiograph of the pelvis should be obtained. In most cases this film will give sufficient information to make a preliminary diagnosis of pelvic fracture. The exact nature of the injury can be clarified by more detailed radiography once it is certain that the patient can tolerate an extended period of positioning and repositioning on the X-ray table. Five views are necessary: anteroposterior, an inlet view (tube cephalad to the pelvis and tilted 30° downwards), an outlet view (tube caudad to the pelvis and tilted 40° upwards), and right and left oblique views.

If there is any doubt about the integrity of the sacroiliac joint or the bones immediately adjacent to it (often difficult to demonstrate in the plain X-ray), a CT scan is necessary. Especially in displaced single-break injuries, it is essential to exclude a hidden posterior fracture or dislocation.

X-ray of the urinary tract

If there is any evidence of upper abdominal or thoracic trauma, an intravenous urogram is performed to exclude renal injury as a cause for haematuria. This investigation will also exclude ureteric and major bladder damage. In a case of urethral rupture, the base of the bladder may on occasion be riding high (dislocated prostate) or there may be a tear-drop deformity of the bladder owing to compression by blood and extravasated urine (prostate-in-situ) (Fig. 4.3).

When a urethral injury is considered likely, a urethrogram should be undertaken using 25–30 ml of water-soluble contrast agent with suitable aseptic technique. A film must be taken during injection of the contrast agent to ensure that the urethra is fully distended. This technique will confirm a urethral tear and will demonstrate if it is complete or incomplete.

In a patient with possible rupture of the bladder (so long as there is no evidence of a urethral injury) a cystogram must be performed (Fig. 4.4).

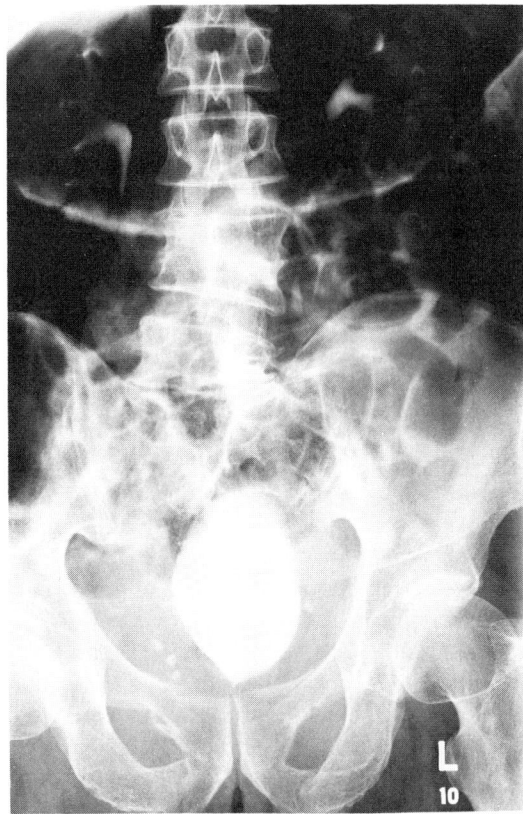

Fig. 4.3 Intravenous urogram outlining the bladder and showing the so-called 'tear-drop' deformity due to compression by blood and extravasated urine. Note that there is also marked gastric dilatation, suggesting the presence of retroperitoneal bleeding.

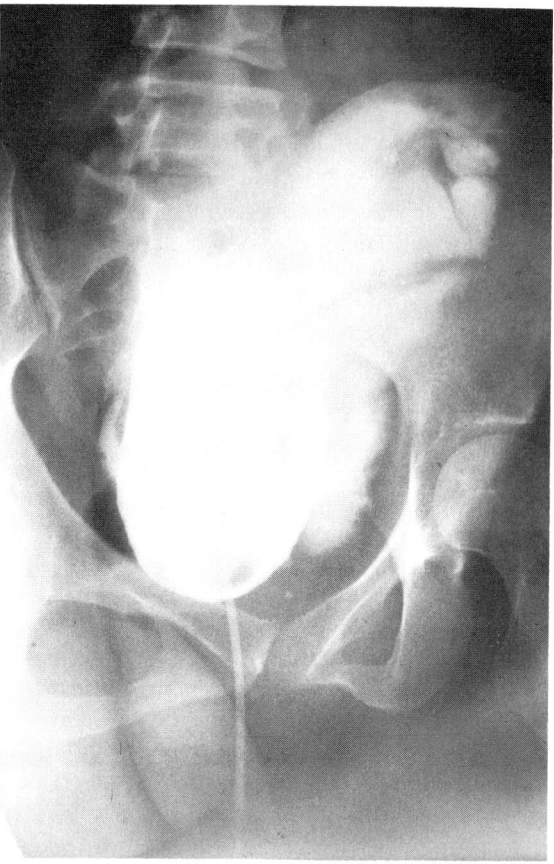

Fig. 4.4 Cystogram showing extravasation of radiopaque material, suggesting intraperitoneal rupture of the bladder.

Adequate contrast medium must be introduced (at least 350 ml is usually required), and radiography should follow micturition, otherwise small extraperitoneal leaks may be missed (Caroll & McAninch 1983).

The role of ultrasound and CT scanning in these injuries has not yet been fully assessed.

Management

Early management

Treatment should not await full and detailed diagnosis. It is vital to keep a sense of priorities and to act on any information that is already available while moving along to the next diagnostic hurdle. 'Management', in this context, is a combination of assessment and treatment.

Six questions must be asked and the answers acted upon as they emerge (see Table 4.1):

1. Is there a clear airway?
2. Are the lungs adequately ventilated?
3. Is the patient losing blood?
4. Is there an intra-abdominal injury?
5. Is there a bladder or urethral injury?
6. Is the pelvic fracture stable or unstable?

With any severely injured patient, the first step is to make sure that the airway is clear and ventilation is unimpaired. Resuscitation must be started immediately and active bleeding con-

Table 4.1 Algorithm for management of patients with pelvic ring fractures

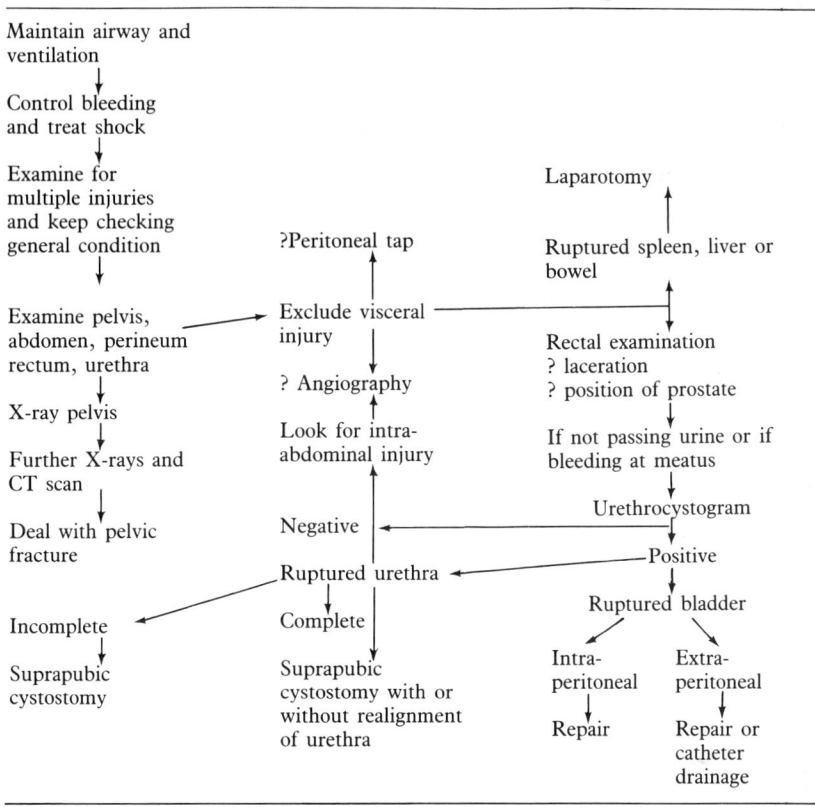

trolled. The patient is rapidly examined for multiple injuries and, if necessary, painful fractures are splinted. A single anteroposterior X-ray of the pelvis is obtained.

A more careful examination is then carried out, paying particular attention to the pelvis, the abdomen, the perineum and the rectum. The urethral meatus is inspected for signs of bleeding. During rectal examination it may be possible to feel the position of the prostate. The lower limbs are examined for signs of nerve injury.

If the patient's general condition is stable, further radiographs can then be obtained. If a urethral tear is suspected, a urethrogram is gently performed. The findings up to that stage may dictate the need for an intravenous urogram.

By now the attendant will have a good idea of the patient's general condition, the extent of the pelvic injury, the presence or absence of visceral injury and the likelihood of continued intra-abdominal or retroperitoneal bleeding. Ideally, a team of experts will be on hand to deal with the individual problems or undertake further investigations.

Management of the fracture

Type I — Undisplaced single break

It is assumed, at least during the early management, that there really is a single break or that, if a second break exists, it is not unstable and will not jeopardise the otherwise favourable prognosis.

Bed rest, either alone or combined with lower limb traction, is usually adequate for these injuries. It is continued until the patient is free of pain, usually 4–6 weeks. Thereafter the patient is allowed up on crutches and slowly resumes normal activity.

Type II — Displaced single break

Displaced fractures through the ipsilateral pubic rami, or separation of the pubic symphysis, must in almost all cases be associated with some disruption of the ring posteriorly. There may be an obvious subluxation of one sacroiliac joint or fracture of the adjacent sacrum or ilium. However, even if the posterior lesion does not show on the plain radiograph, it must be assumed to be present. Fortunately, though, this type of disruption is usually stable.

Ipsilateral pubic rami fractures are usually caused by a lateral compressive force, and it is therefore inappropriate to treat these by using a sling (which exerts a similar force). The patient is nursed supine, if necessary with lower limb traction, until the fractures begin to unite (usually 4–6 weeks).

Wide separation of the symphysis rarely occurs as an isolated injury and is, therefore, more correctly treated as a double break injury.

Type III — Double break

Fracture through both pubic rami on both sides (the 'butterfly injury' or 'straddle fracture') is one of the commoner types of pelvic injury. It is also one of the most serious, with a reported mortality rate of 19% and damage to the abdominal or pelvic viscera in about one third of all cases (Peltier 1965, Conolly & Hedberg 1969). Once the complications have been dealt with, the fracture itself requires little more than prolonged nursing in the supine position.

Disruption of both the anterior and posterior elements of the pelvic ring (Malgaigne fracture) accounts for about 10% of pelvic fractures and is one of the most serious types of injury (Conolly & Hedberg 1969, Slatis & Huittinen 1972). The anterior lesion may be fractures through the pubic rami or separation of the symphysis, while the posterior break is either a separation of the sacroiliac joint or fracture of the adjacent bones or both.

The full extent of the posterior injury is often not apparent on the plain X-rays; it is advisable to obtain a CT scan in all these cases. It is particu-

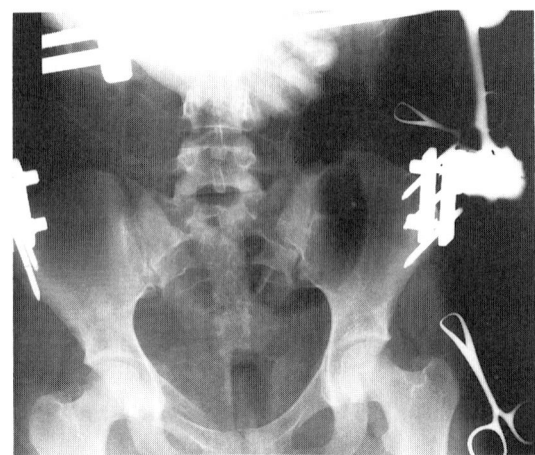

Fig. 4.5 Same case as in Fig. 4.2. The pelvic displacement has been reduced and held by an external fixator attached to the pelvic brim and lower limb traction.

larly important to establish whether there is vertical or backward displacement of the posterior break, because this means that the pelvic ring is unstable; shock and bleeding will be more severe, visceral injury is more likely, and there is a high incidence of late disability due to sacroiliac pain, backache and pelvic asymmetry.

Double break injuries usually require external fixation with iliac pins and a connecting frame (Fig. 4.5) (Slatis & Karaharju 1980). If there is only partial disruption of the posterior elements and the pelvic ring is stable, this manoeuvre will suffice; the external fixator is retained for 6–8 weeks, and during the later stages the patient may even walk about with the frame in place. However, if there is complete disruption of the posterior bridge, external fixation alone will not stabilize the pelvis. If the facilities and expertise are available, the posterior break should be treated by internal fixation; if not, then external fixation should be supplemented by lower limb traction and prolonged bed rest (Tile & Pennal 1980).

Management of severe bleeding

Pelvic injuries may be associated with severe and persistent intraperitoneal or retroperitoneal haemorrhage. Usually the bleeding arises from the fracture itself, but it may be due to visceral injury or arterial damage. It is a sinister complication, and in those cases where the blood volume cannot be maintained by transfusion, the mortality rate is over 50%.

Diagnosis is often difficult, and even when it seems clear that continuing shock is due to haemorrhage, it is not easy to determine the source of bleeding. Signs of hypovolaemic shock may be accompanied by abdominal tenderness and guarding, and in these cases it may be difficult to exclude rupture of the spleen or liver. Patients with suspicious abdominal signs and radiographic evidence of pelvic fracture should be further investigated by peritoneal aspiration or lavage. If there is a negative (or equivocal) tap, the patient should be carefully monitored for 24 or 48 hours in the hope of improvement. If there is a positive diagnostic tap, the abdomen should be explored in an attempt to find the source of bleeding (Hawkins et al 1970). This approach, though it sounds rational, is not without risk. Laparotomy should be undertaken only after very careful evaluation of the patient's overall condition or if the surgeon has arrived at a diagnostic impasse in the face of continuing hypovolaemic shock.

A negative laparotomy with signs of continued blood loss suggests the presence of severe retroperitoneal haemorrhage. Sometimes this can be confirmed at laparotomy, but in other cases it may be extremely difficult to make the diagnosis or to identify the source of bleeding.

CT is helpful, but the use of other procedures such as angiography is highly controversial and may do more harm than good. Moreover, unless a single large vessel rupture is identified, the control of retroperitoneal bleeding is often fruitless because of the extensive collateral supply; worst of all, operative exploration may release the tamponade effect of the haematoma and encourage further bleeding from the torn vascular network. The use of intra-arterial occlusion is equally controversial, but if the appropriate facilities and expertise are available this technique could be considered.

More immediately, and certainly within the scope of the average trauma unit, the pelvic fracture should be stabilized by an external fixator; this will reduce haemorrhage from the fracture and will lessen the chances of further vascular or visceral damage while the patient is being moved about.

Management of the urethra and bladder

Urological injury occurs in about 10% of patients with pelvic ring fractures (Glass et al 1978, Kane 1984). It is a serious complication which calls for expert urological attention. As these patients are often seriously ill from other injuries, a urinary catheter may be required to monitor urinary output, and therefore the urologist is placed under pressure to make a rapid diagnosis of urethral damage.

There is no place for passing a diagnostic catheter as this will most probably convert any partial tear to a complete tear. For an incomplete tear, the insertion of a suprapubic catheter as a formal procedure is all that is required. There is no place for blind percutaneous suprapubic stabs with small-bore catheters. Around half of all incomplete tears will heal and require little long-term management.

The treatment of a complete urethral tear divides urologists into two camps: 1. those who advocate primary realignment of the urethra (Patterson et al 1983) and 2. those who advocate the placement of a suprapubic catheter as popularized by Mitchell in the UK (1968) and Morehouse & Mackinnon in North America (1980).

In the first method an initial suprapubic cystotomy is performed via a lower abdominal incision, at which time the abdominal contents are inspected for further damage. The pelvic haematoma is evacuated, a catheter is passed via a cystotomy through the prostatic urethra to emerge at the proximal end of the damaged urethra. Another catheter is passed up the urethra from the external meatus. The two catheters are found in the pelvis and linked together, then the first catheter is pulled back into the bladder so that the second catheter lies across the injury. One should avoid heavy traction on this urethral catheter as it may well cause pressure necrosis of the bladder neck (Turner Warwick 1973). Instead, the placement of stout nylon sutures through the surface of the lower anterior part of the prostatic capsule has been advocated. These sutures are brought into the perineum on either side of the bulbar urethra and traction is applied to the sutures using elastic bands attached to tape on the inner thigh. This traction must be maintained for 16–18 days (Turner Warwick 1985).

In the second method a suprapubic cystostomy with a diagnostic laparotomy (if needed) is performed at the time of the injury. No attempt is made to drain the pelvis or dissect the urethra. This method is simple and safe and is strongly recommended for those who do not have great expertise in pelvic surgery in these difficult circumstances. This measure decreases the chances of further neurovascular damage and further bleeding, as it does not disrupt the pelvic haematoma. The resulting stricture is then dealt with 4–6 months later. It is usually less than 20 mm long, and the alignment of the two ends is good. The stricture can be treated either by internal urethrotomy or urethroplasty.

Primary realignment of the urethra is indicated in three situations: 1. Severe prostatic dislocation, where it is over-optimistic to expect the haematoma to resolve without leaving a considerable amount of fibrous tissue between the two ends of the urethra. 2. When the rectum has been torn; this greatly increases the risk of sepsis in the pelvic haematoma, which must be drained at the same time as the colostomy is performed. 3. Bladder neck injury, which must be repaired as soon as possible if long-term continence is to be maintained (Webster et al 1983).

Both types of management result in a high incidence of stricture formation, incontinence and impotence. Webster et al (1983) have collated the results of many series: of 301 patients with primary realignment of the urethra, 69% developed strictures requiring repeated dilatations or urethroplasty, 44% were impotent and 20% were incontinent. By contrast, among the 237 who had only suprapubic cystostomy, 12% were impotent and only 4% were incontinent.

Rupture of the bladder in association with a pelvic fracture may lead to either intra- or extraperitoneal extravasation. Intraperitoneal extravasation of urine usually occurs when the bladder is full at the time of trauma. The mechanism of injury is either the bony pelvis or a seat-belt depressing the full bladder or the ligamentous attachments disrupting the bladder. Delayed rupture may occur when the symphysis is split apart and is presumably due to ischaemic necrosis of the bladder wall. Intraperitoneal rupture is commoner in children, because their bladder is an intra-abdominal organ. Extraperitoneal rupture is caused by a spicule or fragment of bone damaging the bladder.

An intraperitoneal tear of the bladder must be repaired immediately. The repair is performed via a midline incision to exclude other abdominal injuries. The edges of the bladder are identified and excised and then closed in two layers, using an absorbable suture.

An indwelling catheter is left in situ for 10 days, when a cystogram is performed to confirm that the bladder has healed. Greater experience of endoscopic surgery has shown that an extraperitoneal leak is not as serious as was once thought. A small tear leading to extraperitoneal leakage of urine can certainly be managed with a period of catheter drainage. A larger tear will also heal so long as the catheter does not become blocked. Thus only a large tear that is bleeding would have to be repaired in order to stop the bleeding; otherwise, a period of catheter drainage (i.e. 10 days) and broad-spectrum antibiotics are sufficient (Richardson & Leadbetter 1975).

In the rare cases where the bladder base becomes separated from the prostate in the male, or from the urethra in the female, it is best not to attempt any primary repair, but rather to wait for the reaction to trauma to settle before undertaking what is often very complex surgery.

REFERENCES

Bucholz R W 1981 The pathological anatomy of Malgaigne fracture — dislocations of the pelvis. Journal of Bone & Joint Surgery 63A: 400–404

Caroll P R, McAninch J W 1983 Major bladder trauma: the accuracy of cystography. Journal of Urology 130: 887–888

Conolly W B, Hedberg E A 1969 Observations on fractures of the pelvis. Journal of Trauma 9: 104–111

Eid A M 1981 Non-urogenital abdominal complications associated with fractures of the pelvis. Archives of Orthopedic & Traumatic Surgery 98: 35–40

Froman C, Stein A 1967 Complicated crushing injuries of the pelvis. Journal of Bone & Joint Surgery 49B: 24–32

Glass R E, Flynn J T, King J B, Blandy J P 1978 Urethral injury and fractured pelvis. British Journal of Urology 50: 578–582

Hawkins L, Pomerantz M, Eiseman B 1970 Laparotomy at the time of pelvic fracture. Journal of Trauma 10: 619–623

Kane W J 1984 Fractures of the pelvis. In: Rockwood C A, and Green D P (eds) Fractures in adults, 2nd edn. Lippincott, Philadelphia, p 1182

Levine J I, Crampton R W 1963 Major abdominal injuries associated with pelvic fractures. Surgery Gynecology & Obstetrics 116: 223–226

Malgaigne J F 1859 Treatise on fractures. Lippincott, Philadelphia

Mitchell J P 1968 Injuries to the urethra. British Journal of Urology 40: 649–670

Morehouse D D, Mackinnon K J 1980 Management of prostatomembranous urethral disruption; 13-year experience. Journal of Urology 123: 173–174

Patterson D E, Barrett D M, Myers R P, De-Weerd J H, Hall B B, Benson R C, Jr 1983 Primary realignment of posterior urethral injuries. Journal of Urology 129: 513–516

Peltier L F 1965 Complications associated with fractures of the pelvis. Journal of Bone & Joint Surgery 47A: 1060–1069

Richardson J R, Leadbetter G W 1975 Non-operative treatment of ruptured bladder. Journal of Urology 114: 213–216

Slatis P, Huittinen V M 1972 Double vertical fractures of the pelvis. Acta Chirurgica Scandinavica 138: 799–807

Slatis P, Karaharju E O 1980 External fixation of unstable pelvic fractures: Experiences in 22 patients treated with a trapezoid compression frame. Clinical Orthopedics 151: 73–80

Tile M, Pennal G F 1980 Pelvic disruption: Principles of management. Clinical Orthopedics 151: 56–64

Turner Warwick R T 1973 Observations on the treatment of traumatic urethral injuries and the value of the fenestrated urethral catheter. British Journal of Surgery 60: 775–781

Turner Warwick R T 1985 In: Whitfield H N, Hendry W R (eds) Textbook of genito-urinary surgery. Churchill Livingstone, Edinburgh pp 865–871

Webster G D, Mathes G L, Selli C 1983 Prostatomembranous urethral injuries: a review of the literature and a rational approach to their management. Journal of Urology 130: 898–902

5

Septicaemic shock

M. S. DAHN and A. J. WALT

Sepsis and its associated sequelae are major causes of death today. Shock complicates the clinical course of approximately 40% of patients suffering from gram negative bacteraemia, and the mortality of the attendant shock ranges from 40–90% (Parker & Parrillo 1983). Ultimately, death results from multiple organ failure in most cases, and considerable effort has been devoted to the understanding of organ dysfunction associated with Gram-negative sepsis. Although the major focus of this chapter will be on the response to endotoxin, a component of all Gram-negative bacteria, it should be understood that many, if not most, of the host responses to infection result from the generation of endogenous mediators. Consequently, the response to Gram-positive agents, fungal and viral infections, exhibits similar physiological and metabolic profiles (Deutschman et al 1987). Investigators have indicated that a non-septic inflammatory stress may precipitate multiple organ failure in humans and experimental models (Goris et al 1985, 1986), suggesting that ongoing sepsis is not essential for the evolution of a septic-like syndrome. Nevertheless, it is generally believed that the systemic response associated with multiple organ dysfunction is at least initiated by microorganisms and most commonly by Gram-negative bacteria, with endotoxin as the active component. Observations such as the absence of detectable blood endotoxin and the occurrence of a hypodynamic circulatory response to injected endotoxin in experimental models (as opposed to the hyperdynamic human septic response) have been used to refute the concept that endotoxin plays a key role in the genesis of the septic syndrome. However, most authors have ascribed these variations to duration of exposure to the initiating events and to the degree of resuscitation that occurs during the active insult. Also, the response to various species of Gram-negative organisms may vary somewhat, probably reflecting variations in the specific molecular structure of the active principle of endotoxin, which is thought to be lipopolysaccharide (LPS). Nevertheless, common response patterns generally characterize infection with a variety of Gram-negative bacterial pathogens, and these patterns will be considered in this chapter.

Definitions and characteristics of septic states

Endotoxaemic and septic shock

Endotoxaemic shock refers most commonly to the metabolic and physiological response patterns associated with exogenous endotoxin infusion in an experimental model. This has been characterized as a hypodynamic model with decreased blood pressure and cardiac output (CO), increased lactate production and hypoglycaemia after a short initial hyperglycaemic phase (Wichterman et al 1980). A number of authors have commented that such a model, commonly used during early studies of septic shock, does not reflect the human septic condition, which is most commonly characterized by normotension, increased CO and total body oxygen consumption (V_{O_2}) and a sustained increase in blood glucose level. Recent studies have indicated that the specific response to endotoxin can be modified to simulate the human condition by smaller doses of endotoxin, slower infusion rates and vigorous volume resuscitation (Houtchens & Westenskow 1984).

Septic shock is the term used most commonly in the clinical sense when an infectious process leads to circulatory insufficiency. The term has also been applied to experimental situations where live Gram-negative bacteria are infused to simulate septicaemia. Clinical as well as experimental circumstances are generally characterized by a hyperdynamic response, which implies that CO and V_{O_2} rise. The differences in this terminology (endotoxaemic vs. septic shock) are ill defined, and the reader should therefore evaluate individual reports based upon the specific haemodynamic and metabolic data. Finally, 'sepsis' or 'the septic syndrome' refers to the clinical response associated with a less severe form of infection, in which no apparent circulatory embarrassment is present. This latter circumstance, however, may not be easily ruled out since occult regional perfusion deficits may coexist with a hyperdynamic circulatory response, thereby masking the distinction between sepsis and septic shock.

Oxygen utilization characteristics

The factors that are usually used to characterize the host response to infection or LPS include their cardiovascular and metabolic response patterns. Oxygen consumption is the most sophisticated parameter in the assessment of the systemic response to sepsis. Abnormally high V_{O_2}, which is usually associated with an elevated cardiac output, reduced peripheral vascular resistance and possibly a mild reduction in mean arterial pressure in response to vasodilatation, has been considered an appropriate and compensated response. This response pattern is thought to enhance substantially the likelihood of survival in contrast to a depressed V_{O_2} and CO. However, even when these parameters appear to reflect a compensated hyperdynamic state, death can ensue within minutes to hours. Consequently, the systemic V_{O_2} is not a reliable prognosticator of outcome (Houtchens & Westenskow 1984, Groeneveld et al 1987).

A number of recent human studies have suggested possible reasons for a poor outcome in the presence of an elevated V_{O_2}. It is believed that V_{O_2} remains constant and independent of oxygen delivery over a broad range unless this transport drops below the 'critical oxygen delivery point' (Mohsenifar et al 1983, Shumacker & Cain 1987). Below this level (Fig. 5.1), which has been estimated at 8.2 ml/kg/min, V_{O_2} is determined by the rate of transport to the tissues, and a decrease below this limiting value suggests tissue oxygen deprivation (Shibutani et al 1983). The critical oxygen delivery point is low enough for flow limitation of V_{O_2} to be uncommon normally. Patients suffering from sepsis, especially those with adult respiratory distress syndrome (ARDS), have been found to exhibit different patterns (Wolf et al 1987, Danek et al 1980). Oxygen consumption is dependent on supply to a much higher level with a transition to transport independence at 21 ml/kg/min. Recent studies on critically ill patients have indicated that those who died exhibited this oxygen transport dependence, whereas survivors resemble unstressed subjects and appear to function at the plateau of the oxygen transport curve (Fig. 5.1). The implication is that

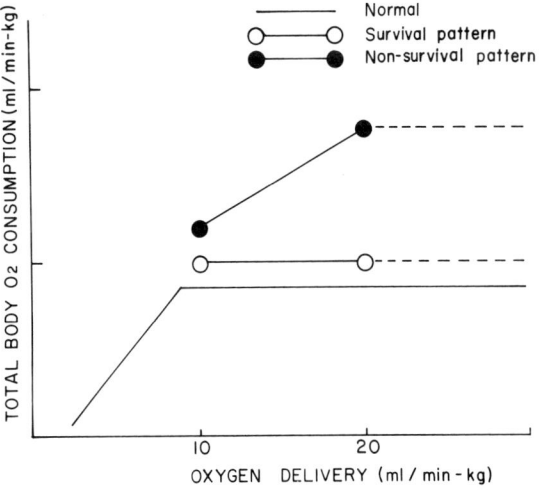

Fig. 5.1 The concept of 'critical oxygen consumption'. Total body oxygen consumption is generally independent of oxygen delivery until a critically low level of transport is reached. Below this level oxygen consumption is delivery-dependent. Surviving patients with sepsis exhibit an oxygen transport dependence similar to normal patients; however, nonsurviving patients exhibit a critical oxygen consumption level which may be much higher than normal, thus making them more subject to occult tissue ischaemia.

occult tissue hypoxia may be present in some seriously septic patients despite an already elevated V_{O_2} which is detectable only by stimulating oxygen transport (usually by increasing cardiac output) and observing the oxygen consumption response (Bihari et al 1987).

The normal range of V_{O_2} (Shoemaker et al 1983) is 100–180 ml/min/m². Although an elevation in V_{O_2} is the most common sequel of sepsis, a decline in oxygen consumption below this range signals hypodynamic sepsis or septic shock (Cerra et al 1979, Bland & Shoemaker 1985) (Fig. 5.2). The progression to this latter state may be quite insidious and occur in the absence of hypotension. Furthermore, it should be kept in mind that the presence of an elevated oxygen consumption does not rule out decompensated sepsis, since (as mentioned previously) a flow-limited oxygen consumption may be observed in hyperdynamic states. The observed range of oxygen consumption (and cardiac index) in a decompensated state is quite broad, and probably reflects multiple mechanisms, with dominance determined by the stage of sepsis.

Major reductions in V_{O_2} usually occur in late or advanced sepsis and if this state persists, mortality is high. Factors postulated to account for a declining oxygen consumption are: 1. flow limitation, i.e., a cardiac output insufficient to meet V_{O_2} needs; 2. arteriovenous shunting, resulting in inadequate nutrient exchange to peripheral tissue; 3. altered oxyhaemoglobin dissociation resulting in poor off-loading of arterial oxygen content; and 4. direct depression of mitochondrial respiration.

The metabolic response to sepsis

Energy needs

The hyperdynamic state associated with sepsis is precipitated by increased peripheral metabolism and liberation of endogenous vasoactive agents. The associated hypermetabolism results from increased activity of a variety of biochemical and transport processes such as increased glucose production by the liver, stimulated protein synthesis, a generalized increase in body protein turnover, stepped up substrate transport across cell membranes and other less clearly evaluated contributions from processes such as futile cycling, increased lipid metabolism and nucleic acid turnover under the stresses of infection. Septic complications may increase metabolic rate by 20–60% above basal needs (Fig. 5.2). The degree of hypermetabolism is directly related to the degree of urinary urea loss (Fig. 5.2) and thus to total body nitrogen loss. From this standpoint, the rate at which lean body mass is lost would therefore depend upon the degree of elevation in metabolic rate and, in highly stressed individuals, early nutritional support would appear to be an urgent issue.

The measurement of gas exchange in order to determine V_{O_2} and carbon dioxide production has been advocated as a guide to the degree of hypermetabolism as well as of caloric requirements for

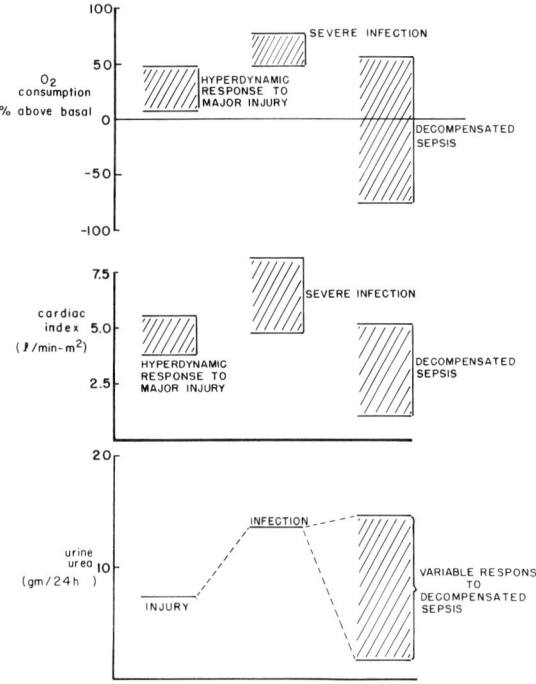

Fig. 5.2 The cardiac index, urea loss and percentage increase of total body oxygen consumption above basal are related to the type and magnitude of the stress event. Sepsis generally increases these parameters to higher levels than injury. Decompensated sepsis manifests as a flow-dependent oxygen-consuming state, and these parameters may exhibit a wide range.

nutritional support purposes. The measurement of energy expenditure (EE) via gas exchange measurements is referred to as indirect calorimetry. Mobile units containing gas analyzers are currently available to determine gas exchange at the patient's bedside. The use of this tool has received a mixed response because some of the shortcomings of this technique in assessing metabolic response have recently become evident. Energy expenditure is determined by at least three components: 1. basal EE; 2. thermogenesis, or heat generated by accelerated metabolic processes of sepsis and injury; and 3. energy of physical activity. Measured resting energy expenditure (REE) (composed of basal EE and thermogenesis) in the critically ill may overestimate or underestimate the true total EE, depending upon the specific state of the subject (Swinamer et al 1987, Weissman et al 1986). Factors such as pain and activity may transiently alter EE and may not be considered during the measurement process. Also, the accurate measurement of oxygen exchange becomes increasingly difficult as airway pressures rise and as the fraction of inspired oxygen required by the patient increases. Therefore, patients who are the most seriously ill, requiring a high fraction of inspired oxygen (FI_{O_2}), benefit least from

this modality. Nevertheless, the most beneficial aspect of this technique is that it provides an estimated range of V_{O_2} and caloric need which may guide the physician in assessing the clinical status and instituting hyperalimentation.

Another approach to estimate total caloric needs includes use of the Harris-Benedict equations (Gray 1985) to calculate unstressed basal requirements, followed by the inclusion of the projected stress contribution (i.e. +20–60% of basal estimate for the infection-induced increase in metabolic rate) to the REE. This approach is obviously heavily dependent on the clinician's guess of the fractional stress contribution. Alternatively, one can simply estimate caloric needs at 35–40 non-protein kcal/kg/day (Cerra 1987) without exceeding 5 mg/kg/min (Wolfe et al 1980) of glucose intake (maximum glucose oxidation rate). All these approaches require sequential nitrogen balance studies to verify the adequacy of therapy.

Glucose metabolism

Following the induction of sepsis, the net balance of glucose metabolism is determined largely by three factors (Fig. 5.3): 1. rate of glucose production by the liver; 2. size of the glucose pool; and 3. rate of peripheral glucose clearance. Hepatic glucose production is substantially increased following injury and infection (Gump et al 1974, Long 1977) due to a combination of glycogenolysis and gluconeogenesis from lactate, amino acids and glycerol mobilized from peripheral body mass. Lactate results from the anaerobic metabolism of glucose and appears to be a dominant feature of sepsis, possibly resulting from inactivation of pyruvate dehydrogenase (PDH), a key enzyme which can either retard or accelerate the entrance of pyruvate into further oxidative metabolic pathways (Fig. 5.3). It has been suggested that as the degree of sepsis worsens, the block associated with PDH inactivity increases, thus forcing more pyruvate to convert to lactate and thereby increasing the level of lactate in the blood. This process may partly be related to insulin depression, which is commonly observed with hypoperfusion (Clowes et al 1974), since PDH activity is sensitive to ambient insulin levels. However, the shock state itself

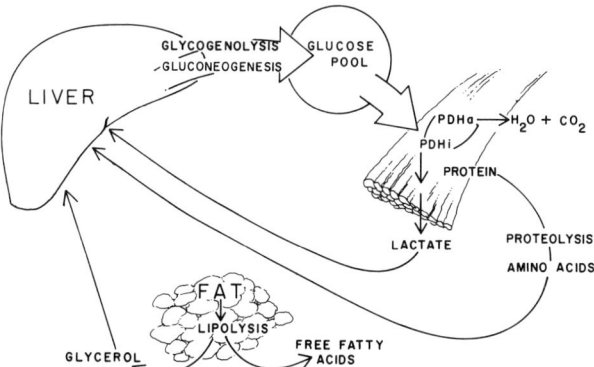

Fig. 5.3 Key aspects of glucose turnover. Plasma glucose level reflects the balance of glucose production from the liver by gluconeogenesis and glycogenolysis, glucose clearance by actively metabolizing tissues such as skeletal muscle, and the distribution of the available glucose to intra- and extravascular body compartments collectively termed the glucose pool. Contributors toward hepatic gluconeogenesis include lactate, amino acids and glycerol. The metabolic fate of glucose that is taken up by skeletal muscle may be heavily dependent upon a key enzyme, pyruvate dehydrogenase (PDH).

seems to influence this metabolic block negatively in an ill-defined manner (Ryan et al 1974a). The presence of large amounts of lactate results in a great availability of gluconeogenic substrate to the liver, thus stimulating hepatic glucose output.

Gluconeogenic substrate for the liver is also provided by the mobilization of peripheral amino acids stemming from the increased rate of proteolysis in the peripheral tissues. This event is particularly important in skeletal muscle, which is the largest reserve of protein in the body. Amino acid transport to the liver may increase three to five times (Clowes et al 1980) following the stress of severe sepsis. The predominant amino acids transported are glutamine and alanine, which are produced at an accelerated rate in skeletal muscle by transamination of pyruvate and alpha-ketoglutarate (to glutamate). The gluconeogenic role of these newly formed amino acids is probably incidental to the need for transporting excess ammonia (linked to a carbon based carrier) to the liver for ureagenesis. It has been suggested that the excess ammonia stems from local skeletal muscle oxidation of amino acids (particularly leucine). Finally, glycerol arises from peripheral lipolysis. Glycerol, which is split from triglycerides cannot be re-utilized locally but undergoes transport to the liver and serves as gluconeogenic substrate.

A notable feature of increased glucose production during sepsis is that it tends to be non-suppressible despite the infusion of hypertonic glucose solutions (Long et al 1976). This finding may in part stem from the need to clear large amounts of lactate. As sepsis progresses to the extreme of septic shock the fraction of glucose oxidized to carbon dioxide gradually declines and the production of lactate markedly increases. This situation may be compounded by the development of liver failure commonly associated with septic shock. Since the liver is the major organ which clears lactate, significant liver dysfunction will rapidly augment lactate accumulation. Specific sites of injury may preferentially use glycolysis as opposed to complete oxidation of glucose. This process has been noted in granulating burn wounds, which exhibit relatively increased glucose uptake and lactate production rates compared with non-burned regions (Aulick et al 1980). Since the rise in the lactate level correlates with the severity

of hypermetabolism, it may serve as an index of the severity of septic stress. Eventually, if the septic process remains unchecked, the ability of the liver to oxidize and/or convert lactate to glucose diminishes and hepatic glucose output declines. This decline is manifested as acute hypoglycaemia and usually indicates advanced liver failure, carrying a dismal prognosis.

Basal glucose clearance is elevated following injury (Thomas et al 1979) and sepsis (Dahn et al 1985, Raymond et al 1985, Lang et al 1987). Compared to normal volunteers, patients suffering from traumatic injury have been observed to exhibit reduced maximal glucose disposal rates in response to elevated insulin concentrations. This phenomenon has been termed insulin resistance, and evidence exists that this response is secondary to increased beta adrenergic (epinephrine) activity which may be present after injury (Bessey & Wilmore 1983, Bessey et al 1983). Experimental studies using maximal insulin stimulations in septic models have yielded variable results, demonstrating or failing to support peripheral insulin resistance (Wichterman et al 1979). These discrepancies possibly relate to specifics in experimental design. Recent studies using the hyperglycaemic glucose clamp technique have indicated that impaired glucose utilization can be demonstrated in septic patients. The reduction in glucose utilization is associated with an increase in fat oxidation (White et al 1987). Observations such as these have fostered the view that lipid is a preferred fuel, especially in seriously septic patients.

Generalizations that probably can be made are that in compensated sepsis, basal metabolic clearance of glucose is elevated and glucose oxidation increases in proportion to glucose infusion (Shaw et al 1984). As the degree of sepsis worsens, glucose oxidation declines (Lang et al 1984a) and lactate production correspondingly increases (Stoner et al 1983), possibly due to PDH inactivation, (Vary et al 1986) but metabolic clearance remains high (Wichterman et al 1979, Lang et al 1984a).

Finally, it has recently been reported that increased non-productive glycolytic–gluconeogenic cycling ('futile cycling') exists in burn patients. Substrate cycling exists when opposing reactions catalyzed by different enzymes are operating simultaneously and consuming ATP. The net result is a wasteful ATP hydrolysis, resulting in increased energy expenditure, approximately 15% above expected levels (Wolfe et al 1987). This response in sepsis has not been studied but since it is thought to involve the counterregulatory hormones, glucogen and catecholamines, which are elevated following trauma and sepsis, it seems likely that it may also contribute to the overall metabolic response following septicaemia.

The clinical use of glucose as the sole source of non-nitrogen caloric support, although once popular, has declined. The factors responsible for this situation are several. We have already indicated that a number of studies using indirect calorimetry have suggested that lipids may be the preferred fuel source in sepsis. Additionally, the use of large glucose loads can stimulate substantial increases of endogenous carbon dioxide production and oxygen utilization (Askanazi et al 1980), resulting in increased stresses being placed on the respiratory and cardiovascular systems. This increased stress may be particularly important during the period of ventilator weaning and in patients with congestive heart failure. Finally, hypertonic glucose has been associated with greater risks of glycaemic related and septic complications (Kirkpatrick et al 1981). Many authorities are recommending a mixed fuel source system containing as much as 60% lipid calories.

Lipid metabolism

Most recently, research on lipid metabolism in sepsis has addressed the issue as to whether the body efficiently utilizes fats, both exogenous and endogenous, as a fuel source during the hypermetabolic response to infection. These studies arose because Gram-negative sepsis has previously been characterized by hypertriglyceridaemia and intolerance to lipid loading (Kaufman et al 1976).

The major relevant avenues of triglyceride metabolism are indicated in Figure 5.4 Plasma triglycerides (TG) associated with chylomicrons (exogenous), or in the form of endogenous lipoprotein lipids, require hydrolysis by peripheral lipoprotein lipase (LPL) prior to being taken up

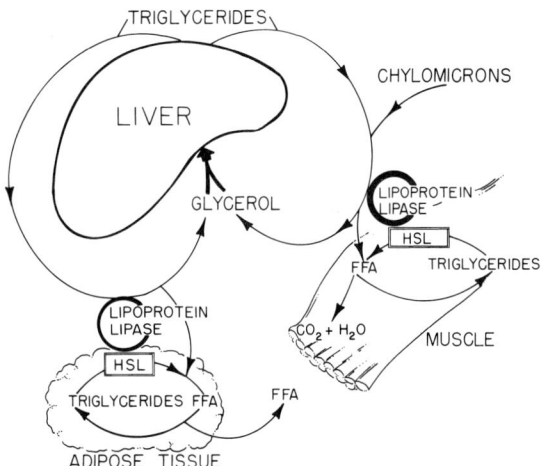

Fig. 5.4 Metabolism of triglycerides and chylomicrons. Lipoprotein lipase is an important and widely distributed enzyme required for the clearance of these substrates: deficiency may result in lipaemia and hypertriglyceridaemia. Hormone-sensitive lipase (HSL) catalyzes the mobilization of fatty acids, which may be utilized for fuel in various tissues or may be converted back to triglycerides by the liver.

into body tissue. LPL is located primarily on endothelial surfaces, and interaction between this enzyme and TG is required in the process of fat metabolism. Following hydrolysis, free fatty acids (FFA) are liberated, enter the tissue and may undergo beta oxidation or re-esterification to TG. Under stressful conditions, an opposing response may be stimulated in order to increase the availability of lipids (Fig. 5.4). Hormone-sensitive lipase (HSL) may be activated by a variety of hormones, including catecholamines, glucagon, and growth hormone, to hydrolyze peripheral TG stores for the purpose of increasing FFA availability to serve as a local or remote fuel source.

The processes most affected by the onset of infection appear to be the rate of mobilization of fatty acids through the stimulation of HSL and the clearance rate of TG by depression of LPL. Observations based on isotopic as well as indirect calorimetric studies (Nordenstrom et al 1983) indicate that septic stress results in an increased lipolysis and FFA turnover. It has been suggested that elevated levels of the counterregulatory hormones (catecholamines, glucagon and cortisol) are responsible for high rates of FFA mobilization.

Stress-induced catecholamines in particular are known to stimulate lipolysis markedly and to inhibit the action of insulin, which normally suppresses HSL. Catecholamine-induced lipolysis is probably the main factor responsible for persistent fat oxidation, which occurs in septic but not normal subjects despite the administration of elevated carbohydrate loads, as might occur during total parenteral nutrition. Experimental studies have also focused on the acute lipolytic action of noradrenaline (norepinephrine) as the dominant factor causing elevation of FFA release. An additional observation in these studies is that the normal antilipolytic action of insulin on adipose tissue becomes attenuated with time, thus contributing to ongoing fat mobilization during glucose infusions (Spitzer & Fish 1986).

Occasionally, patients with severe sepsis exhibit lipaemia. Human as well as experimental studies have demonstrated decreases in LPL activity in muscle and particularly adipose tissue, which probably accounts for this observation (Robin et al 1981, Lanza-Jacoby et al 1982). Despite these findings, a number of clinical reports studying hyperdynamic sepsis have indicated that exogenous lipids are cleared and oxidized in a manner similar to endogenous lipids (Nordenstrom et al 1982). These findings, along with the observation that fat oxidation persists despite hypertonic glucose administration in critically ill septic patients, have stimulated the use of fat emulsions as a caloric source in patients receiving parenteral nutrition. It is suggested that lipaemia and marked depression of lipid clearance occurs only in hypodynamic sepsis. However, this phenomenon, if it occurs, would contraindicate the use of fat emulsions.

Protein metabolism

Net body protein balance results from the difference between whole-body protein synthesis and degradation (Fig. 5.5). Septic human subjects who are not in shock exhibit elevations in both synthesis and breakdown rates (Long et al 1977, Yamamori et al 1987). These observations, therefore, indicate that the mechanism of nitrogen wasting that is observed in septic patients results not from a suppression of protein synthesis (as was

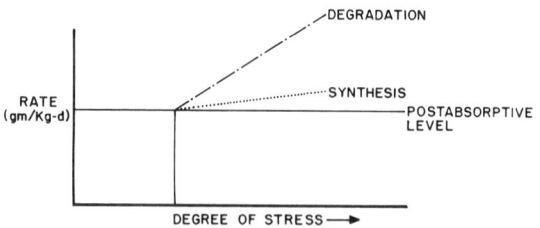

Fig. 5.5 Idealized relative rate of whole-body protein degradation and synthesis, relative to the degree of stress.

once commonly believed) but from the unfavourable balance of synthesis and catabolism. As these results are derived from whole-body turnover measurements, they provide no information on organ-specific events. With the use of incubated biopsy specimens of liver and skeletal muscle from infected human subjects, individual tissue-specific rates of protein synthesis and degradation have been estimated. Liver tissue exhibits increased rates of protein synthesis and decreased rates of protein degradation compared to tissue from elective surgical cases. Skeletal muscle specimens exhibit synthetic rates similar to those of liver tissue, but rates of proteolysis are markedly elevated (Rosenblatt et al 1983). These data indicate that the bulk of stepped-up protein degradation observed in whole-body protein kinetic experiments probably arises from the skeletal muscle mass, the largest protein mass in the body. The net result is an accelerated transfer of amino acids from muscle to viscera for the purpose of protein synthesis. This transfer of amino acids, however, is also associated with an increased oxidation of essential amino acids in the skeletal muscle and increased hepatic ureagenesis, both of which are nitrogen-losing (catabolic) processes. These observations have been made in 'stable sepsis', and relatively little data exist for hypoperfusion states. Experimental late sepsis is probably the most representative model currently available for the study of protein dynamics during septic shock. Such studies have reaffirmed that increases in skeletal muscle proteolytic rates dominate net protein turnover (Hasselgren et al 1986). Hepatic protein synthesis, although generally increased as a result of the large rise in amino acid availability from the periphery, is sensitive to perfusion and declines under ischaemic circumstances (Hasselgren et al 1983). This fact may explain the finding that liver-derived acute-phase plasma proteins are much lower in patients who expire from severe infections than the levels found in survivors (Dominioni et al 1981, 1987). Overall, the events of advanced infection and septic shock are less clearly understood and warrant further study.

A number of factors have been identified as regulators of net protein synthesis. Hormonal effectors of skeletal muscle protein production include insulin, glucocorticoids and the somatomedins. Insulin is known to stimulate protein synthesis as well as inhibit protein degradation and has been shown to attenuate the accelerated release of skeletal muscle amino acids in trauma patients (Brooks et al 1986). Clinical studies demonstrating the net benefit of added insulin above standard nutritional support in non-diabetics are scant. A septic animal model has demonstrated that insulin stimulates muscle protein synthesis (probably by increasing amino acid uptake), but the usual inhibitory action upon proteolysis is lost (Hasselgren et al 1987). The somatomedins are a group of proteins which are growth-hormone-dependent, produced primarily by the liver, which exhibit potent anabolic properties (Froesch et al 1985). They are currently undergoing scrutiny because of the recent availability of biosynthetic growth hormone (Ward et al 1987) and the observation that some critically ill patients exhibit depressed endogenous growth hormone production (Dahn et al 1984b). Currently, there are insufficient data to judge their importance in clinical sepsis. Glucocorticoids (which are elevated in sepsis) have been reported to accelerate the oxidation of branched-chain amino acids in skeletal muscle tissue, thus stimulating the overall rate of amino acid loss by this tissue (Ryan et al 1974b).

Several other modifiers have received considerable attention recently including leucine, interleukin-1 and the prostaglandins E_2 (PGE$_2$) and $F_{2\alpha}$ (PGF$_{2\alpha}$). Leucine, which is an essential amino acid, is known to reduce protein catabolism in muscle, possibly due to its ability to act as a direct local energy source as well as exerting ill-defined hormonal-like properties (Goldberg 1983). This finding has spurred the use of amino acid solutions high in leucine content (high branched-chain amino acid formulas) for providing nutritional support for critically ill patients, particularly highly-stressed septic patients. The clinical efficacy of this approach is currently considered quite controversial, and specific guidelines for the use of these specialized solutions still await formulation (Brennan et al 1986).

Interleukin-1 (IL-1) is a macrophage peptide product released upon stimulation with endotoxin, which apparently exerts its early effects by stimulating the formation of PGE$_2$, resulting in increased lysosomal mediated proteolysis in skeletal muscle and fever production (Baracos et al 1983, Keusch & Farthing 1986). IL-1 is produced as a 17 000 dalton peptide but apparently undergoes extensive proteolysis. A plasma peptide of approximately 4000 daltons has been reported to exhibit properties resembling IL-1 and has been termed 'proteolysis inducing factor' (PIF); it is able to increase the proteolytic rate in skeletal muscle without altering synthetic rate substantially. The net effect is a major amino acid loss by the involved tissue. In addition, in-vivo amino acid loss by skeletal muscle, as well as induction of visceral protein synthesis in septic patients, appear to correlate with PIF activity. This finding supports the view that a humoral agent is responsible for the mobilization of amino acids to vital organ systems in order to increase their protein production, particularly the acute-phase proteins of the liver (Clowes et al 1983, Loda et al 1984).

Although in-vitro experimental models have indicated that PGE$_2$ (produced from arachidonic acid through the action of IL-1) precipitates a markedly increased rate of muscle proteolysis, recent findings using cyclo-oxygenase inhibitors have complicated this issue. In established burn injury, PGE$_2$, but not proteolytic rate, is suppressible (McKinley & Turinsky 1986, Odessey 1985). This fact has led to the hypothesis that PGE$_2$ may be an initiator but does not necessarily maintain proteolysis in muscle. Other studies utilizing acute septic animal models have indicated that prostaglandin cyclo-oxygenase inhibitors exhibit very limited effect on the metabolic response to endotoxin or IL-1 (Hulton et al 1985, Sobrado et al 1983). PGF$_{2\alpha}$, another metabolite of arachidonic acid, has been shown to be directly related to the rate of muscle protein synthesis (Reeds & Palmer

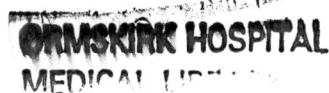

1983), and it has been suggested that the relative balance of these two prostenoids, PGE_2 and $PGF_{2\alpha}$, may determine or reflect the net metabolic balance of protein production in skeletal muscle. Whether these two lipids are effectors or simply reflect epiphenomena awaits further investigation.

Clinical management of patients with severe sepsis consists of providing an adequate non-nitrogen caloric intake and a moderate-to-high intake of amino acids (2–3 gm/kg/day). These levels have been suggested to achieve nitrogen equilibrium. In order to place a patient into positive nitrogen balance, even higher rates (3–4 gm/kg/day) have been recommended (Cerra 1987). Serial nitrogen balance studies should be conducted to determine the effectiveness of therapy.

Intestinal role in sepsis

Recently, it has been suggested that trauma and endotoxaemia may promote the transmural migration or translocation of bacteria across the intact intestinal wall (Deitch et al 1987). The mechanism (Fig 5.6) remains unclear, since disruption of the surface architecture of the intestinal mucosa need not be demonstrated for this process to occur. Several hypotheses have been considered, including: 1. increased gut permeability, which cannot, however, be demonstrated histologically; 2. impaired host immunity, resulting in failure of the usual bacterial clearing mechanisms in the intestinal wall or regional lymphatic network, allowing systemic escape of bacteria; and 3. alteration of the normal ecology of the gut intraluminal bacterial content (through the use of

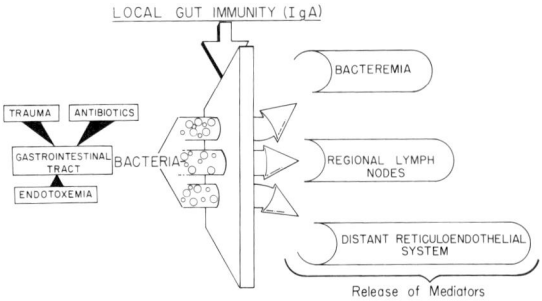

Fig. 5.6   Key features of the gut hypothesis.

broad-spectrum antibiotics), resulting in excessive population levels and associated transmural migration of certain indigenous bacteria (Steffen & Berg 1983). This overall hypothesis suggests that translocation, once initiated by a stressor, may result in metastatic infection due to progressive bacterial involvement of regional mesenteric lymph nodes, culminating in an overflow of bacteria to lymphatics and the blood stream. This sequence leads to the liberation of endogenous inflammatory mediators, resulting in a sustained hypermetabolic state similar or identical to that seen in septicaemia. Most of the evidence supporting this hypothesis stems from animal experiments, and their relevance to the human septic condition still needs to be demonstrated. Nevertheless, the translocation hypothesis does seem to provide a reasonable explanation of the recurrent septic episodes and metabolic alterations noted in patients suffering from severe septic processes for which no distinct focus can be defined.

Parallel to the evolution of the gut hypothesis, studies supporting the use of enteral nutrition to maintain gut wall integrity have arisen. These considerations appear to be complementary to the gut hypothesis and are therefore discussed here. Enteral feeding in experimental animals supports gastrointestinal levels of secretory IgA much better than providing nutrients through the intravenous route. Low levels of IgA have been implicated in increasing the susceptibility to bacterial translocation (Alverdy et al 1985). Other studies have indicated that enteral feedings following burn injury maintain the intestinal integrity and minimize the catabolic hormone response (glucagon, cortisol) to injury (Saito et al 1987). These studies have not yet been duplicated in the septic model. Nevertheless, the inescapable presumption is that support of the intestinal tract through direct enteral nutrition may suppress the adverse metabolic state associated with injury and sepsis, possibly by reducing bacterial translocation.

Mediators of the septic syndrome

Indirect nature of the response to septicaemia

It is generally believed that systemic expression of

invasive infection results, not directly from components of the bacterial organism, but largely from the generation of endogenous mediators (Keusch & Farthing 1986). These mediators are liberated in response to the presence of LPS, the active component of the cell wall from Gram-negative bacteria, and cause major alterations of cardiovascular and metabolic functions. LPS has been subdivided into at least two major components: 1. lipid A and 2. a covalently bound polysaccharide moiety. It has been found that the lipid A component is responsible for the major biological response to endotoxaemia. The polysaccharide portion determines the elimination kinetics, mediates binding with macrophages and lymphocytes and is largely necessary for activation of the alternate pathway of the complement system (Emau et al 1986). Additionally, major differences in the polysaccharide component from different bacterial species may explain, to some degree, variations in biological response patterns to septicaemia.

Endotoxin may elicit a variety of cellular activities by directly interacting with cell membranes, as evidenced by its ability to enhance lysosomal enzyme activities and uncouple mitochondria in the absence of added serum (Bradley 1981). Nevertheless, it is generally felt that the major response to endotoxaemia results from the action of activated serum factors or endogenously produced cellular peptide products. The mediators which are liberated are thought to act in coordination to produce characteristic response patterns. The major groups of responsible mediators include: 1. endocrine hormones; 2. macrophage-derived peptide products; 3. lipid mediators; 4. complement; and 5. opiate mediators.

Endocrine factors

Although a multitude of endocrine effects in sepsis has been identified, the synergistic response pattern associated with the counterregulatory hormones glucagon, adrenaline (epinephrine) and cortisol has received the greatest attention (Dahn et al 1980). Historically, interest in these hormones stems from their known property of regulating the glucose metabolism. Each hormone can stimulate hepatic glucose output, which is also a characteristic feature of septicaemia and human sepsis. However, under experimental conditions, glucagon or adrenaline alone cause only transient increases in hepatic glucose production, and cortisol infusion fails to alter glucose kinetics acutely. It has been noted that multiple-hormone infusions, combining the effects of all the counterregulatory hormones, provide a persistent and synergistic action which is more typical of the septic response (DeFronzo et al 1980). Additionally, physiological infusions of these three 'stress' hormones in humans are able to simulate many of the metabolic responses observed following injury and sepsis, including increased metabolic rate, negative nitrogen balance, glucose intolerance, insulin resistance and peripheral leucocytosis (Bessey et al 1984). Furthermore, increases in whole-body protein turnover can be induced with this hormone 'cocktail', indicating that these hormones play a key role in determining the overall metabolic status in sepsis. Studies on normal human volunteers to determine the relative caloric effects of triple hormone infusions vs. induced interleukin-1 have shown that the greatest contribution to metabolic rate arises from the stress hormones (Watters et al 1986). However, recent studies on seriously septic patients have emphasized other hormone profiles. Glucagon levels were found to be normal and cortisol and noradrenaline levels appeared to be more closely related to the observed metabolic changes (White et al 1987). The reason for these different conclusions remains unclear at present. This fact may indicate that hypermetabolism of sepsis may arise through multiple mediator pathways, or that the initial hormonal response to infection arises from the typical triple hormone response modelled above, but that these hormones are not required for perpetuation of this response.

Insulin and growth hormone are probably the most important anabolic hormones interacting with the stress response to limit the counterregulatory catabolic state. Variable insulin responses to infection have been reported. Patients and experimental models with stable or mild sepsis exhibit normal insulin levels (Dahn et al 1980, Neufeld et al 1980). In sepsis with low cardiac output, and hypotensive septic shock, insulin production by the pancreatic islet cells is markedly depressed, resulting in low plasma insulin levels (Clowes et al 1978). This decreased output results from reduced blood flow to the endocrine pancreas and a direct suppressive effect of the sympathetic nervous system as well as increased suppressive alpha adrenergic activity from circulating noradrenaline. However, in intermediate degrees of sepsis, the absolute insulin levels have been reported not to correlate with the relative pancreatic output of insulin. Consequently, insulin levels must be interpreted with caution (Dahn et al 1987a).

Growth hormone levels are generally considered to rise in response to stress. Recently, patients exhibiting complicated and severely septic hospital courses have been reported to exhibit depressed growth hormone production, which may be significant in accelerating increased body nitrogen loss (Dahn et al 1984b). Growth hormone is thought to mediate its anabolic properties via stimulation of a group of proteins known as the somatomedins, or sometimes called 'insulin-like growth factors'. The anabolic activity of plasma somatomedins is depressed immediately after in-

jury, and this may play a role in the susceptibility of injured patients to infection (Coates et al 1981, Dahn et al 1987b), although this area is not well explored yet. Significantly, the availability of recombinant human growth hormone may magnify the importance of these observations since this agent may provide a simple pharmacological approach to improve a depressed anabolic hormone profile.

Macrophage-derived peptides

Monokines are polypeptide products from activated monocytes and macrophages. These agents have become recognized as powerful mediators of the haemodynamic, metabolic and immunological events surrounding septicaemia and septic shock. Activation of these cells results from the interaction of macrophages with antigen–antibody complexes, traumatized tissue and microorganisms. The most potent stimulus resulting in the liberation of these monokines is endotoxin (Fig. 5.7), and at least one of them (tumour necrosis factor) is thought to be the principal mediator of endotoxin-induced shock.

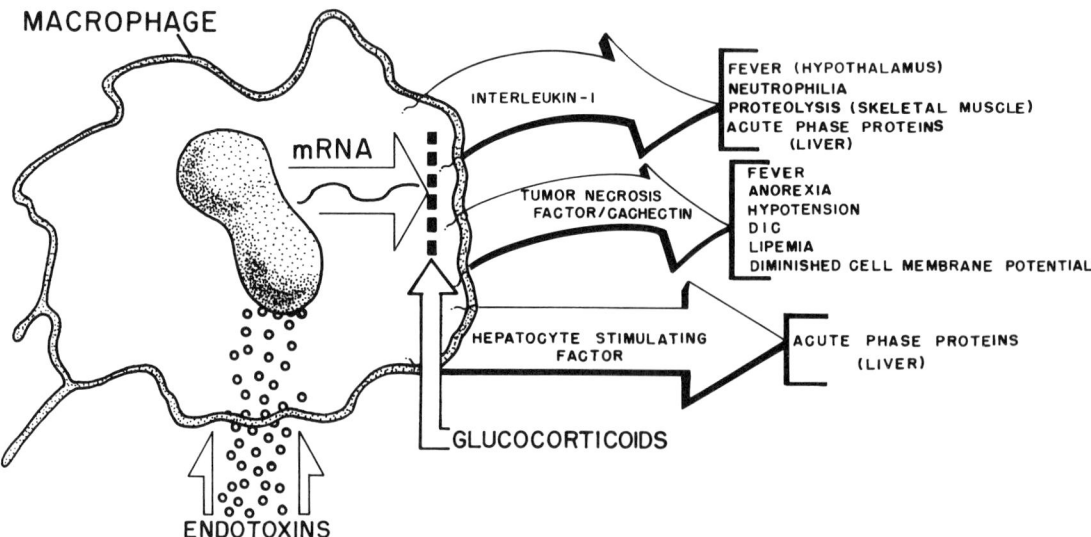

Fig. 5.7 The macrophage is the source of at least three groups of peptide products (monokines) which are major mediators of the host response to invasive infection. Bacterial endotoxin is a potent stimulus for the production of interleukin-1, tumour necrosis factor/cachectin and hepatocyte stimulating factor.

Interleukin-1 (IL-1)

Of the macrophage-derived mediators, inter-leukin-1 enjoyed the earliest attention in the pathophysiology of injury and sepsis. IL-1 was originally defined in terms of its biological activity and therefore went under a variety of names including endogenous pyrogen (EP) for its ability to induce fever and leucocyte endogenous mediator (LEM) because of its ability to cause characteristic changes of inflammatory states, such as stimulation of acute-phase protein production, granulocytosis, hypoferraemia and hypozincaemia (Keusch & Farthing 1986, Dinarello & Mier 1986). Eventually, it became clear that these agents, as well as the lymphocyte activating factor (LAF) which activates T-lymphocytes and causes proliferation of B-lymphocytes, were all the same polypeptide or a closely related family of polypeptides now termed IL-1. The major sources of IL-1 are blood monocytes, phagocytic cells lining the liver (Kupffer cells) and splenic sinusoids, lymphocytes, keratinocytes, brain astrocytes and others (Dinarello 1984). IL-1, which is produced by macrophages or other phagocytic cells, may act locally or enter the circulation to stimulate a systemic response. Fever associated with an infectious process is believed to be the response to the IL-1 initiated production of prostaglandin E_2 (PGE_2) in the hypothalamus. Also, induction of IL-1 in normal human subjects results in leucocytosis, which predominantly stems from increased neutrophils (Bessey et al 1984). Several reports have indicated that IL-1 may modulate some of its actions through its stimulatory function on the endocrine pancreas. Insulin and glucagon output is increased markedly in experimental animals treated with IL-1 (George et al 1977). As a consequence, hepatic carbohydrate and lipid metabolism may be significantly affected by this monokine.

Most notably, IL-1 added to normal skeletal muscle in vitro results in a markedly increased rate of proteolysis via induction of PGE_2 synthesis (Baracos et al 1983). Also, a small plasma peptide taken from septic human patients can induce an increase in muscle proteolytic rate (Clowes et al 1983). It is thought that this soluble peptide is a proteolytic cleavage fragment (proteolysis-inducting factor) of IL-1 which retains its metabolic activity.

Additionally, IL-1 is able to stimulate the production of liver-derived acute-phase proteins. The mechanism is probably twofold: 1. by increasing the availability of amino acids from peripheral proteolysis; and 2. by directly stimulating specific acute-phase protein gene expression in liver cells (Gauldie et al 1987). The acute-phase proteins are produced by the liver in increased amounts in response to various stimuli such as tissue injury and infection. They include C-reactive protein, haptoglobin, transferrin, alpha-1 antitrypsin, caeruloplasmin and others (Stahl 1987). Increased production of these plasma proteins in response to stress is thought to be appropriate and carry survival value. For example, C-reactive protein may play an important role as an opsonin. Haptoglobin and transferrin bind haemoglobin and iron respectively, thus possibly reducing the availability of iron which is required for bacterial proliferation. Alpha-1 antitrypsin may control excessive protease activity in the post-injury and septic state, thus inhibiting excessive mediator activation. These protective mechanisms are hypothetical and their relative significance remains uncertain. From the practical standpoint, however, the level of the acute-phase proteins serves as a good indicator of the extent of an inflammatory or septic process.

Although the actions of IL-1 generally appear beneficial to the host in withstanding the septic insult, it also stimulates the formation of other vasoactive substances, such as arachidonic acid metabolites, which may contribute to the overall circulatory instability observed in septic shock. Also, IL-1 can stimulate endothelial prostacyclin formation and activity of procoagulant resembling tissue factor (Bevilacqua et al 1985). These are two opposing actions, with prostacyclin acting to inhibit platelet aggregation and procoagulant activity stimulating localized intravascular coagulation. Because of the latter action, IL-1 could promote DIC or contribute to a DIC-type syndrome.

Hepatocyte stimulating factor, a 30 000 dalton polypeptide, is another monokine produced by the activated macrophage. It appears to be able to stimulate the liver acute phase response (Stahl 1987) in the same way as IL-1. Possibly, in a particular acute circumstance the specific response may be regulated by both monokines. Many fewer data are currently available on this protein product.

Tumour necrosis factor/cachectin (TNF)

It has become clear that the macrophage is a key target cell for endotoxin in precipitating shock and other metabolic phenomena. Like IL-1, tumour necrosis factor (TNF) is produced by the macrophage upon stimulation by endotoxin. This polypeptide gained its name through its ability to induce necrosis in certain tumour cell lines (TNF) and wasting and lipaemia in experimental animals (cachectin).

Current interest in TNF centres on its remarkable ability to reproduce the sequelae of endotoxaemia including shock, massive extravascular fluid sequestration, hypergylcaemia and subsequent hypoglycaemia, DIC (Beutler & Cerami 1986, Morrison & Ryan 1987). One of TNF's most prominent features is its ability to cause lipaemia through the suppression of adipocyte lipoprotein lipase activity. This experimental observation is reminiscent of findings in septic human and animal studies of lipid metabolism. Additionally, glucocorticoids can strongly inhibit the production of TNF by inhibition of gene transcription and translation, a possible explanation for the protection that steroids afford experimental animals when given prior to endotoxin injection. However, post-endotoxaemia steroid treatment is ineffective in curtailing TNF production as well as limiting the evolution of the septic shock syndrome (Beutler & Cerami 1987). TNF is thought to participate in the induction of extravascular fluid sequestration which accompanies septic shock, in part through its ability to induce a reduction of skeletal muscle transmembrane potential. Additionally, TNF precipitates a marked stress hormone response characterized by increased catecholamines, cortisol and glucagon levels, which is a hormone profile similar to the acute metabolic response to septicaemia (Tracey et al 1987). Although TNF shares some metabolic actions with IL-1, it is not structurally related. Some of the apparent shared activities such as stimulation of fever may result from the fact that TNF induces IL-1 formation and the joint action of both monokines may be difficult to differentiate. In summary, TNF has been suggested as a likely candidate responsible for most of the biological responses associated with endotoxaemia (Beutler & Cerami 1986).

Lipid mediators of endotoxic and septic shock

A number of endogenously synthesized lipid materials are formed and released by various tissues of the body in response to a shock-inducing stimulus or endotoxaemia. Marked increases in levels of arachidonic acid metabolites (Fig. 5.8) are present following endotoxin infusion in septic animal models (Morrison & Ryan 1987). Each of these lipid products exhibits diverse biological activities but also reflects the events of septic shock.

Arachidonic acid metabolites

Following the induction of endotoxic or septic stress, arachidonic acid production is increased by the action of phospholipase A_2 on cell membrane phospholipids. This process provides substrate for the cyclo-oxygenase or lipoxygenase cascades (Fig. 5.8). The relative preponderance of a specific pathway is determined by the relative activity of key enzymes in the biosynthetic pathways, which depend largely on the tissue and the physiological state. The products of these pathways serve as direct effector agents as well as modulators of other physiological functions (Morrison & Ryan 1987).

The products of the cyclo-oxygenase pathway stimulated by Gram-negative bacterial endotoxins include the E- and F-series prostaglandins, thromboxane A_2 (TxA_2) and prostacyclin (PGI_2). TxA_2 and PGI_2 are currently thought to be the most important members of this group because of their very potent effects on the circulatory system and platelet function. TxA_2 is a powerful vasoconstrictor and mediator of platelet aggregation, whereas PGI_2 is a vasodilator and has a platelet antiaggregating effect (Feuerstein & Hallenbeck 1987). Both agents are quite unstable, and are assayed by measuring their inactive stable metabolites throm-

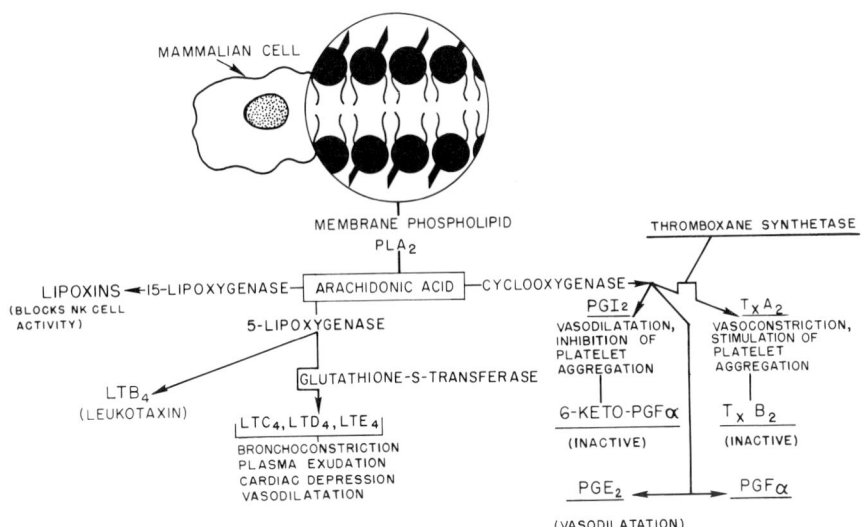

Fig. 5.8 Membrane-derived arachidonic acid is a precursor of at least three major classes of vasoactive and metabolically active lipids, including the prostaglandins, leukotrienes and lipoxins.

boxane B_2 (TxB$_2$) and 6-keto-prostaglandin F_α (6-keto-PGF$_\alpha$) respectively.

Plasma TxB$_2$ levels are elevated following traumatic conditions in patients, and some investigators have found a further rise when sepsis is superimposed. A very high TxB$_2$ level in sepsis may forecast an unfavourable prognosis (Reines et al 1982), but this is not a uniform observation (Ball et al 1986). This variability probably reflects species differences and the timing of these studies. TxB$_2$ tends to be higher in septic shock then in early sepsis (Yellin et al 1986). TxA$_2$ may result in diminished organ perfusion in septic conditions (Ball et al 1986). Associated responses to endotoxaemia and sepsis that have been related to TxA$_2$ include pulmonary artery hypertension, hypoxaemia and thrombocytopenia.

The significance of elevated prostaglandin and TxB$_2$ plasma levels has been investigated extensively using cyclo-oxygenase and selective TxA$_2$ synthetase inhibitors. Selective inhibition of the latter enzyme, leading to diminished TxA$_2$ formation, substantially attenuates many of the cardiopulmonary responses associated with endotoxin shock. Improvements are seen in arterial P_{O_2}, arterial pressure and CO, and reductions may be noted in pulmonary artery pressure and degree of acidosis. Survival rates have been variable in experimental models with these selective agents.

Cyclo-oxygenase blockers appear to fare better in this latter regard, and this has suggested that limiting production of PGI$_2$ and other PGs may play a vital role in survival (Ball et al 1986). However, the data relating PGI$_2$ to other PGs are confusing and very difficult to rationalize at present. It has been noted that selective inhibition of thromboxane synthetase results in reduced 6-keto-PGF$_\alpha$ formation, suggesting that inhibition of TxA$_2$ may reduce ischaemic tissue damage. Also, non-surviving septic shock patients exhibit significantly higher TxB$_2$ and 6-keto-PGF$_\alpha$ levels than survivors, indicating that increased prostacyclin formation signals a poor outcome (Halushka et al 1985). On the other hand, patients exhibiting elevated PGI$_2$ levels appeared to be protected from development of acute respiratory failure following trauma (Slotman et al 1985), and PGI$_2$ infusion into endotoxin-treated animals affords protection against acute lung failure (Demling et al 1981). A reasonable interpretation of these studies might be that in the late stages of septic shock, 6-keto-PGF$_\alpha$ formation is increased and simply reflects the pathophysiology of tissue damage, whereby early and intermediate septic shock may be benefited by the vasoactive and cellular actions of prostacyclin. This sequence is however entirely hypothetical and requires further study.

The leukotrienes (LTs) are formed from arachidonic acid by the action of 5-lipoxygenase to yield 5-hydroperoxyeicosatetraenoic acid, which is unstable and converts to the stable products LTB_4, LTC_4, LTD_4 and LTE_4. Evidence for their role in the haemodynamic and respiratory responses to endotoxaemia and systemic sepsis arises from the findings: 1. that exogenous LTC_4 and LTD_4 can induce characteristic features of sepsis in a variety of animal models; 2. that increased levels of LTE_4 and its metabolite may be found in models of endotoxaemia; and 3. that LT antagonists can attenuate the noxious actions of endotoxin (Feuerstein & Hallenbeck 1987, Pacitti et al 1987).

Several of the biological effects attributed to LTC_4 and LTD_4, including long-lasting hypotension, probably arise from two sources. LTC_4 can induce a generalized plasma leakage resulting in hypovolaemia, and LTC_4 and LTD_4 reduce myocardial contractility, probably by decreasing coronary blood flow. Additionally, a marked increase in interstitial lung water may be precipitated by the LTs in endotoxic shock. It is suspected that they play a role in adult respiratory distress syndrome of human sepsis but this is unproven. LT antagonists have also been shown to increase survival in some lethal endotoxin models, but a major difficulty is that LT antagonists in current use may not be specific and may inhibit the cyclo-oxygenase pathway in addition to LT formation.

LTB_4 does not exhibit a direct effect on blood flow but stimulates leucocyte margination and efflux from the vascular compartment, and thereby may play a role in regulating the neutrophil-mediated inflammatory response to sepsis. Lipoxins result from the metabolism of arachidonic acid through the 15-lipoxygenase pathway. They have only recently been discovered and their significance in septic models is unknown. However, since this class of compounds exhibit chemotactic properties for neutrophils, it is possible they may play a role in sepsis.

Complement activation

Many studies have demonstrated that complement

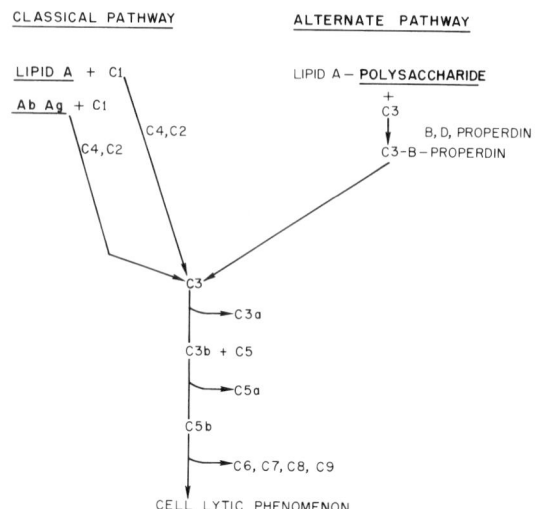

Fig. 5.9 The classical and alternate complement cascades may be activated by lipopolysaccharide (LPS) or antibody–antigen complexes. LPS is thought to activate the classical pathway mainly through its lipid A component and the alternate pathway through the polysaccharide moiety.

activation is a usual response to invasive infection and endotoxaemia. The complement activation scheme (Fig. 5.9) has been divided into a classical pathway, which has been ascribed to a mechanism mediated by the antibody-antigen complex, and an alternate pathway which results from a direct lipopolysaccharide-complement component (C_3) activation mechanism. It has been shown, however, that endotoxin can activate complement by interaction of the lipid A portion of lipopolysaccharide with C_1 complex directly, and also activate the alternate pathway through the polysaccharide portion. Both of these mechanisms are antibody-independent (Fine 1985).

The activation of complement results in the generation of three main functions: 1. release of the so-called anaphylatoxins, C_{5a} and C_{3a} fragments, resulting from the activation of C_5 and C_3 complement components; 2. liberation of C_{3b} which acts as a major opsonin, binding its targets and making them more readily engulfed by phagocytic cells; and 3. generation of C_{5a}, and to a lesser extent C_{3a}, which act as chemotactic factors attracting leucocytes to the area of infection.

The components C_{5a} and C_{3a} stimulate histamine release from basophils and mast cells early following endotoxaemia. This action may contribute to the early hypotension noted from rapidly progressing sepsis. Histamine can lead to acute vasodilatation in animal models of endotoxaemia where it is initially released in large quantities (Krause & Hess 1979). Histamine infusion in experimental animals made endotoxaemic will also increase lung lymph flow (Brigham et al 1980). Pretreament of experimental animals with the antihistamine, diphenhydramine, attenuates these responses. Other experiments have indicated that histamine has a vasodilatory role in the coronary bed and causes a positive inotropic effect. However, these are early and transient effects of histamine, and this compound may not be important in the intermediate and late phase of sepsis and septic shock. The relative importance of histamine in sepsis and septic shock is still considered uncertain. It is generally believed that the specific actions of the arachidonic acid metabolite thromboxane A_2 and the leukotrienes are more important to the lung and heart than histamine.

With ongoing sepsis, continued complement activation occurs. However, due to wide variations in levels, particularly of C_3 and C_{3a}, these parameters do not serve as good predictors of the degree of sepsis or lung failure (Hallgren et al 1987), except possibly in patients in severe septic shock where C_3 levels are abnormally low (Fine 1985).

Endorphins in septic shock

Endorphins are neuropeptides produced endogenously in response to stress, with morphine-like or analgesic properties. Their relevance in septic shock arises from suggestions that these opiates mediate cardiovascular dysfunction by interacting with specific central nervous system and peripheral opiate receptors. The best studied members of this group of agents include β-endorphin and the enkephalins, which arise in two forms according to whether C-terminal amino acid is leucine or methionine — leu-enkephalin and met-enkephalin (Gurll 1985). These peptides are distributed widely in the brain and pituitary gland (β-endorphin) and the brain, sympathetic ganglia and adrenal medulla (enkephalins). In particular, opioid peptides and receptors are found in

hypothalamic and brain stem nuclei which are known to control haemodynamic functions. Intravenous or intracisternal injection of these substances is followed by hypotension and tachycardia, which may be preceded by a short period of hypertension. The hypotensive period can be attenuated or blocked entirely by pretreatment with an opiate receptor antagonist such as naloxone (Gurll 1985). Experimental studies have shown substantial improvement in the overall haemodynamics and survival of some animal models subjected to endotoxic and bacteraemic shock, resulting from the use of naloxone. Hypotension, depressed cardiac output and ventricular function can be reversed with this opiate antagonist. No significant effect of naloxone is noted in normal animals.

The use of naloxone in human septic shock has yielded variable results, with some studies showing substantial haemodynamic improvement (Peters et al 1981) and others showing no benefit (Bonnet et al 1985). Several reasons for failure to show efficacy have been cited, including: 1. the need for adequate albeit high, doses (1–2 mg/kg) when injected into the peripheral venous system; 2. the need to use this agent early in the course of septic shock (<8 hours from onset of shock); and 3. variability in selection, with the best results obtained in patients who exhibit increased arousal or pain in response to naloxone (Gurll 1985, Bonnet et al 1985). This latter factor implicates the pain response as having a significant role in the action of opiate receptor antagonists. In this regard another neuropeptide, thyrotopin-releasing hormone (TRH), is of considerable interest since it may exhibit a pressor response in septic shock similar to naloxone without undermining the analgesic properties of opiates. TRH is a tripeptide pyroglutamyl-histidyl-prolineamide widely distributed in the brain and spinal cord which antagonizes the cardiovascular depressant actions of endogenous opioids. TRH has been reported to reverse hypotension, improve ventricular contractility and decrease mortality in experimental endotoxaemic models. Additional TRH exerts benefit when injected peripherally or into the cerebral ventricle, although the specific mechanism of action remains unknown (McIntosh & Faden 1986).

Organ failure in sepsis and endotoxaemic shock

Overview

Persistent sepsis is generally accepted to be the most common cause of death in the surgical intensive care unit. The ill-defined syndrome of multiple system organ failure (MSOF), presenting as sequential organ dysfunction and usually associated with uncontrolled infection, is a frequent mode of death for patients who require extended intensive care following surgical complications. Infection appears to be a common initiating feature, but several additional factors have been cited as contributing to the severity of this syndrome including: 1. inadequate control of infection (Fry et al 1980a); 2. presence of a substantial amount of necrotic tissue (Fry et al 1980a); 3. pre- or postoperative episodes of shock (Pine et al 1983) causing inadequate oxygen transport and perfusion deficits; and 4. unrecognized or uncompensated malnutrition, which may impair endogenous protective mechanisms (Cerra 1987, Watson & Petro 1982). A drawback in the management of organ dysfunction is our limited understanding of the genesis of multiple organ failure. It has been noted that the sequential organ failure due to septicaemia has a temporal pattern, with pulmonary insufficiency arising first, followed by hepatic dysfunction, stress bleeding and renal failure (Fry et al 1980b). The interval between the onset of pulmonary failure and failure of other organ systems may be several weeks. Because of the diversity of organ systems affected and the extended time scale of the evolution of the entire syndrome, a single therapeutic approach cannot be successful in managing this complex sequence of events. In practice, the onset of MSOF frequently signals the presence of previously unsuspected sepsis (Polk & Shields 1977) and should always precipitate a diligent search for infection. The source of infection may be remote from the organ system involved.

Lung failure

Acute respiratory insufficiency is commonly as-

sociated with severe sepsis and is often its first manifested complication (Hyers & Fowler 1986). The most severe form has been termed the adult respiratory distress syndrome (ARDS), which is characterized by hypoxaemia, diffuse pulmonary infiltrates visible on the chest radiograph and the presence of a normal or low pulmonary capillary wedge pressure. It appears likely that subclinical forms of this syndrome escape detection and that many clinical studies of ARDS catalogue only the most severe forms of this disorder. Careful distinction must be made from other causes of acute pulmonary insufficiency such as aspiration, bronchopneumonia, pulmonary embolism and left ventricular failure with cardiogenic pulmonary odema. Pulmonary artery catheterization may aid in making this distinction by measurement of the pulmonary capillary wedge pressure, which is elevated in cardiac failure. However, a feature of ARDS is decreased lung compliance associated with progressive hypoxaemia requiring assisted mechanical ventilation. Attendant high airway pressures may give a falsely high estimate of left atrial pressure and incorrectly suggest a cardiogenic source of oedema.

Experimental studies have indicated that there are two phases in the effect of endotoxin on the

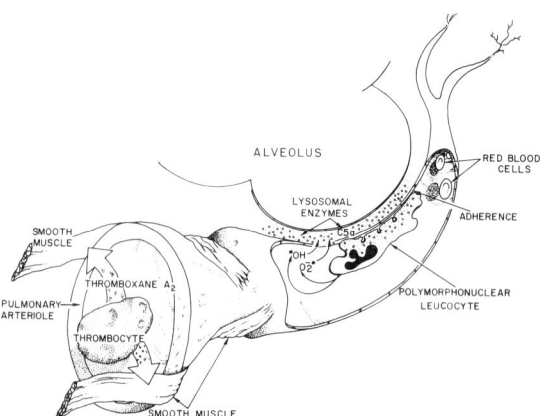

Fig. 5.10 Factors that appear to contribute to sepsis-induced noncardiogenic pulmonary oedema. Thromboxane A_2 arises from a variety of sources including thrombocytes, and causes pulmonary artery hypertension and ventilation/perfusion mismatch. Marginated and activated neutrophils liberate toxic oxygen radicals and proteolytic enzymes which interfere with the alveolar/capillary membrane integrity.

lung Fig. 5.10). The most prominent features of the early phase include pulmonary artery hypertension, increased lung lymph flow and a granulocytopenia. This phase is thought to arise from altered vasomotor tone associated with the liberation of TxA_2 from thrombocytes and neutrophils trapped in the pulmonary vascular bed. Furthermore, the accumulation of formed blood elements in the microvasculature of the lung may contribute to this pulmonary hypertension by decreasing the cross-sectional area of the perfusion bed. It is likely, however, that their main role is in the liberation of proximate mediators of lung injury. Experimentally, cyclo-oxygenase inhibitors have been able to attenuate or prevent these early pulmonary changes. Notably, hypoxaemia precedes the development of radiographic changes, suggesting that TxA_2 may be a major contributor to early ventilation-perfusion mismatch causing reduced arterial oxygen tension (Slotman et al 1986). Although pulmonary hypertension is commonly observed in animal studies, it is not a major feature of early human ARDS except in very rapidly progressing sepsis (Judges et al 1986).

Other derivatives of the cyclo-oxygenase pathway, PGI_2 and PGE, are produced, and the increased availability of these agents may exert some protective effect on the lung, possibly by depressing the degree of pulmonary hypertension through their action as vasodilators or by reducing platelet and neutrophil microaggregation. On the other hand, they may also be partly responsible for the development of hypotension due to the concomitant peripheral vasodilatation commonly observed during the early period of ARDS (Slotman et al 1986). Because of their potential benefit to the lung, several investigators have studied the effects of PGI_2 and PGE_2 infusions in animal studies (Demling et al 1981) and in human subjects (Shoemaker & Appel 1986, Holcraft et al 1986) suffering from ARDS. These infusions have resulted in a temporary reduction in the severity of lung injury. The general application of PGI_2 and vasodilator prostaglandins is not yet established.

The second phase of ARDS is characterized by the development of noncardiogenic pulmonary oedema due to increased capillary permeability (Fig. 5.10). At least two and probably three factors are responsible for this permeability phenomenon: 1. increased availability of chemotactic factors activating and attracting neutrophils to the lung; 2. neutrophil adherence to the pulmonary microvasculature, with subsequent release of toxic oxygen radicals and lysosomal enzymes (Worthen et al 1986); and 3. possibly direct pulmonary endothelial injury due to the action of LPS (Meyrick 1986). Acute pulmonary injury depends on the availability of both complement and neutrophils. The generation of C_{5a}, a known chemotactic agent for neutrophils, results from endotoxin activation of serum complement, which subsequently activates and increases sequestration of granulocytes in the lung. The endotoxin-primed neutrophils respond with enhanced release of oxygen radicals (superoxide anion and hydroxyl radical) and lysosomal enzymes to produce an endothelial cell injury manifested as increased lung water. Additionally, damage to type II pneumocytes and proteolytic damage to pulmonary elastin decreases surfactant production and pulmonary compliance respectively. Evidence exists that ARDS resulting from a non-septic mechanism is a less severe syndrome and that the presence of endotoxin exerts a direct toxic effect on the pulmonary endothelium, thereby enhancing the lung damage induced by the former two factors (Meyrick 1986).

Several other mediators may compound the injury produced by the neutrophil. In particular, the leukotrienes are currently receiving considerable attention in this regard. Elevated levels of lipoxygenase products are detectable in lung lymph just prior to the increase in vascular permeability which occurs in ARDS. Infusions of LTD_4 cause increases in extravascular lung water in animals (Shapiro et al 1987). Further work is required to define their relative role in ARDS.

Therapy of ARDS is currently nonspecific and supportive. The goals are to correct hypoxaemia ($Pa_{O_2} > 70$ torr, $FI_{O_2} < 0.5$) with assisted mechanical ventilation, maintain oxygen transport, provide nutritional support and, most of all, locate and treat the precipitating source of infection. Respiratory support is most commonly supplemented with positive end expiratory pressure to increase lung volume and reduce FI_{O_2} levels. Evidence exists that FI_{O_2} levels as low as 0.5 can result in worsening of lung function (Register et al

1987). Therefore, the general approach in respiratory support for these patients has been to reduce the FI_{O_2} as low as it is compatible with the maintenance of oxygen transport. In this regard, patients requiring the use of moderate-to-high levels of positive end-expiratory pressure (PEEP) should generally undergo pulmonary artery catheterization for the purpose of monitoring cardiac output and oxygen transport.

Several additional approaches for the management of ARDS are presently viewed as experimental and unproven, such as extracorporeal membrane oxygenation (ECMO) and high-frequency jet ventilation. ECMO has previously been shown not to increase survival in adult patients with ARDS but is currently undergoing re-evaluation (Gattinoni et al 1986). High-frequency jet ventilation has been advocated as it can provide ventilatory support with lower mean airway pressures than in conventional assisted ventilation. The main theoretical advantages include reduced barotrauma and a decreased negative effect on cardiac output. Clinical studies have not generally supported these potential benefits (Carlon & Howland 1983). Corticosteroids have generally been ineffective in the prevention or treatment of ARDS. Other pharmacological therapy undergoing evaluation includes pulmonary surfactant replacement (Taeusch et al 1983), administration of superoxide scavengers (Freeman et al 1985) and proteolytic enzyme inhibitors (Vered et al 1985). Whether these agents will improve survival remains to be seen.

Liver dysfunction

Altered liver function test results are commonly observed in the seriously ill surgical patient. Due to the multitude of causes of hyperbilirubinaemia and lack of specificity of biochemical tests, interpretation is difficult. Separation of these factors involves a painstaking analysis of potential causes and the use of a variety of diagnostic tests, with no guarantee that this evaluation will alter management or outcome (Table 5.1). Probably the most critical assessment involves identifying those causes of liver dysfunction that require operative intervention or specific medical therapy, such as

Table 5.1 Causes of hyperbilirubinaemia which may arise in the critically ill surgical patient

Potential causes	Diagnostic/therapeutic consideration
● Hepatic ischaemia due to hypotension	Optimize oxygen transport
● Hepatitis: viral/toxic	Serological evaluation; anaesthetic/drug history
● Cholestatic jaundice: Starvation or TPN-induced	Reduce excessive caloric and glucose intake and/or convert to enteral feeding; CCK trial to alleviate cholestasis
● Septic liver failure	Locate and treat septic focus
● Extrahepatic cause: Biliary obstruction/leak	Re-evaluation of an operative site and procedure by noninvasive or invasive test (i.e. ERCP)
● Acalculous cholecystitis	Physical examination, ultrasound, HIDA scan
● Prehepatic jaundice due to extravascular blood sequestration or haemolysis	Bilirubin fractionation
● Pre-existing disease such as cirrhosis or metastatic disease	Re-evaluation of clinical history and evidence of pre-existing liver disease

biliary obstruction or leak, acalculous cholecystitis or an occult septic process requiring drainage or specific antibiotic therapy.

It is generally believed that sepsis can precipitate liver failure in the absence of septic shock or direct anatomical involvement of the organ itself. The specific mechanisms remain controversial. The most fundamental abnormality which may result in liver damage arises from flow abnormalities. The splanchnic bed may experience a disproportionate increase in regional vasoconstriction in response to acute reductions in cardiac output (Bailey et al 1987). Also, a number of experimental studies in which normal cardiac output is maintained have indicated that hepatic perfusion is diminished following endotoxaemia, and this reduction in flow correlates with decreased liver function (Schirmer et al 1987b). Factors that may be responsible for these observations include: 1. angiotensin II, which is elevated after endotoxaemia and appears to be a more potent vasoconstrictor in the splanchnic vascular bed than concomitant adrenergic mechanisms (Bailey et al 1987); 2. thromboxane A_2, which is known to be elevated in endotoxaemic conditions (Schirmer et al 1987a); and 3. microaggregates due to fibrin, platelets and leucocyte fragments, which may produce partial obstruction of the hepatic sinusoidal bed, resulting in a diminished effective hepatic blood flow (Asher et al 1986). A notable feature of these studies is that cardiac output may be normal while regional hypoperfusion precipitates functional and ultimately anatomical abnormalities of the hepatic parenchyma.

Hepatic injury due to insufficient blood flow, may occur in two phases (Hasselgren 1987). The first phase results from the ischaemic period during which oxygen delivery is inadequate to maintain cellular energy levels and functions. As a result, mitochondrial and peripheral cell membrane functions are impaired. At least two processes have been proposed. Shock produces a progressive loss of phospholipids from the ischaemic cells, possibly through the activation of endogenous phospholipase A_2. This phenomenon results in altered cellular permeability to calcium ions, which eventually damages cellular organelles irreversibly if accumulation occurs in excessive amounts (Chien et al 1977). Alternatively, it has been reported that endotoxaemia will cause lipid peroxidation, probably due to free radical formation. Mitochondrial membranes appear to be most dramatically affected by these endogenously generated oxidants. Administration of free radical scavengers such as α-tocopheral and coenzyme Q_{10} can suppress lipid peroxide formation and preserve high-energy phosphate levels and energy metabolism in the liver. In addition, these agents can enhance survival in endotoxic experimental animals (Sugino et al 1986).

The second phase of injury results from reperfusion due to resuscitation if frank hypotensive shock should be present. Reperfusion has been associated with the generation of free radicals resulting in associated tissue injury. These radicals arise from the oxidative conversion of tissue hypoxanthine (derived from adenosine diphosphate) to xanthine by tissue xanthine oxidase. This reaction will generate superoxide anions (O_2^-) which are toxic to tissue.

$$\text{ATP} \rightarrow \text{ADP} \xrightarrow[\text{Shock}]{\text{Xanthine oxidase}} \text{Hypoxanthine} \rightarrow \text{Xanthine} + O_2^-$$

In addition to free radical scavengers, allopurinol, which is an inhibitor of tissue xanthine oxidase, has been used to diminish the generation of toxic oxygen free radicals (Nordstrom et al 1985). The relative importance of these experimentally determined mechanisms in the genesis of septic liver failure in the clinical situation is not yet known.

The major drawback of these experimental observations is that splanchnic and hepatic blood flow in seriously septic human subjects is elevated, not depressed as the above studies have indicated (Dahn et al 1987c). Septic patients may exhibit two to three times the normal liver blood flow (Wilmore et al 1980). An interesting observation is that splanchnic and liver oxygen consumption may increase to such disproportionately high levels that even a supranormal liver blood flow may be inadequate to support all the liver's vital metabolic processes. Additionally, a very high regional metabolic rate may make this organ bed particularly sensitive to transient episodes of hypoxaemia and hypotension.

Finally, a mechanism for the induction of hepatic failure has been proposed which does not necessarily depend upon the regional blood flow characteristics of the splanchnic bed. Kupffer cells, which are resident macrophage/reticuloendothelial cells in the liver, may respond to circulating bacterial products by elaborating locally active substances that regulate liver function. It has been shown that Kupffer cell products can dramatically depress hepatocyte protein synthesis (West et al 1985). Although the specific mechanisms of this action remain obscure, these findings have generated considerable interest in view of the multitude of bioactive mediators known to be expressed by the macrophage cell line.

Myocardial function in sepsis

The normal circulatory response to bacterial sepsis (Fig. 5.11) is an increased cardiac output (CO), reduced total peripheral vascular resistance and a mean arterial blood pressure near normal (Lang et al 1984a, b). In contrast, acute endotoxaemia, where the severity of insult may be greater over a shorter period of time, is characterized by a progressively declining cardiac output and increased

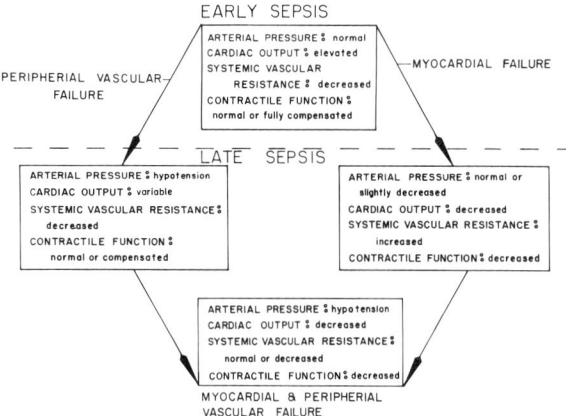

EARLY SEPSIS

ARTERIAL PRESSURE ↕ normal
CARDIAC OUTPUT ↕ elevated
SYSTEMIC VASCULAR
    RESISTANCE ↕ decreased
CONTRACTILE FUNCTION ↕
normal or fully compensated

PERIPHERIAL VASCULAR
FAILURE

MYOCARDIAL FAILURE

LATE SEPSIS

ARTERIAL PRESSURE ↕ hypotension
CARDIAC OUTPUT ↕ variable
SYSTEMIC VASCULAR RESISTANCE↕
    decreased
CONTRACTILE FUNCTION ↕
    normal or compensated

ARTERIAL PRESSURE ↕ normal or
    slightly decreased
CARDIAC OUTPUT ↕ decreased
SYSTEMIC VASCULAR RESISTANCE ↕
    increased
CONTRACTILE FUNCTION↕ decreased

ARTERIAL PRESSURE ↕ hypotension
CARDIAC OUTPUT ↕ decreased
SYSTEMIC VASCULAR RESISTANCE↕
    normal or decreased
CONTRACTILE FUNCTION↕ decreased

MYOCARDIAL & PERIPHERIAL
VASCULAR FAILURE

Fig. 5.11 The two major components of circulatory insufficiency due to septicaemia are myocardial and peripheral vascular failure. The clinical state depends on the stage of sepsis as well as on the particular component which dominates at a given time period.

peripheral vascular resistance. The latter profile most closely models a late form of clinical septic shock.

It is a commonly held but probably fallacious belief that because cardiac output may double or triple during sepsis, cardiac depression does not exist. In fact, a substantial body of experimental and clinical data now exists to indicate that myocardial dysfunction may coexist with an elevated cardiac output. Consequently, an increased CO should not be used to exclude the presence of cardiac failure. It is believed that early in sepsis when cardiac function does not meet in-vivo demand, cardiac reserve is mobilized by the actions of the sympathetic nervous system to bring cardiac function up to more acceptable levels (Shepherd et al 1986). In this manner, myocardial dysfunction may be masked, particularly by an increase in heart rate.

Impaired cardiovascular performance during septicaemic shock has been attributed to a failure of the peripheral vasculature (Groeneveld et al 1986) or to an intrinsic dysfunction of the myocardium (Shepherd et al 1986). More likely, both mechanisms play a role (Fig. 5.11), but one mechanism dominates in any specific clinical or experimental situation. Alternatively, one mechanism may precede the other.

Evidence for myocardial contractile dysfunction includes: 1. increased coronary vascular resistance

due to humoral substances, resulting in myocardial ischaemia (Artman et al 1986); 2. decreased response to adrenergic compensatory mechanisms (Shepherd et al 1986); and 3. contractile depression due to endogenous opiates (Tuggle & Horton 1986) or cardiodepressant peptides (Sagher et al 1986).

Decreased coronary blood flow may be attributed to a variety of circulatory vasopressors such as catecholamines, TxA_2 and leukotrienes, which are known to be elevated in septic shock and may exert their action upon the coronary bed. Coronary blood flow, however, has been found to be normal or elevated in hyperdynamic septic models, and myocardial high-energy phosphate levels are reportedly in the normal range (Mc-Donough et al 1986). It remains unclear as to how these findings may be rationalized. Decreased sensitivity of the myocardium in sepsis to beta-adrenergic agonists has been observed, and has its clinical counterpart in septic patients who respond poorly to inotropic agents. The presence of cardiodepressant agents that exert a direct myocardial action has been postulated. Recently, a clinical study has supported this hypothesis by noting that serum obtained from patients exhibiting depressed left ventricular ejection fractions during the acute septic shock phase could depress the velocity of isolated myocardial cell shortening during contraction in an in-vitro assay (Parrillo et al 1985). Additionally, minor depression in the ejection fraction seems to exist in some groups of septic patients even in the absence of septic shock. The importance of these findings has been questioned by clinical studies showing that many patients in septic shock die as a result of peripheral vascular, rather than cardiac failure since persistent vasodilation, irrespective of cardiac index, has been found to be a major haemodynamic determinant in nonsurviving patients until shortly before death (Groeneveld et al 1986). From this broad array of findings in sepsis and septic shock, the most reasonable generalizations are indicated in Figure 5.11.

Specific clinical management is complicated by the difficulty in demonstrating contractile dysfunction. No practical solution currently exists to this problem. A reasonable approach to management of the circulatory status in sepsis is to institute monitoring of the pulmonary capillary wedge pressure and cardiac output when oxygen transport is suspected to be inadequate as manifested by hypotension, lactic acidaemia, reduced mixed venous oxygen saturation or diminished end-organ function (i.e. decreased urine output). When these factors are not improved by ensuring adequate preload (PCWP = 10–15 mm Hg), the use of vasodilators and inotropic agents is indicated. Finally, one must ensure that extramyocardial factors are not responsible for decreased right or left ventricular function, e.g. high airway pressures during assisted mechanical ventilation resulting in right heart failure, pleural effusions or increased intra-abdominal pressure.

Stress gastric ulceration

Acute upper gastrointestinal ulcerations associated with sepsis are regarded as another component of the multiple organ failure syndrome. Although a clear pathogenetic mechanism of stress gastritis is still not available, several interesting observations have been made which are worthy of review.

Experimental studies have indicated that the development of mucosal ulcers is dependent upon the presence of at least three factors — mucosal ischaemia, luminal acid and bile (Payne & Bowen 1981). The most important determinant producing a defect in mucosal defence appears to be hypoxia of the surface epithelium during septicaemic shock or sepsis (Rees & Bowen 1982). Stress lesions are more prone to occur in the body or fundus of the stomach than in the antrum, presumably due in part to the relatively better blood flow that the antrum enjoys during sepsis (Nilsson et al 1983). Regional hypoxia may result from gastric vasoconstriction during frank shock, but it appears that decreased perfusion is an unlikely mechanism for the production of stress ulcers in hyperdynamic sepsis. It has been noted that even in the presence of normal gastric blood flow, a reduction in surface mucosal oxygen tension occurs in response to septic challenge, reflecting an impairment of nutrient subepithelial microcirculatory blood flow. The basis of this finding remains unclear but it has been postulated to result from the presence of functional arteriovenous shunting in the microcirculation of the stomach mucosa. These shunts enhance the susceptibility of the surface epithelium to acute ulceration by acid and bile, although total gastric blood flow is undiminished (Payne & Bowen 1981). Surface hypoxaemia has been noted in animal and human studies and has been associated with a reduction in intramural pH (Fiddian-Green et al 1983). In the presence of an inadequate energy supply, the gastric mucosa is not capable of handling the high flux of back-diffusing hydrogen ions (Rees & Bowen 1982). Accumulation of hydrogen ions in the mucosal cells will finally destroy them.

Recent experiments have also indicated that free radical scavengers can attenuate gastric mucosal damage associated with *Escherichia coli* sepsis. This finding suggests that free oxygen radicals may be of at least partial importance in the development of sepsis-induced gastric ulceration (Arvidsson et al 1985).

The approach to acute erosive gastritis is largely prophylactic. Prevention of septic complications through the use of good surgical technique, proper selection of patients for surgical procedures and judicious use of antibiotics are of paramount importance. In the event of systemic sepsis, early identification and elimination of the focus provides the best prophylaxis. A recent decline in the incidence of stress gastritis has been attributed to improved care of the circulatory and respiratory system, thus avoiding states of hypoxaemia and deficient oxygen transport. Additionally, increased awareness of the syndrome, with greater attention being paid to gastric alkalinization with antacid and histamine-blocking agents, has contributed to a reduced incidence of stress bleeding. Histamine-blocking agents, however, have been reported to exhibit a high failure rate in controlling gastric pH when used alone. If they are used, regular pH monitoring is essential to detect clinical failure of these drugs (More et al 1985). Rarely, aggressive surgical management may be required to control major gastric haemorrhage.

Acute renal failure

A number of factors influence the development of

acute renal failure (ARF) in sepsis, particularly ischaemia and the presence of nephrotoxic agents. Sepsis and septic shock can induce a number of prerenal factors that produce ischaemic injury, such as hypovolaemia from extravascular volume sequestration, hypotension due to diffuse vasodilatation (increase in vascular capacitance) and cardiac dysfunction resulting from severe sepsis or extracardiac factors (i.e. unrecognized pneumothorax). Compounding these factors are additional renal changes, which have been noted to cause an ischaemic injury despite the presence of a hyperdynamic septic state. Investigators have noted that the glomerular filtration rate (GFR) may decline markedly in sepsis despite the maintenance of CO and only mild decreases in total renal blood flow (Haybron et al 1987). This fact has suggested that a cortical-medullary flow redistribution occurs, resulting in glomerular ischaemia and medullary hyperperfusion. Additional renal factors that may contribute to the evolution of ARF include tubular backleak, i.e. glomerular filtrate leaking into the peritubular spaces, causing reabsorption of excretory products, and tubular obstruction from sloughed tubular epithelial cells or precipitated proteins (Sillix & McDonald 1987). An important clinical observation is that renal damage associated with sepsis does not necessarily produce major functional impairment unless volume contraction is allowed to occur (Richmond et al 1985), thus emphasizing the need to control prerenal factors. Additional phenomena that may contribute to the overall incidence of ARF include toxic nephropathies due to aminoglycosides, cephalosporins, Amphoterocin B, myoglobin and radiological contrast agents which are commonly used during the care of septic patients. Thus, ARF resulting from septicaemia is better considered a multifactorial phenomenon.

Management of renal dysfunction consists of limiting the ischaemic injury by identifying and controlling inadequate CO, use of diuretics if CO has already been optimized and vigorous supportive care consisting of dialysis and nutritional support if ARF occurs. Nevertheless, eradication of the septic focus remains the key factor in eventual recovery. Because of the approximately 90% mortality rate associated with established renal failure induced by sepsis, the best opportunity for

survival lies in early identification of prerenal factors responsible for acute oliguria. Analysis of urinary sediment for casts, sodium content (fractional sodium excretion) and invasive cardiac monitoring (pulmonary capillary wedge pressures and CO) are probably the best diagnostic indices in the renal management of the critically ill septic patient.

Host defence mechanisms

Overview

The most important host defence factors responsible for protection against invasive infection are schematically indicated in Fig. 5.12. These factors will be briefly reviewed from the standpoint of mechanisms that may be responsible for the development or progression of serious septic processes.

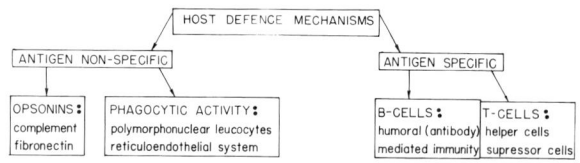

Fig. 5.12 Endogenous host defence mechanisms may be subdivided into nonspecific and specific groups.

The occurrence of sepsis correlates positively with the extent of traumatic injury (Yurt et al 1984), degree of wound contamination (Lewis & Klein 1979), presence of malnutrition (Watson & Petro 1982), advanced age (Fry et al 1980a) and a recent history of hypotension (Pine et al 1983). Several of these states have been shown to impact on particular areas of the host defence schema in Fig. 5.12, and these will be commented on specifically.

Opsonins

Certain plasma components assist in host defence because they are deposited on particles such as bacteria, making them more easily engulfed by polymorphonuclear leucocytes, macrophages, B-lymphocytes and other phagocytic cells. This coating process is known as opsonization, and the plasma components that have received the greatest attention in septic conditions are complement, plasma fibronectin and immunoglobulins.

Activation of the complement cascade (Fig. 5.9) results in the generation of intermediates such as C_{3b} which may bind to target elements, thereby acting as a major opsonin. Proteolytic removal of a portion of C_{3b} converts it to iC_{3b}, which also acts as an opsonin. These opsonic proteins act as bifunctional ligands, offering a point of association with specific C_{3b} and iC_{3b} receptors (also known as complement receptors type 1 and 3 or CR1 and CR3) present on phagocytic cells (Frank 1987) as well as binding to microorganisms and other particulate matter (Fig. 5.13). Human studies have indicated that complement levels are quite variable in sepsis, and overall may offer relatively little prognostic information. A few reports have indicated decreased levels of C_3 and properdin in patients with Gram-negative shock, suggesting preferential activation of the alternate complement pathway (Fearon et al 1975). Other authors have noted decreases in classical complement pathway components prior to and during septic episodes

(Bjornson et al 1978). These observations indicate that either pathway may be activated during septicaemia. Sepsis-associated complement consumption or decreased opsonin synthesis due to hepatic failure, although probably uncommon, may reduce the opsonic capacity of a patient's serum and thereby place the patient at an increased risk of disseminated septicaemia (Larcher et al 1982).

Fibronectin is a circulating plasma protein that acts as a nonimmune circulatory opsonin. It is thought to act by mediating the internalization of bound targets by neutrophils and macrophages and possibly by increasing the cellular surface expression of C_{3b} and IgG receptors on some phagocytic cells (Doran et al 1986). Some authors have noted a depletion of plasma fibronectin in association with organ failure and sepsis and have suggested a causal relationship (Lanser et al 1980). As a result, fibronectin repletion therapy with plasma cryoprecipitate for septic patients has been advocated. Cryoprecipitate is a plasma protein concentrate enriched in fibronectin, and infusion should theoretically augment or restore the bacterial clearance mechanisms of the body. Clinical studies, although still inconclusive, have not indicated significant benefits from this therapeutic

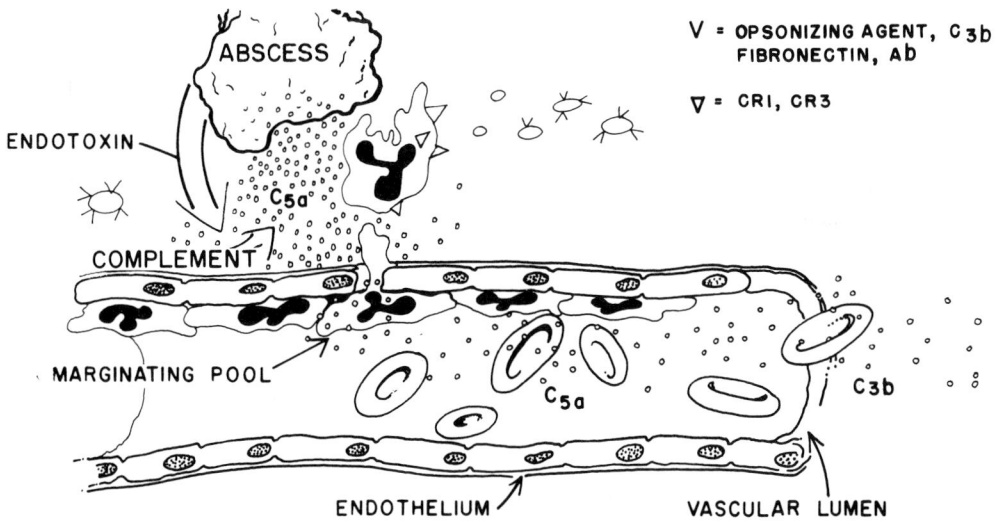

Fig. 5.13 Summary of events leading to activation of host defence mechanisms. Endotoxin derived from an infectious process activates the complement cascade. Opsonizing agents such as the complement activation product C_{3b} will coat particulate matter such as bacteria, preparing them for neutrophil engulfment. Local C_{5a} formation provides a chemotactic stimulus for neutrophils and increases neutrophil surface complement receptor proteins (CR_1, CR_3), which improve phagocytic capability.

approach (Doran et al 1986). Further studies are proceeding.

Phagocytic activity

Neutrophil activity and function is commonly divided into at least four aspects: 1. cell activation; 2. chemotaxis; 3. phagocytosis; and 4. lysosomal degranulation. The endotoxin–neutrophil interaction may result from a direct or an indirect (mainly complement-mediated) effect (Wilson 1985), and almost every aspect of the neutrophil response has been reported to be negatively affected by sepsis and endotoxaemia.

Early experimental burn models have indicated that neutrophil adherence and chemotaxis is defective post-injury, and this may account for an increased incidence of burn wound infection (McManus 1983). More recent work, however, has shown that endotoxin in low doses can directly increase the neutrophil cell surface C_{3b} and iC_{3b} receptors (CR1 and CR3, respectively), which are the receptors for the complement protein opsonins generated by the complement cascade (Fig. 5.9). This response occurs in the absence of complement activation. An additional effect results from the generation of C_{5a} due to complement activation, also causing an increase in CR1 and CR3. These actions prime neutrophils for phagocytosis because of the large number of surface opsonin receptors (Moore et al 1987, Davis et al 1987). Other in-vitro experiments also indicate that bacterial endotoxins can directly stimulate neutrophil adherence. In addition to the role of CR3 in phagocytosis, this receptor appears to function in the process of cell adhesion, which is therefore increased in sepsis.

Endotoxin depression of chemotaxis has been noted repeatedly and appears to exhibit selectivity depending on the specific chemoattractant (Wilson 1985). A potent endogenous chemoattractant arises from C_{5a} liberation, particularly in proximity to an infectious process (Fig. 5.13). Migration of the neutrophil is dependent upon a gradient of C_{5a} acting as a chemical signal. However, in the presence of large amounts of C_{5a}, as may occur following severe bacterial invasion or massive tissue injury, neutrophils may be overwhelmed and selectively lose their responsivity to this chemoattractant while retaining their locomotor properties for other agents. This phenomenon of selective desensitization of circulating neutrophils to C_{5a} resulting from excessive complement activation (Davis et al 1987, Solomkin et al 1984) is probably the most prominent alteration in neutrophil function to gain attention in recent years. It is thought possibly to account for the apparently 'depressed' neutrophil activity following trauma and sepsis.

Studies on the effects of sepsis on neutrophil degranulation, phagocytosis, oxidative capacity and microbicidal activity have yielded variable results. It is clear that endotoxins can precipitate lysosomal degranulation and stimulate oxygen consumption of the neutrophil, but results appear to be dependent upon specific experimental circumstances (Wilson 1985). Further studies in this area are required.

Reticuloendothelial system

The reticuloendothelial system (RES) comprises cellular and tissue elements that mainly serve a phagocytic function in the body. The major constituents include macrophages, Kupffer cells, splenic and alveolar macrophages. The Kupffer cells of the liver are the major functional component of the fixed RES. It has been suggested that a vital function of this system is to scavenge and mediate the clearance of micro-organisms, toxins, immune complexes and particulate matter in the vascular stream. Depression of the RES has been associated with various forms of shock, including endotoxic shock, but may also follow the injection of large doses of particulate matter, simulating tissue destruction with the formation of collagenous tissue debris. This depression generally resolves in a matter of days after the precipitating event has ceased. During this early period, the host is thought to be at an increased risk for infectious complications (Schildt 1975).

Several mechanisms have been proposed as responsible for RES depression (Schildt 1975) following sepsis and septicaemic shock, including: 1. hepatic ischaemia, since the liver contains the largest fraction of fixed RES tissue (Olcay et al 1974); 2. toxicity due to endotoxaemia and septicaemia (Loegering 1986); and 3. opsonin deficiency (Kiener et al 1986). Reduced liver blood flow resulting in decreased delivery of material to Kupffer cells has not been shown to be an important factor in RES depression; however, ischaemic hepatic injury is likely to be associated with RES dysfunction. Ischaemic and endotoxin-induced RES depression probably results from a decrease in complement receptor function. It has been shown that Kupffer cell clearance of intravascular foreign materials is mediated by complement receptors, whose role is similar to their role in the engulfing of bacteria by neutrophils. Interaction of the complement fragments C_{3b} (and iC_{3b}) with Kupffer cell receptors CR1 (and CR3) augments the clearance of undesirable blood constituents. A large body of data exists indicating that receptor-ligand interaction failure is a major factor explaining RES depression associated with septicaemia. The specific mechanism for this failure is unknown.

Opsonin deficiency can theoretically cause RES dysfunction. The commonly accepted opsonins (fibronectin, complement and IgG) have been considered, and experimental evidence exists that marked decreases in the plasma concentration of these proteins may increase susceptibility to the lethal effects of bacterial infection. Impaired opsonization has been reported in patients suffering from Gram-negative septicaemia (Weinstein & Young 1976), but several studies have suggested that this is probably uncommon (Taeusch et al 1983, Alexander et al 1978).

Other than replacement therapy, which has uncertain benefit, nutritional support and control of the source of infection are the most important therapies that can be provided under these circumstances. Depressed complement levels, neutrophil and macrophage phagocytic function (Dionigi et al 1977) have been associated with inadequate nutrition, supporting the need to maintain a positive nitrogen balance in sepsis.

Immunoglobulins and B-cell function

Immunoglobulins commonly decline following trauma, and gradually recover to normal levels during convalescence (Alexander et al 1978,

Munster et al 1970, Faillace et al 1982). This observation applies to all major classes of immunoglobulins. Relatively little data are available on the immunoglobulin response to infection; most of the existing data refer to the septic burn patient. No major differences have been noted in IgG levels comparing septic and non-septic burn patients; however, non-surviving septic patients have been found to exhibit lower levels than survivors. Causes for these low levels are multifactorial, including consumption and decreased production on a nutritional basis. Evidence does exist that no intrinsic B-lymphocyte functional abnormality leading to infection is present in burn patients. It is known that polyclonal activation of B-lymphocytes to produce immunoglobulin requires support from helper T-lymphocytes, whose function appears to be altered following injury and sepsis. Interleukin-2 production by helper cells has been reported to be depressed and has been suggested to account for decreased T-cell dependent secretion of antibody by B cells (Wood et al 1984, 1986).

T-lymphocytes and cell-mediated immunity

A detailed review of lymphoctye function following injury and sepsis is beyond the scope of this chapter, but a general understanding of this area may be of value. As few data describing the immune response to septic shock exist, immune factors related to the septic syndrome will be considered.

The presence of anergy or failure of delayed cutaneous hypersensitivity response to standard recall antigens has been associated with an increased risk of sepsis and death. This increased risk has been documented for pre- and postoperative patients and has most commonly been related to deficiencies in nutritional status. In some studies, the maintenance of body cell mass using parenteral nutrition has been associated with reversal of the anergic state and improved prognosis. However, the source of anergy may be quite variable, stemming from causes such as old age, cancer, sepsis, shock and major trauma, making interpretation of this finding difficult (Meakins et al 1977, 1979). Anergic patients have exhibited decreased total lymphocyte counts (particularly T-lymphocytes), depressed T-cell mitogenic responses and abnormal neutrophil chemotaxis, which may be reversed by correcting the precipitating event such as drainage of a septic focus or control of a surgical emergency (Lewis & Klein 1979, Meakins et al 1979, Dominioni & Dionigi 1987). Consequently, the specific management of the anergic state must be tailored to the cause and not limited to nutritional considerations (Meakins et al 1979).

A number of additional alterations in cellular immune function have been related to the occurrence of sepsis. T-lymphocytes and their peptide products (mediators) called lymphokines appear to be important for classical cell-mediated responses. Figure 5.14 may be helpful in appreciating some of the key aspects of the cellular response to foreign antigen. Following phagocytosis by the macrophage, antigen is partially digested, modified and presented to a recognition cell such as a T- or B-lymphocyte. T-lymphocytes may be characterized, on the basis of their cell surface markers, into helper/inducer cells, which assist in amplification of the antigen recognition response, and suppressor T-cells, which inhibit the T-cell-dependent inflammatory response. Under the influence of antigen presentation (and IL-1 production by the macrophage), the T-helper cell produces interleukin-2 (IL-2) which is a lymphocyte growth factor/peptide resulting in T- and B-cell clonal expansion. Depressed IL-2 production has been reported in burn and trauma patients, and levels appear to be particularly low in patients who develop sepsis (O'Mahoney et al 1985). Since reduction in IL-2 is related to extent of injury, it is possible that diminished IL-2 production predisposes to sepsis. Additionally, septic patients, especially non-survivors, exhibit significantly depressed helper T-cell subset levels (O'Mahoney et al 1985, Williams et al 1983, Dahn et al 1988) which are probably related to depressed IL-2 levels. The likely sequence of events is that under the influence of depressed IL-2, T- and B-cell populations may decline, resulting in a further depression of humoral and cell-mediated immunity.

Other findings that may contribute to post-traumatic immunosuppression include decreased IL-2 receptor expressing cells (Teodorczyk-Injeyan et al 1986) and increased T-suppressor cell activity, which may lower resistance to bacterial infection (Kupper et al 1985). Further experimental work is required in these areas.

Conclusion

Septicaemic shock remains a frequent cause of death in surgical patients. Although the origins and responsible micro-organisms may vary widely, the pathophysiological disruption has a broad common pathway. While the anatomical, physiological, metabolic, endocrinological and immunological changes are still relatively poorly understood, enough is now known to enable the clinician to correlate changing physical signs and laboratory values with the fundamental cellular changes that are associated with sepsis, and to do so with fair accuracy.

As sepsis is a systemic disease, virtually all organs and organ systems are affected from the start. Successful treatment is rooted in early recognition of the pathophysiological changes and reversal of these before the multiple organ failure syndrome supervenes. Identification and elimination of the source of sepsis is always vital but may not be enough unless the wide array of functional changes

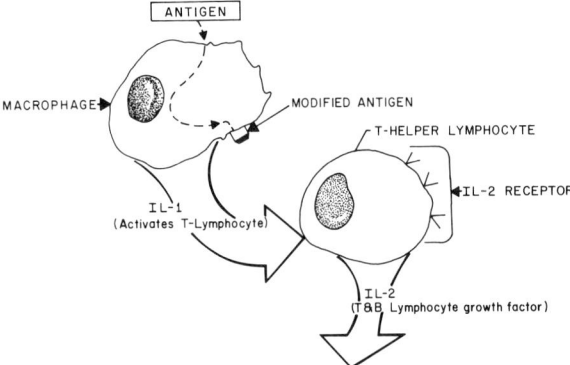

Fig. 5.14 Antigen specific immunity is dependent upon a series of key processes, some of which are illustrated. Antigen is engulfed and processed (modified) by the macrophage and presented to a lymphocyte, which under the influence of a variety of cytokines such as IL-1 may liberate interleukin-2 (IL-2). IL-2 then stimulates T- and B-lymphocyte clonal expansion.

set into motion by the sepsis are restored towards normal. Specific rational therapeutic manipulations in the modern critical care unit may make the differences between life and death.

Some accepted mechanisms and a few speculative hypotheses on the basic changes have been delineated together with selected clinical manifestations. Septicaemic shock remains the fear of every surgeon.

Acknowledgement. The authors would like to express their appreciation to Matthew L. Guilford for preparing the graphics used in this chapter.

REFERENCES

Alexander J W, Ogle C, Stinnett J D, MacMillan B G 1978 A sequential prospective analysis of immunologic abnormalities and infection following severe thermal injury. Annals of Surgery 188: 809–816

Alverdy J, Chi H S, Sheldon G F 1985 The effect of parenteral nutrition on gastrointestinal immunity. Annals of Surgery 202: 681–684

Artman M, Jackson J D, Boucek R J, Graham T P, Boerth R C 1986 Effects of endotoxin on coronary vascular resistance in the isolated blood-perfused rabbit heart. Circulatory Shock 19: 13–22

Arvidsson S, Falt K, Marklund S, Haglund U 1985 Role of free oxygen radicals in the development of gastrointestinal mucosal damage in *Escherichia coli* Sepsis. Circulatory Shock 16: 383–393

Asher E F, Rowe R L, Garrison R N, Fry D E 1986 Experimental bacteremia and hepatic nutrient blood flow. Circulatory Shock 20: 43–49

Askanazi J, Carpentier Y A, Elwyn D H et al 1980 Influence of total parenteral nutrition on fuel utilization in injury and sepsis. Annals of Surgery 191: 40–46

Aulick L H, Baze W B, McLeod C G, Wilmore D W 1980 Control of blood flow in a large surface wound. Annals of Surgery 191: 249–258

Bailey R W, Bulkley G B, Hamilton S R, Morris J B, Haglund U H, Meilahn J E 1987 The fundamental hemodynamic mechanism underlying gastric "Stress Ulceration" in cardiogenic shock. Annals of Surgery 205: 597–612

Ball H A, Cook J A, Wise W C, Halushka P V 1986 Role of thromboxane, prostaglandins, and leukotrienes in endotoxic and septic shock. Intensive Care Medicine 12: 116–126

Baracos V, Rodemann H P, Dinarello C A, Goldberg A L 1983 Stimulation of muscle protein degradation and prostaglandin E$_2$ release by leukocytic pyrogen (Interleukin-1). New England Journal of Medicine 308: 553–558

Bessey P, Wilmore D W 1983 β-adrenergic regulation of glucose disposal: A reciprocal relationship with insulin release. Journal of Surgical Research 34: 404–414

Bessey P Q, Brooks D C, Black P R, Aoki T T, Wilmore D W 1983 Epinephrine acutely mediates skeletal muscle insulin resistance. Surgery 94: 172–179

Bessey P Q, Watters J M, Aoki T T, Wilmore D W 1984 Combined hormone infusion simulates the metabolic response to injury. Annals of Surgery Research 200: 264–281

Beutler B, Cerami A 1986 Cachectin and tumor necrosis factor as two sides of the same biological coin. Nature 320: 584–588

Beutler B, Cerami A 1987 Cachetin: More than a tumor necrosis factor. New England Journal of Medicine 316: 379–385

Bevilacqua M P, Pober J S, Wheeler M E, Cotran R S, Gimbrone M A 1985 Interleukin-1 activation of vascular endothelium. Effects on procoagulant activity and leukocyte adhesion. American Journal of Pathology 121: 394–403

Bihari D, Smithies M, Gimson A, Tinker J 1987 The effects of vasodilation with prostacyclin on oxygen delivery and uptake in critically ill patients. New England Journal of Medicine 317: 397–403

Bjornson A B, Altemeier W A, Bjornson H S, Tang T, Iserson M L 1978 Host defense against opportunistic microorganisms following trauma. Annals of Surgery 188: 93–101

Bland R D, Shoemaker W C 1985 Common physiologic patterns in general surgical patients: hemodynamic and oxygen transport changes during and after operations in patients with and without associated medical problems. Surgical Clinics of North America NA 65: 793–809

Bonnet F, Bilaine J, Lhoste F, Mankikian B, Kerdelhue M, Rapin M 1985 Naloxone therapy of human septic shock. Critical Care Medicine 13: 972–975

Bradley S G 1981 Direct action of bacterial endotoxin on cells, mitochondria, and lysosomes. In: Majde J A, Person R J (eds) Pathophysiological effects of endotoxins at the cellular level. Alan R Liss, New York, pp 3–14

Brennan M F, Cerra F, Daly J M et al 1986 Report of a research workshop: branched chain amino acids in stress and injury. Journal of Parenteral and Enteral Nutrition 10: 446–452

Brigham K L, Padove S J, Bryant D, McKeen C R, Bowers R E 1980 Diphenhydramine reduces endotoxin effects on lung vascular permeability in sheep. Journal of Applied Physiology 49: 516–526

Brooks D C, Bessey P Q, Black P R, Aoki T T, Wilmore D W 1986 Insulin stimulates branched chain amino acid uptake and diminishes nitrogen flux from skeletal muscle of injured patients. Journal of Surgical Research 40: 395–405

Carlon G C, Howland W S 1983 Clinical experience with high frequency jet ventilation. International Anesthesiology Clinics 21(3): 99–123

Cerra F B 1987 Hypermetabolism, organ failure, and metabolic support. Surgery 101: 1–14

Cerra F B, Siegel J H J, Border J R, Wiles J, McMenamy R R 1979 The hepatic failure of sepsis: cellular vs. substrate. Surgery 86: 409–422

Chien K R, Abrams J, Pfau R G, Farber J L 1977 Prevention by chlorpromazine of ischemic liver cell death. American Journal of Pathology 88: 539–558

Clowes G H A, O'Donnell T F, Ryan N T, Blackburn G L

1974 Energy metabolism in sepsis: treatment based on different patterns in shock and high output stage. Annals of Surgery 179: 684–96

Clowes G H A, Randall H T, Cha C J 1980 Amino acid and energy metabolism in septic and traumatized patients. Journal of Parenteral and Enteral Nutrition 4: 195–205

Clowes G H A, Martin H, Walji S, Hirsch E, Gazitua R, Goodfellow R 1978 Blood insulin responses to blood glucose levels in high output sepsis and septic shock. American Journal of Surgery 135: 577–582

Clowes G H A, George B C, Villee C A, Saravis C A 1983 Muscle proteolysis induced by a circulating peptide in patients with sepsis or trauma. New England Journal of Medicine 308: 545–552

Coates C L, Burwell R G, Carlin S A, Milligan G F 1981 The somatomedin activity in plasma from patients with multiple mechanical injuries: with observations on plasma cortisol. Injury 13: 100–107

Dahn M S, Kirkpatrick J R, Bouwman D L 1980 Sepsis, glucose intolerance and protein malnutrition: a metabolic paradox. Archives of Surgery 115: 1415–1418

Dahn M S, Kirkpatrick J R, Blasier R 1984a Alterations in the metabolism of exogenous lipids associated with sepsis. Journal of Parenteral and Enteral Nutrition 8: 169–173

Dahn M S, Mitchell R A, Smith S, Lange M P, Whitcomb M P, Kirkpatrick J R 1984b Altered immunologic function and nitrogen metabolism associated with Depression of plasma growth hormone. Journal of Parenteral and Enteral Nutrition 8: 690–694

Dahn M S, Jacobs L A, Smith S, Hans B, Lange M P, Mitchell R A, Kirkpatrick J R 1985 The relationship of insulin production to glucose metabolism in severe sepsis. Archives of Surgery 120: 166–172

Dahn M S, Lange M P, Mitchell R A, Lobdell K, Wilson R F 1987a Insulin production following injury and sepsis. Journal of Trauma 27: 1031–1038

Dahn M S, Lange M P, Mitchell R A, Jacobs L A, Kololgi S 1987b The response of post-surgical subjects to exogenous growth hormone. Federation Proceedings 46: 601

Dahn M S, Lange P, Lobdell K, Hans B, Jacobs L A, Mitchell R A 1987c Splanchnic and total body oxygen consumption differences in septic and injured patients. Surgery 101: 69–80

Dahn M S, Whitcomb M P, Lange M P, Jacobs L A 1988 Altered T-lymphocyte subsets in severe sepsis. American Surgeon 54: 450–455

Danek S J, Lynch J P, Weg J G, Dantzker D R 1980 The dependence of oxygen uptake on oxygen delivery in the adult respiratory distress syndrome. American Review of Respiratory Disease 122: 387–395

Davis C F, Moore F D, Rodrick M L, Fearon D T, Mannick J A 1987 Neutrophil activation after burn injury contribution of the classic complement pathway and of endotoxin. Surgery 102: 477–483

DeFronzo R A, Sherwin R S, Felig P 1980 Synergistic interactions of counterregulatory hormones: a mechanism for stress hyperglycemia. Acta Chirurgica Scandinavica (Suppl) 498: 33–42

Deitch E A, Berg R, Specian R 1987 Endotoxin promotes the translocation of bacteria from the gut. Archives of Surgery 122: 185–190

Demling R H, Smith M, Gunther R, Gee M, Flynn J 1981 The effect of prostaglandin infusion on endotoxin-induced lung injury. Surgery 89: 257–263

Deutschman C S, Konstantinides F N, Tsai M, Simmons R L, Cerra F B 1987 Physiology and metabolism in isolated viral septicemia. Further evidence of an organism-independent, host-dependent response. Archives of Surgery 122: 21–25

Dinarello C A 1984 Interleukin-1. Review of Infectious Disease 6: 51–95

Dinarello C A, Mier J W 1986 Interleukins. Annual Review of Medicine 37: 173–178

Dionigi R, Zonta A, Dominioni L, Gnes F, Ballabio A 1977 The effect of total parenteral nutrition on immunodepression due to malnutrition. Annals of Surgery 185: 467–474

Dominioni L, Dionigi R 1987 Immunological function and nutritional assessment. Journal of Parenteral and Enteral Nutrition 11: 70S–72S

Dominioni L, Dionigi R, Jemos V 1981 The acute phase response of plasma proteins in surgical patients. In: Wesdorp R I C, Soeters P G (eds) Clinical Nutrition '81. Churchill Livingstone, Edinburgh, pp 239–259

Dominioni L, Dionigi R, Zanello M et al 1987 Sepsis score and acute-phase protein response as predictors of outcome in septic surgical patients. Archives of Surgery 122: 141–146

Doran J E, Lundsgaard-Hansen P, Rubli E 1986 Plasma fibronectin: relevance for anesthesiology and intensive care. Intensive Care Medicine 12: 340–349

Emau P, Giri S N, Bruss M L 1986 Comparative effects of smooth and rough *Pasteurella hemolytica* lipopolysaccharides on arachidonic acid, eicosanoids, serotonin and histamine in calves. Circulatory Shock 20: 239–253

Faillace D F, Ledgerwood A M, Lucas C E, Kithier K, Higgins R F 1982 Immunoglobulin changes after varied resuscitation regimens. Journal of Trauma 22: 1–5

Fearon D T, Ruddy S, Schur P H, McCabe W R 1975 Activation of the properdin pathway of complement in patients with Gram-negative bacteremia. New England Journal of Medicine 292: 937–940

Feuerstein G, Hallenbeck J M 1987 Prostaglandins, leukotrienes, and platelet activating factor in shock. Annual Review of Pharmacology and Toxicology 27: 301–313

Fiddian-Green R G, McGough E, Pittenger G, Rothman E 1983 Predictive value of intramural pH and other risk factors for massive bleeding from stress ulceration. Gastroenterology 85: 613–620

Fine D P 1985 Role of complement in endotoxin shock. In: Hinshaw L B (ed) Handbook of endotoxin, Vol. 2: Pathophysiology of endotoxin. Elsevier, New York, pp 129–144

Frank M M 1987 Complement in the pathophysiology of human disease. New England Journal of Medicine 316: 1525–1530

Freeman B A, Turrens J F, Mirza Z, Crapo J D, Young S L 1985 Modulation of oxidant lung injury by using liposome-entrapped superoxide dismutase and catalase. Federation Procedings 44: 2591–2595

Froesch E R, Schmid C, Schwander J, Zapf J 1985 Actions of insulin-like growth factors. Annual Review of Physiology 47: 443–467

Fry D E, Garrison R N, Heitsch R C, Calhoun K, Polk H C 1980a Determinants of death in patients with intraabdominal abscess. Surgery 88: 517–523

Fry D E, Pearlstein L, Fulton R L, Polk H C 1980b

Multiple system organ failure: the role of uncontrolled infection. Archives of Surgery 115: 136–140

Gattinoni L, Pesenti A, Mascheroni D et al 1986 Low-frequency positive pressure ventilation with extracorporeal CO_2 removal in severe acute respiratory failure. Journal of the American Medical Association 256: 881–886

Gauldie J, Sauder D N, McAdams K P W J, Dinarello C A 1987 Purified interleukin-1 (IL-1) from human monocytes stimulates acute-phase protein synthesis by rodent hepatocytes in vitro. Immunology 60: 203–207

George D T, Abeles F B, Mapes C A, Sobocinski P Z, Zenser T V, Powanda M C 1977 Effect of leukocytic endogenous mediator on endocrine pancreas secretory responses. American Journal of Physiology 233: E240–E245

Goldberg A C 1983 Factors affecting protein balance in skeletal muscle in normal and pathological states. In: Blackburn G C, Grant J P, Young V R (eds) Amino acids: metabolism and medical applications. John Wright, Boston, pp 201–211

Goris R J A, te Bockhorst T P A, Nuytinck J K S, Gimbrere J S F 1985 Multiple-organ failure. Generalized autodestruction inflammation? Archives of Surgery 120: 1109–1115

Goris R J A, Boekholtz W K F, van Bebber I P T, Nuytinck J K S, Schillings P H M 1986 Multiple-organ failure and sepsis without bacteria. An experimental model. Archives of Surgery 121: 897–901

Gray D S 1985 Energetics. In: Kaminski M V (ed) Hyperalimentation: a guide for clinicians. Marcel Dekker, New York, p 17

Groeneveld A B J, Bronsveld W, Thijs L G 1986 Hemodynamic determinants of mortality in human septic shock. Surgery 99: 140–153

Groeneveld A B J, Kester A D M, Nauta J J P, Thijs L G 1987 Relation of arterial blood lactate to oxygen delivery and hemodynamic variables in human shock states. Circulatory Shock 22: 35–53

Gump F E, Long C, Killian P, Kinney J M 1974 Studies of glucose intolerance in septic injured patients. Journal of Trauma 14: 378–388

Gurll N J 1985 Endorphins in Endotoxin shock. In: Hinshaw L B (ed) Handbook of endotoxin, Vol. 2: Pathophysiology of endotoxin. Elsevier, New York, pp 299–337

Hallgren R, Samuelsson T, Modig J 1987 Complement activation and increased alveolar-capillary permeability after major surgery and in adult respiratory distress syndrome. Critical Care Medicine 15: 189–192

Halushka P V, Reines H D, Barrow S E et al 1985 Elevated plasma 6-keto-prostaglandin $F_{1\alpha}$ in patients in septic shock. Critical Care Medicine 13: 451–453

Hasselgren P O 1987 prevention and treatment of ischemia of the liver. Surgery, Gynecology and Obstetrics 164: 187–196

Hasselgren P O, Biber B, Fornander J 1983 Improved blood flow and protein synthesis in the postischemic liver following infusion of dopamine. Journal of Surgical Research 34: 44–52

Hasselgren P O, Talamini M, James J H, Fischer J E 1986 Protein metabolism in different types of skeletal muscle during early and late sepsis in rats. Archives of Surgery 121: 918–923

Hasselgren P O, Warner B W, James J H, Takehara H, Fischer J F 1987 Effect of insulin on amino acid uptake and protein turnover in skeletal muscle from septic rats. Archives of Surgery 122: 228–233

Haybron D M, Townsend M C, Hamptom W W, Schirmer W J, Schirmer J M, Fry D E 1987 Alterations in renal perfusion and renal energy charge in murine peritonitis. Archives of Surgery 122: 328–331

Holcraft J W, Vassar M J, Weber C J 1986 Prostaglandin E_1 and survival in patients with adult respiratory distress syndrome. Annals of Surgery 203: 371–378

Houtchens B A, Westenskow D R 1984 Oxygen consumption in septic shock: collective review. Circulatory Shock 13: 361–384

Hulton N R, Johnson D J, Wilmore D W 1985 Limited effects of prostaglandin inhibitors in *Escherichia coli* sepsis. Surgery 98: 291–297

Hyers T M, Fowler A A 1986 Adult respiratory distress syndrome: causes, morbidity, and mortality. Federation Proceedings 45: 25–29

Judges D, Sharkey P, Cheung H et al 1986 Pulmonary microvascular fluid flux in a large animal model of sepsis: evidence of increased pulmonary endothelial permeability accompanying surgical induced peritonitis in sheep. Surgery 99: 222–234

Kaufmann R L, Matson C F, Rowberg A H, Beisel W R 1976 Defective lipid disposal mechanisms during bacterial infection in rhesis monkeys. Metabolism 25: 615–624

Keusch G T, Farthing M J G 1986 Nutrition and infection. Annual Review of Nutrition 6: 131–154

Kiener J L, Cho E, Saba T M 1986 Comparative effect of circulating bacterial or nonbacterial particulates on plasma fibronectin: relationship to lung deposition of blood-borne foreign particles. Circulatory Shock 19: 357–370

Kirkpatrick J R, Dahn M S, Hynes M J, Williams D G 1981 The therapeutic advantages of a balanced nutritional support system. Surgery 89: 370–374

Krause S M, Hess M L 1979 Diphenhydramine protection of the failing myocardium during Gram-negative endotoxemia. Circulatory Shock 6: 75–78

Kupper T S, Baker C C, Ferguson T A, Green D R 1985 A burn induced Ly-2 suppressor T cell lowers resistance to bacterial infection. Journal of Surgical Research 38: 606–612

Lang C H, Bagby G J, Spitzer J J 1984a Carbohydrate dynamics in the hypermetabolic septic rat. Metabolism 33: 959–963

Lang C H, Bagby G J, Ferguson J C, Spitzer J J 1984b Cardiac output and redistribution of organ blood flow in hypermetabolic sepsis. American Journal of Physiology 246: R331–R337

Lang C H, Bagby G J, Blakesley H L, Spitzer J J 1987 Inhibition of eicosanoid production by BW755C does not attenuate sepsis-induced alterations in glucose kinetics. Circulatory Shock 22: 105–113

Lanser M E, Saba T M, Scovill W A 1980 Opsonic glycoprotein (plasma fibronectin) levels after burn injury. Annals of Surgery 192: 776–782

Lanza-Jacoby S, Lansey S C, Cleary M P, Rosato F E 1982 Alterations in lipogenic enzymes and lipoprotein lipase activity during gram negative sepsis in the rat. Archives of Surgery 117: 144–147

Larcher V F, Wyke R J, Mowat A P, Williams R 1982 Bacterial and fungal infections in children with fulminant hepatic failure: possible role of opsonisation and complement deficiency. Gut 23: 1037–1043

Lewis R T, Klein H 1979 Risk factors in postoperative

sepsis: significance of preoperative lymphocytopenia. Journal of Surgical Research 26: 365–371

Loda M, Clowes G H A, Dinarello C A, George B C, Lane B, Richardson W 1984 Induction of hepatic protein synthesis by a peptide in blood plasma of patients with sepsis and trauma. Surgery 96: 204–213

Loegering D J 1986 Kupffer cell complement receptor clearance function and host defense. Circulatory Shock 20: 321–333

Long C L 1977 Energy balance and carbohydrate metabolism in infection and sepsis. American Journal of Clinical Nutrition 30: 1301–1310

Long C L, Kinney J M, Geiger J W 1976 Nonsuppressibility of gluconeogenesis in septic injured patients. Metabolism 25: 193–201

Long C L, Jeevanandam M, Kim B M, Kinney J M 1977 Whole body protein synthesis and catabolism in septic man. American Journal of Clinical Nutrition 30: 1340–4

McDonough K H, Henry J J, Lang C H, Spitzer J J 1986 Substrate utilization and high energy phosphate levels of hearts from hyperdynamic septic rats. Circulatory Shock 18: 161–170

McIntosh T K, Faden A I 1986 Thyrotropin-releasing hormone (TRH) and circulatory shock. Circulatory Shock 18: 241–258

McKinley C J, Turinsky J 1986 Prostaglandin E_2 and muscle proteolysis: effect of burn injury and cycloheximide. American Journal of Physiology 250: R207–210

McManus A T 1983 Examination of neutrophil function in a rat model of decreased host resistance following burn trauma. Review of Infectious Disease 5: S898–S907

Meakins J L, Pietsch J B, Bubenick O, Kelly R, Rode H, Gordon J, MacLean L D 1977 Delayed hypersensitivity: indicator of acquired failure of host defense in sepsis and trauma. Annals of Surgery 186: 241–250

Meakins J L, Christou N V, Shizgal H M, MacLean L D 1979 Therapeutic approaches to anergy in surgical patients. Annals of Surgery 190: 286–296

Meyrick B O 1986 Endotoxin-mediated pulmonary endothelial cell injury. Federation Proceedings 45: 19–24

Mohsenifar Z, Goldbach P, Tashkin D P, Campisi D J 1983 Relationship between O_2 delivery and O_2 consumption in the adult respiratory distress syndrome. Chest 84: 267–271

Moore F D, Moss N A, Revhaug A, Wilmore D, Mannick J A, Rodrick M L 1987 A single dose of endotoxin activates neutrophils without activating complement. Surgery 102: 200–205

More D G, Roper R F, Munro J A, Watson C J, Boutagy J S, Shenfield G M 1985 Randomized, prospective trial of cimetidine and ranitidine for control of intragastric pH in the critically ill. Surgery 97: 215–223

Morrison D C, Ryan J L 1987 Endotoxins and disease mechanisms. Annual Review of Medicine 38: 417–432

Munster A M, Hoagland H C, Pruitt B A 1970 The effect of thermal injury on serum immunoglobulins. Annals of Surgery 172: 965–969

Neufeld H A, Pace J G, Kaminski M V, George D T, Jahrling P B, Wannemacher R W, Beisel W R 1980 A probable endocrine basis for the depression of ketone bodies during infections of inflammatory states in rats. Endocrinology 107: 596–601

Nilsson L O, Stone A M, Stein T A, Wise L 1983 Indomethacin and the gastric mucosal blood flow changes of sepsis. Annals of Surgery 198: 592–595

Nordstrom G, Seeman T, Hasselgren P O 1985 Beneficial effect of allopurinol in liver ischemia. Surgery 97: 679–684

Nordenstrom J, Carpentier Y A, Askanazi J et al 1982 Metabolic utilization of intravenous fat emulsions during total parenteral nutrition. Annals of Surgery 196: 221–231

Nordenstrom J, Carpentier Y A, Askanazi J et al 1983 Free fatty acid mobilization and oxidation during total parental nutrition in trauma and infection. Annals of Surgery 198: 725–735

Odessey R 1985 Effect of inhibitors of proteolysis and arachidonic acid metabolism on burn-induced protein breakdown. Metabolism 34: 616–620

Olcay I, Holper K, Kitahama A, Miller R H, Drapanos T, Trijo R A, DiLuzio N R 1974 Reticuloendothelial function: determinant for survival following hepatic ischemia in the baboon. Surgery 76: 643–653

O'Mahoney J B, Wood J J, Rodrick M L, Mannick J A 1985 Change in T-lymphocyte subsets following injury. Annals of Surgery 202: 580–586

Pacitti N, Bryson S E, McKechnie K, Rodger I W, Parsatt J R 1987 Leukotriene antagonist FPL57231 prevents the acute pulmonary effects of *Escherichia coli* endotoxin in cats. Circulatory Shock 21: 155–168

Parker M M, Parrillo J E 1983 Septic shock. Hemodynamics and pathogenesis. Journal of the American Medical Association 250: 3324–3327

Parrillo J E, Burch C, Shelhamer J H, Parker M M, Natason C, Schuette W 1985 A circulatory myocardial depressant substance in humans with septic shock. Journal of Clinical Investigation 76: 1539–1553

Payne J G, Bowen J C 1981 Hypoxia of canine gastric mucosa caused by *Escherichia coli* sepsis and prevented with methylprednisolone therapy. Gastroenterology 80: 84–93

Peters W P, Johnson M W, Friedman P A, Mitch W E 1981 Pressor effect of naloxone in septic shock. Lancet 1: 529–532

Pine R W, Wertz M J, Lennard E S, Dellinger E P, Carrico C J, Minshew B H 1983 Determinants of organ malfunction or death in patients with intra-abdominal sepsis. Archives of Surgery 118: 242–249

Polk H C, Shields C L 1977 Remote organ failure: A valid sign of occult intra-abdominal infection. Surgery 81: 310–313

Raymond R M, Klein D M, Gibbons D A, Jacobs H K, Emerson T E 1985 Skeletal muscle unresponsiveness during chronic hyperdynamic sepsis in the dog. Journal of Trauma 25: 845–855

Reeds P J, Palmer R M 1983 The possible involvement of prostaglandin $F_{2\alpha}$ in the stimulation of muscle protein synthesis by insulin. Biochemical and Biophysical Research Communications 116: 1084–1087

Rees M, Bowen J C 1982 Stress ulcers during live Escherichia coli sepsis. The Role of Acid and Bile. Annals of Surgery 195: 646–652

Register S D, Downs J B, Stock M C, Kirby R R 1987 Is 50% oxygen harmful? Critical Care Medicine 15: 598–601

Reines H D, Halushka P V, Cook J A, Wise W C, Rambo W 1982 Plasma thromboxane concentrations are raised in patients dying with septic shock. Lancet 2: 174–175

Richmond J M, Walker J F, Avila A et al 1985 Renal and cardiovascular response to nonhypotensive sepsis in a large animal model with peritonitis. Surgery 97: 205–213

Robin A P, Askanazi J, Greenwood M R C, Carpentier Y A, Gump F E, Kinney J M 1981 Lipoprotein lipase activity in surgical patients: influence of trauma and infection. Surgery 90: 401–408

Rosenblatt S, Clowes G H A, George B C, Hirsch E, Lindberg B 1983 Exchange of amino acids by muscle and liver sepsis. Archives of Surgery 118: 167–175

Ryan N T, Blackburn G L, Clowes G H A 1974a Differential tissue sensitivity to elevated endogenous insulin levels during experimental peritonitis in rats. Metabolism 23: 1081–1089

Ryan N T, George B C, Odessey R, Egdahl R 1974b Effect of hemorrhagic shock, fasting and corticosterone administration on leucine oxidation and incorporation into protein by skeletal muscle. Metabolism 23: 901–904

Sagher U, Rosen H, Sarel O, Becker Y 1986 Studies on a pancreatic cardiodepressant factor. Circulatory Shock 19: 319–327

Saito H, Trocki O, Alexander J W, Kopcha R, Heyd T, Joffe S N 1987 The effect of route of nutrient administration on the nutritional state, catabolic hormone secretion, and gut mucosal integrity after burn injury. Journal of Parenteral and Enteral Nutrition 11: 1–7

Schildt B E 1975 The present view of RES and shock. Advances in Experimental Medicine and Biology 73A: 375–387

Schirmer W J, Schirmer J M, Townsend H C, Fry D E 1987a Imidazole and indomethacin improve hepatic perfusion in sepsis. Circulatory Shock 21: 253–259

Schirmer W J, Townsend M C, Schirmer J M, Hampton W W, Fry D E 1987b Galactose elimination kinetics in sepsis. Correlation of hepatic blood flow with function. Archives of Surgery 122: 349–354

Shapiro J M, Mihm F G, Trudell J R, Stevens J H, Feeley T W 1987 Leukotriene D$_4$ increases extravascular lung water in the dog. Circulatory Shock 21: 121–128

Shaw J H F, Klein S, Wolfe R R 1984 Assessment of alanine, urea, and glucose interrelationships in normal subjects and in patients with sepsis with stable isotopic tracers. Surgery 97: 557–567

Shepherd R E, McDonough K H, Burns A H 1986 Mechanism of cardiac dysfunction in hearts from endotoxin-treated rats. Circulatory Shock 19: 371–384

Shibutani K, Komatsu T, Kubal K, Sanchala V, Kumar V, Bizzarri D V 1983 Critical level of oxygen delivery in anesthetized man. Critical Care Medicine 11: 640–643

Shoemaker W C, Appel P L 1986 Effects of prostaglandin E$_1$ in adult respiratory distress syndrome. Surgery 99: 275–283

Shoemaker W C, Appel P, Bland R 1983 Use of physiologic monitoring to predict outcome and to assist in clinical decisions in critically ill postoperative patients. American Journal of Surgery 146: 43–49

Shumacker P T, Cain S M 1987 The concept of a critical oxygen delivery. Intensive Care Medicine 13: 223–229

Sillix D H, McDonald F D 1987 Acute renal failure. Critical Care Clinics 3: 909–925

Slotman G J, Burchard K W, Gann D S 1985 Thromboxane and prostaglandin in clinical acute respiratory failure. Journal of Surgical Research 39: 1–7

Slotman G J, Yellin S A, Handy J R, Hulstyn M, Husain S E, Gann D S 1986 Thromboxane A$_2$ mediates hemodynamic and respiratory dysfunction in graded bacteremia. Surgery 100: 214–221

Sobrado J, Moldawer L L, Bistrian B R, Dinarello C A, Blackburn G L 1983 Effects of ibuprofen on fever and metabolic changes induced by continuous infusion of leukocytic pyrogen (Interleukin-1) or endotoxin. Infection and Immunity 42: 997–1005

Solomkin J S, Nelson R D, Chenoweth D E, Solem L D, Simmons R L 1984 Regulation of neutrophil migratory function in burn injury by complement activation products. Annals of Surgery 200: 742–746

Spitzer J A, Fish R E 1986 Lipolytic patterns in isolated adipocytes of continuously endotoxemic rats. Circulatory Shock 18: 21–29

Stahl W M 1987 Acute phase protein response to tissue injury. Critical Care Medicine 6: 545–550

Steffen E K, Berg R D 1983 Relationship between cecal population levels of indigenous bacteria and translocation to the mesenteric lymph nodes. Infection and Immunity 39: 1252–1259

Stoner H B, Little R A, Frayn K N, Elebute A E, Tresadern J, Gross E 1983 The effect of sepsis on the oxidation of carbohydrate and fat. British Journal of Surgery 70: 32–35

Sugino K, Dohi K, Yamada K, Kawasaki T 1986 The role of lipid peroxidation in endotoxic-induced hepatic damage and the protective effect of antioxidants. Surgery 101: 746–751

Swinamer D L, Phang P T, Jones R L, Grace M, King E G 1987 Twenty-four hour energy expenditure in critically ill patients. Critical Care Medicine 15: 637–643

Taeusch H W, Clements J, Benson B 1983 Exogenous surfactant for human lung disease. American Review of Respiratory Disease 128: 791–794

Teodorczyk-Injeyan J A, Sparkes B G, Mills G B, Peters W J, Falk R E 1986 Impairment of T cell activation in burn patients: a possible mechanism of thermal injury — induced immunosuppression. Clinical and Experimental Immunology 65: 570–581

Thomas R, Aikawa N, Burke J F 1979 Insulin resistance in peripheral tissues after a burn injury. Surgery 86: 742–747

Tracey K J, Lowry S F, Fahey T J et al 1987 Cachectin//tumor necrosis factor induces lethal shock and stress hormone responses in the dog. Surgery, Gynecology and Obstetrics 164: 415–422

Tuggle D W, Horton J W 1986 Cardiocirculatory effects of physiological doses of beta-endorphin. Circulatory Shock 18: 215–225

Vary T C, Siegel J H, Nakatani T, Sato T, Aoyama H 1986 Effect of sepsis on activity of pyruvate dehydrogenase complex in skeletal muscle and liver. American Journal of Physiology 250: E634–E640

Vered M, Dearing R, Janoff A 1985 A new elastase inhibitor from *Streptococcus Pneumoniae* protects against acute lung injury induced by neutrophil granules. American Review of Respiratory Disease 131: 131–133

Ward H C, Halliday D, Sim A J W 1987 Protein and energy metabolism with biosynthetic human growth hormone after gastrointestinal surgery. Annals of Surgery 206: 56–61

Watson R R, Petro T M 1982 Resistance to bacterial and parasitic infections in the nutritionally compromised host. CRC Critical Reviews in Micobiology 10: 297–314

Watters J M, Bessey P Q, Dinarello C A, Wolff S M, Wilmore D W 1986 Both inflammatory and endocrine mediators stimulate host responses to sepsis. Archives of Surgery 121: 179–190

Weinstein R J, Young L S 1976 Neutrophil function in Gram-negative rod bacteremia. Journal of Clinical Investigation 58: 190–199

Weissman C, Kemper M, Elwyn D H, Askanazi J, Hyman A I, Kinney J M 1986 The energy expenditure of the mechanically ventilated critically ill patient. An analysis. Chest 89: 254–259

West M A, Keller G A, Hyland B J, Cerra F B, Simmons R L 1985 Hepatocyte function in sepsis: Kupffer cells mediate a biphasic protein synthesis response in hepatocytes after exposure to endotoxin or killed Escherichia coli. Surgery 98: 388–395

White R H, Frayn K N, Little R A, Threlfall C J, Stoner H B, Irving M H 1987 Hormonal and metabolic responses to glucose infusion in sepsis studied by the hyperglycemic glucose clamp technique. Journal of Parenteral and Enteral Nutrition 11: 345–353

Wichterman K A, Chaudry I H, Baue A E 1979 Studies of peripheral glucose uptake during sepsis. Archives of Surgery 114: 740–745

Wichterman K A, Baue A E, Chaudry I H 1980 Sepsis and septic shock — a review of laboratory models and a proposal. Journal of Surgical Research 29: 189–201

Williams R C, Koster F T, Kilpatrick K A 1983 Alterations in lymphocyte cell surface markers during various human infections. American Journal of Medicine 75: 807–816

Wilmore D W, Goodwin C W, Aulick L H, Powanda M C, Mason A D, Pruitt B A 1980 Effect of injury and infection on visceral metabolism and circulation. Annals of Surgery 192: 491–504

Wilson M E 1985 Effects of bacterial endotoxin on neutrophil function. Review of Infectious Disease 7: 404–418

Wolf, Y G, Cotev S, Perel A, Manny J 1987 Dependence of oxygen consumption on cardiac output in sepsis. Critical Care Medicine 15: 198–203

Wolfe R R, O'Donnell T F, Stone M D, Richmond D A, Burke T F 1980 Investigation of factors determining optimal glucose infusion rate in total parenteral nutrition. Metabolism 29: 892–900

Wolfe R R, Herndon D N, Jahoor F, Miyoshi H, Wolfe M 1987 Effect of severe burn injury on substrate cycling by glucose and fatty acids. New England Journal of Medicine 317: 403–408

Wood J J, Rodrick M L, O'Mahoney J B et al 1984 Inadequate interleukin-2 production. A fundamental immunological deficiency in patients with major burns. Annals of Surgery 200: 311–320

Wood J J, O'Mahoney J B, Rodrick M L, Eaton R, Demling R H, Mannick J A 1986 Abnormalities of antibody production after thermal injury. Archives of Surgery 121: 108–115

Worthen G S, Haslett C, Smedly L A et al 1986 Lung vascular injury induced by chemotactic factors: enhancement by bacterial endotoxin. Federation Proceedings 45: 7–12

Yamamori H, Tashiro T, Mashima Y, Okui K 1987 Effects of severity of surgical trauma on whole body protein turnover in patients receiving total parenteral nutrition. Journal of Parenteral and Enteral Nutrition 11: 454–457

Yellin S A, Nguyen D, Quinn J V, Burchard K W, Crowley J P, Slotman G J 1986 Prostacyclin and thromboxane A_2 in septic shock: species differences. Circulatory Shock 20: 291–297

Yurt R W, McManus A T, Mason A D, Pruitt B A 1984 Increased susceptibility to infection related to extent of burn injury. Archives of Surgery 119: 183–188

6

Peptic ulcer haemorrhage

K. E. WHEATLEY and M. R. B. KEIGHLEY

Upper gastrointestinal bleeding from peptic ulceration remains a major clinical problem, accounting for over 15 000 admissions per annum in the UK (Salmon 1986) and between 1 and 2% of all medical and surgical admissions in the USA (Pingleton 1987). Overall mortality rates of over 10% are regularly reported in the literature (Clason et al 1986), and the operative mortality rates range from 10 to 35% (Madden & Griffith 1986). Within specialist units these mortality rates can be substantially reduced to less than 5% for overall deaths and less than 10% for operative deaths (Hunt et al 1983, Rofe et al 1985) by means of aggressive surgical management and modern conservative methods, although this centralised approach has been criticised by some (Dronfield 1987). Fibroptic endoscopy is accepted as the major diagnostic modality, but the selection of patients for surgery and the type of operation employed are still subject to controversy. The role of pharmaceutical agents is also open to question, despite many drug trials. During the last decade, various per-endoscopic therapeutic techniques have evolved. Although the Nd:YAG laser is associated with a reduction in rebleeding rates, the place of laser therapy is not defined. Hence for most patients with life-threatening upper gastrointestinal bleeding, surgical control of the bleeding vessel is the only definitive therapy.

In this chapter we will concentrate on the indications for emergency surgery in bleeding peptic ulcer disease, the timing of this surgery, and the type of operation performed. Complications from surgery will be reviewed. Factors associated with high risk of rebleeding and with death will be outlined.

Presentation and the role of endoscopy

Upper GI haemorrhage from peptic ulceration presents acutely as haematemesis and melaena. Bright red PR bleeding may be due to upper GI causes but requires rapid blood loss of 500–1000 ml (Pingleton 1987). Peptic ulceration usually accounts for about 50% of all acute admissions with upper GI haemorrhage, duodenal ulcers being more common than gastric ulcers (Schiller et al 1970). There is often a pre-existing history of dyspepsia, but in our experience nearly one-third of patients have no dyspeptic history, or have had symptoms for less than a week. Over 30% of our patients with ulceration are taking non-steroidal anti-inflammatory medication at the time of admission, a similar proportion to that in other series (Somerville et al 1986). Haematemesis may be obvious enough, but it is important to differentiate melaena from lower GI bleeding and black faeces secondary to iron administration. Melaena has a characteristic appearance and odour and implies a source of bleeding proximal to the ileocaecal valve. Clues to the source of the bleeding may be obtained from assessment of the patient, e.g. previous history of duodenal ulcer, or anti-inflammatory drug therapy, but history is unreliable and diagnosis is dependent on skilled endoscopy.

It is especially important to assess the patient's cardiorespiratory status, as cardiorespiratory failure is a major determinant of death and can markedly affect the management of the patient. Initial assessment of haemoglobin is necessary, but because of haemodilution it may give a misleading picture. Blood urea levels may be a useful guide to the source of GI bleeding (Mailer et al 1965). Recent work by Snook et al (1986) has demonstrated that the admission plasma urea-to-creatinine ratio may be an even more sensitive guide, particularly in clinically difficult cases of GI bleeding, a ratio of over 100 being strongly associated with an upper GI cause and a lower ratio with a lower GI lesion. It is our practice to cross-match patients with a clinically significant bleed for a minimum of four units of whole blood.

All patients presenting with an upper GI bleed require an upper GI endoscopy. Other investigations such as barium meal or angiography are required in less than 5% of our patients and are always second-line procedures. Endoscopy may need to be repeated on one or more occasions to obtain a diagnosis, especially if the initial view is obscured by blood or gastric contents (Cotton et al 1973). Nevertheless, the initial endoscopy will nearly always give information about the site of bleeding. Endoscopy has been shown to be more accurate than barium meal for diagnosis, with a yield of 85% or more in several series (Stevenson et al 1976, Zambertas et al 1982). Although this figure can be approached by double-contrast barium meal in the best hands, as in the study by Stevenson et al (1976), endoscopy has the great advantage of being able to identify the actual source of bleeding in most cases and provide important prognostic information (Foster et al 1978). Important causes of blood loss other than ulceration include gastro-oesophageal varices, severe gastritis with erosions and mucosal tears. In some cases these disorders may coexist. Endoscopy in experienced hands can be very accurate, and figures from our own unit indicate a diagnostic accuracy of 95% in patients ultimately requiring surgery or necroscopy in whom the actual cause of blood loss could be verified (Morris 1983). In patients with GI haemorrhage, there is a small risk from endoscopy of aspiration pneumonia and cardiovascular emergencies. A large series of over 2300 endoscopies performed in patients with acute upper GI haemorrhage, however, showed an overall complication rate of 0.9%, of which only half were judged to be potentially serious, e.g. perforation, aspiration and haemorrhage. Only two deaths were attributable to the endoscopy, an incidence of 0.09% (Gilbert et al 1981). However, it is import-

ant to bear the potential risks of endoscopy in mind when assessing the role and timing of these procedures.

Risk factors for rebleeding and mortality

It has been known for three decades, since the work of Avery Jones (1956), that rebleeding is the most important single factor adversely affecting prognosis: it increases the risk of death by about 12 times (Clason et al 1986). Mortality is also dependent on age, with few deaths recorded in patients under 60 years, and the presence of shock on admission (Hunt 1987). Concurrent disease, especially cardiorespiratory problems and pre-existing anaemia, is also an important risk factor (Hunt 1987), but it is very hard to quantify the contribution of this factor. Peptic ulcer bleeding carries a mortality risk that is much lower than either variceal bleeding or bleeding from gastric and oesophageal carcinomas, but because it is a much commoner condition it is responsible for a large percentage of GI bleeding deaths as shown in a 6-year audit from our own unit (Table 6.1).

Table 6.1: 1001 admissions with upper GI bleeding at The General Hospital, Birmingham, 1980–1986

Diagnosis	Admissions	Deaths	Mortality rate, %
Varices	67	32	48
Carcinomas	41	16	39
Duodenal ulcers	359	15	4
Gastric ulcers	188	11	6
(Total peptic ulcer	547	26	4.8)
Oesophagitis	85	0	0
Mallory-Weiss	47	1	2
Others	119	4	3
No diagnosis	95	2	2
Total	1001	81	8

Peptic ulcers were responsible for 32% of the deaths from upper GI haemorrhage, with carcinoma and varices being responsible for another 59%. Despite the increased prevalence of varices in some large series, peptic ulceration is still a major cause of mortality from upper GI haemorrhage. Other causes of bleeding such as oesophagitis, erosions and tears, generally carry a very low mortality.

Rebleeding

It is perhaps more logical to concentrate on risk factors for rebleeding, as it is in this area that therapeutic intervention can have the greatest effect in reducing the risk of death. Independent factors for the prediction of rebleeding have been established from regression analyses of clinical series. Age over 60 was identified by Clason et al (1986) and Brearley et al (1987b), although Hunt (1987) and Northfield (1971) found no effect of age on rebleeding. Gastric rather than duodenal ulceration, shock or anaemia on admission and certain stigmata of recent haemorrhage seen at endoscopy have been consistently reported as good predictive factors of increased rebleeding rates (Wara 1985, Hunt 1987, Clason et al 1986, Brearley et al 1987a, b). Important stigmata include a spurting vessel seen at endoscopy, the 'visible vessel' and adherent clot, which carry risks of rebleeding of 80–100%, 50% and about 25% respectively (Foster et al 1978, Cotton et al 1973, Storey et al 1981). Black or red spots alone appear to carry no increased risk of rebleeding. Per-endoscopic Doppler techniques have been shown by Beckly and Casebow (1986) to increase the accuracy of predicting rebleeding but have not become widely used. Conversely, the risk of rebleeding in the absence of these stigmata is small, of the order of 5%.

It has not been shown that endoscopy per se has any beneficial effect on mortality rates (Stevenson et al 1976, Dronfield et al 1982, Peterson et al 1981), and it does carry a small risk of its own. Nevertheless, endoscopy has an important role in defining the optimum management of patients with bleeding peptic ulcers. Rational treatment demands accurate, early diagnosis. The timing of endoscopy may be controversial, but most units would recommend that it is performed within 24 h of admission, as the yield of prognostic information usually diminishes after that time (Bown et al 1981, Nilsson & Wahlberg 1981). If endoscopic therapy is to be employed, it must be performed as soon as possible after adequate resuscitation of the patient. Patients at high risk of dying may also require endoscopy somewhat earlier than younger and fitter patients, because they may need earlier surgical intervention.

Conservative management

About 70–80% of peptic ulcers stop bleeding spontaneously (Schiller et al 1970) and do not therefore require any urgent surgical intervention, although a small proportion of patients may have an indication for later, elective, surgery. Only about 5% of patients will require immediate operation to control exsanguinating haemorrhage, and only 20–25% will require urgent surgery for continued or recurrent haemorrhage, usually within 48 h of admission (Hunt 1987). Thus conservative management is the mainstay of treatment for the majority of patients, and most patients ultimately requiring surgery will be offered an initial period of conservative management.

There is debate as to whether patients are better managed in special GI bleeding 'units', on general wards, or even in intensive therapy units. There is no agreement as to whether patients should be admitted initially under the care of surgeons or physicians. The best results reported in the literature come from centres with these special 'units' (Murray et al 1986, Hunt et al 1979, 1983), where there is close cooperation between gastroenterologists and surgeons. As long as cooperation and communication are good, it seems fatuous to argue over the type of specialist in overall change, as both groups have an important input in the care of the patient. Hunt and others (1979) aptly stated when commenting on improved mortality figures: 'Possibly the most important factor has been the formation of a unit with a combined medical and surgical approach in which patients are cared for by the same personnel familiar with all aspects of upper GI haemorrhage'. Dronfield (1987) criticizes this approach because of the small numbers of patients seen at any one time in a particular hospital. We admit all patients with acute upper gastrointestinal bleeding to a designated gastroenterology ward with up to four beds set aside for the management of patients with gastrointestinal bleeding. We do not use a high dependency ward or an intensive care unit, except for the most seriously ill patients and those with very limited cardiac reserve; such patients are admitted direct to the intensive therapy unit and represent less than 10% of our admissions. Cotton & Russell (1977), on the other hand, believe that all patients with severe bleeding should be admitted to an intensive care unit for 2–3 days.

Resuscitation is the cornerstone of successful management. Restoration of circulating blood volume with colloid solutions and whole blood should be performed as soon as possible after admission. In most patients, fluid requirements can be assessed accurately enough by simple clinical observations such as pulse rate, blood pressure, urine output and assessment of the peripheral circulation. Blair and others (1986) have suggested that blood transfusion can increase the risks of rebleeding by affecting systemic thrombolytic activity, but we believe that the known benefits of rapid restoration of blood volume to maintain adequate tissue perfusion outweigh any theoretical disadvantages of transfusion. Devitt et al (1966) showed that delayed or inadequate blood transfusion was a major factor in 88% of deaths associated with upper gastrointestinal haemorrhage. On the other hand, unnecessary transfusion or overtransfusion is a practice to be disparaged, both in view of the undesirable effects on the cardiovascular system and the possibility of transmitting infection or antibody production rendering further transfusion more difficult. In our unit, patients are transfused if they show clinical signs of hypovolaemia and for anaemia if the haemoglobin level is below 10 g/dl. Some centres routinely employ invasive monitoring for patients who are shocked on admission, using central venous pressure monitoring or even a Swann-Ganz catheter in patients with established cardiorespiratory disease. Raimes & Venables (1987) believe that central venous pressure monitoring is an essential guide to volume replacement, although they do recognize its limitations. In practice central venous pressure readings can be difficult to interpret and can lead to overtransfusion despite a normal blood volume. Our practice is therefore to reserve invasive monitoring for the few patients (less than 10% of admissions) who have severely compromised myocardial func-

tion. We also believe that such patients require intensive care nursing. In our experience, the more invasive monitoring techniques, such as pulmonary wedge pressure measurements, are seldom if ever needed.

Pharmacological therapy

The place of pharmacological therapy is unclear. It is usual to prescribe anti-ulcer therapy, usually in the form of H2 receptor antagonists, although there is very little definite evidence from single studies that they are of value. In an analysis of several published trials, Collins & Langman (1985) suggested that H2 receptor antagonists might reduce the rate of rebleeding by 10% and the need for surgical intervention by 20%. It was even suggested that mortality rates might be reduced by 30%. It is difficult to derive useful clinical information when the data have been culled from 27 trials, and we believe that the place of these agents is still uncertain. From a comprehensive review of the American literature, Pingleton (1987) suggests that H2 receptor antagonists may confer moderate protection against rebleeding, although she believes that their administration via infusion deserves further assessment.

Somatostatin and tranexamic acid have been extensively investigated in trials, but to date results are inconclusive. Using a longer-acting analogue, somatostatin was found to reduce rebleeding in a small trial reported by Christiansen & Yotis (1986). A recent well-designed study from Spain also appeared to support its use in bleeding peptic ulcer disease (Torres et al 1986). There have been six important trials to assess the use of tranexamic acid in the last 15 years. Results are difficult to interpret because of the different design of the studies, but Cormack et al (1973), Biggs et al (1976) and Stael von Holstein et al (1987) all demonstrated a reduction in blood transfusion requirements, and the latter two studies also reported a reduced operation rate in the treated group (Table 6.2). Two further studies (Engqvist et al 1979, Bergqvist et al 1980) failed to confirm these findings, but Barer et al (1983), in a large study involving over 700 patients, demonstrated a significantly reduced mortality rate with tranexamic acid yet no difference in transfusion requirements or need for surgery. As far as rebleeding is concerned, only one trial (Biggs et al 1976) was able to show a significant decrease amongst patients receiving tranexamic acid. Both somatostatin and tranexamic acid require further evaluation, therefore.

Table 6.2   Effect of tranexamic acid on rebleeding rates

Authors		Rebleeding rates, %	
		Controls	Treated group
Cormack et al[1]	1973	27	20 n.s.
Biggs et al[1]	1976	19	7 p<0.005
Engqvist et al[2]	1979	40	30 n.s.
Bergqvist et al[2]	1980	18	18 n.s.
Barer et al	1983	20	24 n.s.
Stael von Holstein et al	1987	26	17 n.s.

[1] Rebleeding rate includes continued bleeding
[2] Rebleeding rates estimated from number of patients requiring surgery in first 48 h.
n.s. = not significant

Published reports using prostaglandins give equivocal results (Levine et al 1985, Lauritsen et al 1985). At the present time, no pharmacological preparation has consistently been associated with a reduced incidence of rebleeding, a lower operation rate, or a significantly reduced mortality rate. Nevertheless, it still seems prudent to initiate ulcer-curative therapy as early as possible, using an H2 receptor antagonist. Other agents must still be regarded as experimental and should probably not be used outside the confines of a clinical trial.

Endoscopic therapy

Endoscopic therapy aimed at reducing rebleeding is still not widely available throughout Europe or North America. Swain et al (1986) have demonstrated that therapy with the Nd:YAG laser can significantly reduce the incidence of further bleeding and thus the need for surgery. Laser therapy requires an initial capital outlay, and some ulcers (at least 10%) are inaccessible for endoscopic treatment. There are claims that laser therapy is cost-effective; nevertheless many gastroenterologists consider that it has limited application in the near future. The use of the Nd:YAG laser is expanding at a rapid rate in the USA, from three centres in 1979 to over 300 in 1985, despite the lack of convincing evidence that it is cost-effective or clinically efficacious (Fleischer 1986). Kiefhaber et al (1986) were able to publish their experience with the Nd:YAG laser in over 1000 patients and claimed remarkable efficacy for control of bleeding and prevention of rebleeding, but unfortunately they had no non-treated patients for comparison.

Other methods of endoscopic therapy have not been shown to reduce rebleeding. Bipolar diathermy coagulation has been associated with equivocal effects on rebleeding rates in clinical trials (Brearley et al 1987a, Kernohan et al 1984, O'Brien et al 1986, Laine 1987). On the other hand, injection sclerotherapy around the bleeding vessel may prove more effective, and preliminary results suggest a reduction in rebleeding rates (Panes et al 1987). The heater probe may reduce rebleeding, but is probably inferior to Nd:YAG laser therapy (Matthewson et al 1987). Other endoscopic techniques such as application of clips or use of topical vasoactive agents must be regarded as purely experimental (Hajiro et al 1986).

Indications for emergency surgery

It is important to differentiate emergency or urgent surgery, required to save life, from elective treatment of peptic ulceration. Elective surgery may be indicated for patients presenting with upper GI bleeding, particularly if there is a previous history of peptic ulceration and even more so if there have been previous episodes of bleeding due to peptic ulceration. Decisions to undertake a prophylactic operation are usually deferred until the risk of rebleeding from the ulcer is negligible and the patient is in optimum condition for surgery. By contrast, emergency surgery is required to stem life-threatening haemorrhage, often amongst very unfit, elderly and ill-prepared patients, who carry a high risk of complications and death (Table 6.3). It is largely the increasing age of patients with peptic ulceration that is responsible for the unchanged mortality rates from bleeding peptic ulcers over the last three decades, despite advances in medical management, anaesthesia and surgery (Swain et al 1986).

Table 6.3: Relationship between increase in age of patients and mortality from upper GI haemorrhage in different centres.

Author	Centre	Period	Mortality %	% of patients over 60 years
Bulmer 1927, 1932	Birmingham	1926–1931	22	6
Lewin & Truelove 1949	Oxford	1938–1947	19	28
Schiller et al 1970	Oxford	1953–1967	7	47
Allan & Dykes 1976	Birmingham	1970–1973	10	48
Hunt et al 1979	Melbourne	1972–1977	13	40
Hunt et al 1983	Melbourne	1977–1982	6	55
Clason et al 1986	Bangor	1980–1983	12	56
Present authors	Birmingham	1983–1987	8	60

Although indications for surgery and the timing of operation may be considered separately for many conditions, we believe that in upper GI bleeding both aspects are interrelated. The aim of emergency surgical intervention is to save life by controlling blood loss, cure of the ulcer and prevention of further ulceration being of secondary importance. The problem, however, is to define when bleeding is life-threatening, when a patient can safely be managed conservatively and when conservative therapy has failed. In considering these factors, risk factors for mortality play a major role in surgical decision-making. It follows that surgery will mainly be required for the control of rebleeding, especially in elderly patients and those with concomitant disease. Surgery is of course required for control of exsanguinating haemorrhage, but this leaves the question of how much bleeding is a risk to life, i.e. at what point does surgical intervention become essential? Most deaths in this condition are not in fact due to exsanguination (Allan & Dykes 1976), but rather to cardiovascular complications associated with

impaired tissue perfusion following major haemorrhage, e.g. myocardial infarction, cerebrovascular accidents and pulmonary emboli. It is therefore important to intervene before bleeding is sufficient to cause these problems. It is generally accepted that mortality is substantially increased in older patients who require transfusion with more than 3 or 4 units, because of poor cardiac reserve and a reduced ability to cope with rapid blood volume changes (Devitt et al 1966). We believe that transfusion requirements in excess of 3 units of blood indicate the need for urgent surgical intervention in patients over the age of 60 years. Younger patients on the other hand can tolerate larger transfusions, hence it is reasonable to delay operative intervention in this group, particularly to reduce the incidence of unnecessary emergency operations.

The exact indications for surgery in bleeding peptic ulcer (PU) disease remain controversial. Murray (1986) commented that 'A reduction in overall mortality from PU haemorrhage has been associated with: no change in the incidence of surgery, a reduction in the incidence of surgery and an increased incidence of surgery.' Should operations be performed before or after rebleeding has occurred? The difficulty here lies in predicting the natural history of rebleeding in a particular patient. For instance, if a visible vessel is seen in an ulcer base, we expect about half of these patients to sustain a further bleed (Storey et al 1981). A blanket policy to operate on all elderly patients with a visible vessel would result in a large number of unnecessary emergency operations. On the other hand waiting, until patients have a second bleed may carry the risk of death from hypotension and impaired tissue perfusion as a result of a further major haemorrhage. The only group definitely requiring early intervention are those in whom a spurting vessel is seen at endoscopy. Almost all of these patients will rebleed, and some form of immediate therapy is therefore indicated. In some centres this may be possible using some form of endoscopic therapy, but for most patients surgery will be the only option available.

Optimum timing of surgery

In 1980 we mounted a trial to investigate the optimum timing of operative intervention for bleeding peptic ulcers in this unit (Morris et al 1984). Patients were grouped into those above and below the age of 60 years and were randomized to receive either early or delayed operative intervention according to the following precisely defined criteria.

Early surgery

4 units blood or plasma expander required to correct acute blood loss in 24 h.
One rebleed
Endoscopic SRH (active bleeding, visible vessel, adherent clot, spots)
Previous upper GI haemorrhage plus two year history of dyspepsia

Late surgery

8 units blood or plasma expander required to correct acute blood loss in 24 h.
Two rebleeds in hospital
Persistent bleeding requiring transfusion of 12 units/48 h

In younger patients earlier operation was not found to have any advantages, and an operation rate of 50% in the early group was thought to be excessive, but in the older group mortality was significantly lower in patients receiving early surgery, being 5% compared with 15% in patients having delayed surgery. We adopted these criteria for all patients following the trial and have continued to audit our admissions. Since 1983, however, we have removed the presence of stigmata of recent haemorrhage alone as an indication for surgery, with no adverse effect on mortality rate and a significant reduction in operation rates. Our revised criteria for early operation in patients over 60 years of age are given below.

Transfusion requirement of more than 3 units blood or colloid for volume replacement
Spurting vessel bleeding seen at endoscopy
One rebleed in hospital
Continued slow ooze

We have therefore maintained a consistently low overall mortality and operative mortality over these four years (Table 6.4). Further work from

Table 6.4 Outcome of patients admitted with bleeding peptic ulcer disease to the General Hospital Birmingham, 1984–1987

Age group	No. of admissions	Deaths	Operations	Operative mortality
Under 60 y	124	1 (1%)	17 (14%)	1 (6%)
Over 60 y	183	11 (6%)	50 (27%)	1 (2%)
Total	307	12 (4%)	67 (22%)	2 (3%)

this department by Brearley et al (1987b) has produced a formula for the selection of patients for surgery, based upon a regression analysis of risk factors for rebleeding. This formula identifies the following parameters as risk factors for rebleeding: 1. age; 2. endoscopic stigmata; 3. transfusion requirements; 4. past history; and 5. haemoglobin levels at admission. While application of this formula seems to accurately predict the patients requiring surgery, it is rather a cumbersome procedure and unlikely to produce any more benefit than more simple and conventional criteria. It may perhaps have greater application in units with comparatively little experience in GI haemorrhage, rather than the more specialist departments. Other units, however, have reported low mortality rates using much less aggressive policies, albeit with small numbers of patients (Rofe et al 1985). Progressively lower operation rates have been a feature of many series in the last decade, with no apparent deleterious effect on mortality (Vellacott et al 1982). Nevertheless, we believe that operative mortality rates can be kept below 10% using an aggressive surgical policy in older patients.

Type of surgery

Duodenal ulceration

Over the last decade Proximal Gastric Vagotomy (PGV) has become the preferred elective operation for duodenal ulcers (DU). In many units truncal vagotomy with a drainage procedure (TV&P) has been relegated to emergency use for bleeding or perforation. Protagonists of PGV have also recommended its use for selected patients with bleeding duodenal ulcers, although it loses many, if not all, its advantages if the pyloric mechanism has to be destroyed to achieve control of bleeding. Although Johnston et al (1973) reported a series of 26 patients treated by this method with no deaths, there have been few reports of its use since then (Hoffman et al 1987). PGV in most hands is a more lengthy procedure, and unless performed meticulously by an experienced surgeon may be associated with a high rate of recurrent ulcer. For these reasons, TV&P combined with underrunning of the bleeding vessel remains the operation of choice in most cases (Venables 1981, Steger et al 1987). There remains a good case, however, for use of PGV and underrunning in younger and fitter patients who can withstand longer operative procedures, and in whom the adverse affects of TV&P may not be acceptable. For large duodenal ulcers a gastrectomy of the Polya type may be required both to control haemorrhage and to prevent rebleeding. In our experience (Table 6.5) this surgical option is indicated in about 15% cases, although Hunt (1985) finds this procedure necessary in up to a third of patients. It is also the safest method of controlling early rebleeding after a more conservative operation.

Table 6.5   Type of surgery for bleeding duodenal ulcer and outcome at The General Hospital Birmingham, 1984–1987

Procedure		Deaths	Rebleeds
Vagotomy and pyloroplasty	20	0	1
Underrunning alone	4	0	0
Highly selective vagotomy	1	0	1
Polya gastrectomy	4	0	0
Vagotomy and antrectomy	3	0	0
Total	32	0	2

A recent development in surgical management for high risk patients is that of simply controlling bleeding by underrunning the bleeding vessel alone, without performing any definitive procedure. Ulcer healing is then achieved by administration of H2 receptor antagonists. Ideally underrunning can be performed via a duodenotomy, thus leaving the pylorus intact, but the pyloric mechanism may have to be divided to obtain sufficient access to the ulcer base. This approach has the advantage of being relatively simple, quick, and within the compass of most junior surgeons in training. Limiting the length of the operations probably minimizes the postoper-

ative morbidity, and the avoidance of vagotomy, pyloric division or gastrectomy probably prevents diarrhoea, dumping, bile vomiting and long-term metabolic sequelae. Against this, however, is the need for continued anti-ulcer therapy, possibly for life, with the risk of ulcer relapse in noncompliant patients, and the potentially higher risk of early rebleeding necessitating further operative intervention. These fears must be tempered by the knowledge that over 30% of patients with bleeding peptic ulcers in the UK take non-steroidal anti-inflammatory drugs: an ulcer history is often lacking and it is presumed that many ulcers are drug-induced. Under these circumstances an operation to prevent peptic ulceration may be unnecessary. Underrunning of the vessel with medical ulcer therapy has mainly been reserved for patients at extremely high risk from any surgery (Dronfield et al 1979) and has not been studied in fitter patients.

Mortality rates for all types of surgery vary very widely in the literature from 5 to 30% for TV&P and 5 to 35% for less radical surgery. Venables (1981) reviewed several series of standard operative procedures and found an average mortality of 13% for gastric ulcer and 10% for duodenal ulcer, which seemed independent of whether a gastric resection or a vagotomy had been performed. Little information is available on the mortality rate or long-term results of underrunning the vessel alone. Many of the differences between series must be due to the selection of patients, and little useful information can be drawn from the literature. A randomized trial to compare conventional surgery with the conservative approach of merely underrunning the vessel with defined preoperative criteria seems essential before any definite recommendations can be made.

Gastric ulceration

The standard operation for a bleeding gastric ulcer (GU) has been gastrectomy, usually of the Billroth 1 type (Rogers et al 1988). This is associated with a low risk of rebleeding, low risk of ulcer recurrence, and in good hands a low mortality rate (Herrington & Davidson 1987). However, since many operations for bleeding gastric ulcers are performed on high-risk elderly patients, often by comparatively inexperienced surgeons, gastrectomy can carry a very high morbidity and a mortality rate of well over 20% (Rogers et al 1988). Furthermore, high gastric ulcers may present technical difficulties if treated by partial gastrectomy. Largely for these reasons, rather than any doubts of its effectiveness in achieving haemostasis and cure, the practice of gastrectomy has been diminishing over recent years, and truncal vagotomy with excision of the ulcer or underrunning of the vessel and biopsy, combined with a drainage procedure, has become more widely used (Rogers et al 1988). Partial gastrectomy may have the advantage of adequately treating unsuspected gastric carcinomas at the initial operation (Hunt et al 1982), but the standard Billroth 1 procedure is not regarded as an adequate resection for malignancy. In any event, the prognosis for bleeding malignancies is very poor (Allum et al 1989).

PGV probably has little to offer for bleeding gastric ulcers. Underrunning and biopsy or excision of ulcer without any attempt at an ulcer-curative procedure have in the past been reserved for high-risk patients, but more recently some units have been advocating a more widespread use of this approach. Early results from Rogers et al in Glasgow (1988) have been impressive, with an operative mortality rate of 10% for underrunning alone, compared with 26% for partial gastrectomy and the very high figure of 45% for vagotomy and underrunning. This was an uncontrolled report using these different approaches over eight years, which may account for the reported differences in mortality rate. Over the last five years we have become increasingly conservative in the surgical treatment of bleeding gastric ulcer, and currently over two-thirds of patients will not receive a gastrectomy (Table 6.6). We believe that this helps to account for our low operative mortality rate. Again, a controlled trial of the traditional approach and more conservative procedures is required to answer this question more definitely.

The operative approach in the USA to bleeding peptic ulcers is very different from that in the UK. A recent comprehensive review of surgical strategy for bleeding peptic ulceration (Herrington &

Table 6.6 Type of surgery for bleeding gastric ulcer and outcome at The General Hospital Birmingham, 1984–1987.

Procedure		Deaths	Rebleeds
Partial gastrectomy	14	0	0
Underrunning/excision with vagotomy	13	1	0
Underrunning/excision alone	8	1	0
Total	35	2	0

Davidson 1987) recommended Billroth 1 gastrectomy for both bleeding DU and bleeding GU, reserving TV&P for extremely high-risk patients, and saw little if any place for less aggressive operations. This approach may be based on the fear of early rebleeding and ulcer recurrence leading to malpractice litigation, as well as the continued cost of medical therapy for ulcer healing and prevention.

Postoperative complications

Wound infection and dehiscence

Wound infection is quite common after surgery for upper GI bleeding. In our experience it occurs in about 10% of patients, despite the use of prophylactic antimicrobial agents (usually a cephalosporin). Wound infection probably remains a common problem due to the altered gastric flora in patients with bleeding peptic ulcers (Gatehouse et al 1978) and the fact that many patients are elderly and in poor general condition from disease or malnutrition. Haemorrhage itself can also adversely affect the mechanisms of wound healing, predisposing to sepsis (Taylor et al 1987, Stephan et al 1987). With modern methods of closure, wound dehiscence is an uncommon problem after any abdominal operation, and we have not seen a single case following upper GI haemorrhage over the last seven years.

Anastomotic breakdown major intra-abdominal sepsis

Anastomotic breakdown is a serious problem, carrying an extremely high mortality rate. It is very uncommon after TV&P, but is a well-known complication of gastrectomy, particularly at the gastroduodenal anastomosis in a Billroth 1 procedure. Major intra-abdominal sepsis is fortunately rare, but may be seen after breakdown of an anastomosis or leakage from the duodenal stump after a Polya gastrectomy. We have not seen major sepsis in our last 67 cases. These problems can be minimized by confining operations to experienced surgeons and by avoidance of gastrectomy in favour of non-resectional surgery. If the duodenal stump is difficult to close after Polya gastrectomy, it is wise to insert a duodenostomy tube into the second part of the mobilized duodenum, which is sutured to the abdominal wall at the exit site of the tube prior to closure of the abdomen.

Recurrent haemorrhage

The figures available in the literature on this topic are difficult to interpret. The reported rates following TV&P are 5–26% and following gastrectomy 8–33% (Venables 1981). These ranges are enormous and must reflect both inclusion of patients with gastric erosions and poor surgical technique. We have seen 2 cases of recurrent haemorrhage following non-resectional surgery in our last 46 cases (4%) and none following gastrectomy. Both these rebleeds were from duodenal ulcers: one settled with conservative management, the other required a Polya gastrectomy. In the last four years we have had no postoperative rebleeds in 21 patients receiving non-resectional surgery for GU. The mortality rate from recurrent bleeding is generally accepted to be about 30%.

Cardiovascular complications

Myocardial infarction, pulmonary embolism, cerebrovascular accidents and cardiac failure secondary to ischaemic heart disease are amongst the most serious postoperative problems and are important causes of death (Allan & Dykes 1976). In our series, one of our two postoperative deaths in the last four years was in a patient who developed a perioperative cerebral thrombosis. We feel that our policy of early surgery in older

patients is responsible for the low mortality rate from cardiovascular causes, and prophylactic heparin may have helped to prevent any patients developing a pulmonary embolus in this time. However, we still see a 10–15% incidence of postoperative cardiac failure in patients with ischaemic heart disease.

Respiratory complications

The commonest postoperative complication in our unit is chest infection, which occurs in almost one-third of our patients, due to a combination of the frequency of pre-existing pulmonary disease and an upper abdominal operation. Chest infection and respiratory failure caused our other postoperative death during the last four years, occurring in a patient with severe ankylosing spondylitis who had been turned down for elective surgery because of his cardiorespiratory status. Most cases will respond satisfactorily to physiotherapy with or without antibiotics, but a few cases require assisted ventilation and, on occasion, tracheostomy.

Renal failure

Acute tubular necrosis is well recognized as a complication of massive haemorrhage, and many patients requiring surgery have pre-existing renal impairment. Fortunately, this complication is uncommon with modern resuscitation techniques, but it still occurs from time to time and haemodialysis will be required until the kidneys recover. We have only seen one case from the last 67 patients undergoing surgery, with an ultimately satisfactory outcome after a period of dialysis.

Other acute complications

Jaundice is a well recognized complication of operation for bleeding ulcer, either as a result of major sepsis or related to haemolysis. Small rises in postoperative bilirubin are commonly seen, but a clinically important degree of jaundice is rare in our practice.

Disseminated intravascular coagulation related

to either sepsis or haemorrhage is another serious (though uncommon) problem affecting patients postoperatively. We have not seen a case following operation for bleeding peptic ulcer, possibly because we have tried to avoid the need for massive transfusion.

Long-term complications

The long-term adverse effects of both truncal vagotomy and gastrectomy have been well described. They include dumping, bile vomiting, diarrhoea, nutritional deficiencies, metabolic sequelae and, in the case of a partial gastrectomy, the possible risk of malignancy. We believe these factors provide further reasons to avoid vagotomy, resection and pyloric division if feasible and safe.

Management of peptic ulcer bleeding at The General Hospital, Birmingham

Over the last decade we have evolved a policy for the management of bleeding peptic ulcers, associated with a very low overall mortality rate, an acceptable rate for operative intervention and a low postoperative mortality rate. There are many facets to this policy. We believe that no one factor is responsible for these good results — rather, that the combination of the many features is important. Some features have already been mentioned, but they will all be listed here for convenience. We believe that wider adoption of these methods could reduce by at least 50% the number of patients dying from bleeding peptic ulcers, with little or no extra costs in equipment or nursing or medical care, and little or no need for extra training.

1. *All patients are admitted under the care of the receiving medical and surgical teams of the day.* We do not have a policy of only admitting such patients under the care of medical or surgical gastroenterologists, as we feel it is important that all junior doctors should be experienced in the care of this condition. Both medical and surgical

skills are required for many of these patients, and both groups of doctors should be involved.

2. *All patients are referred early to the on-call endoscopist*, who forms part of the team responsible for subsequent patient management. Only endoscopists with specific training and experience in this area are involved, as we believe that emergency endoscopy is a more difficult procedure than elective endoscopy.

3. *Early endoscopy is performed.* Virtually all patients admitted with an upper GI bleed are endoscoped within 24 h of admission, and any patient who has had a major bleed with haemodynamic disturbance is investigated as soon as their condition allows. Endoscopy is normally performed in the endoscopy unit, but if the condition of the patient is critical, it can be carried out in the intensive therapy unit or in the operating theatre immediately prior to surgical intervention. A small percentage of our admissions proceed directly to operation because bleeding is too vigorous to allow time for endoscopy. This eventuality accounts for only 1–2% of all admissions with bleeding peptic ulcers.

4. *Admission to designated ward.* We believe that the best results are obtained when these patients are cared for in a specific area of a ward, with nurses experienced in looking after such cases and especially in the early recognition of rebleeding.

5. *Strict criteria for timing of surgical intervention.* Based on the results of our earlier trial, we have adopted the criteria laid down in the trial except that we no longer use stigmata of recent haemorrhage as an indication in the older age group. These criteria are adhered to as far as possible, but it must be admitted that it can be difficult to decide whether a patient requires 3 or 4 units of blood/colloid to restore circulatory volume on clinical grounds. If there is doubt, we would tend to opt for surgical rather than conservative management. The actual type of operation is left up to the surgeon, but there is a

trend towards less radical operations, especially for gastric ulcers.

6. *Prophylactic heparin and antibiotics*. All patients undergoing surgery for GI haemorrhage receive subcutaneous heparin and intravenous antibiotics immediately before operation to reduce the likelihood of postoperative pulmonary embolus and wound infection. In the last five years, we have only had one postoperative death from pulmonary embolism, and that occurred in a patient in whom the prophylactic heparin had been omitted because of an administrative error.

7. *Experienced surgeons and anaesthetists*. In our unit all operations on bleeding ulcers are performed by surgeons of senior registrar or consultant grade, with an anaesthetist of commensurate experience.

8. *Combined medical and surgical postoperative care*. As already mentioned, patients with a high risk of death are usually elderly with concomitant disease, and such problems require the involvement of both specialties for optimum results.

9. *Continuing audit*. All patients presenting with upper GI haemorrhage are presented each week to a combined medical/surgical gastroenterology meeting, and details are recorded in a prospective clinical audit. Management decisions can be rigorously examined, and problems of communication between medical and nursing staff are brought to light.

10. *Follow-up*. In past years follow-up of patients who have had bleeding from peptic ulcers has been far from ideal, and there is very little adequate information on this topic in the literature (Smart & Langman 1986, Murray et al 1986, Duggan 1986). We have recently established a separate follow-up clinic for all patients treated both conservatively and by operation, who have been admitted with bleeding peptic ulcers. We feel it is important to ensure ulcer healing in patients treated medically or in those who have received surgery for haemostasis only, and this requires endoscopic follow-up.

11. *Awareness and communication*. These two attributes of our overall management policies are the hardest to quantify and to establish, but they are crucially important. We feel that a large part of our success is due to the awareness of all doctors involved in care of such patients regarding potential clinical and management problems and policies. Overall results are presented to all medical staff on an annual basis, and all junior doctors are closely involved in care of patients with upper GI haemorrhage. The problems of communication cannot be overstated. Good communication between several doctors and nurses is a prerequisite of any successful management policy and can be the hardest objective to achieve and maintain. Constant reinforcement is required to ensure that communication between all the different personnel is satisfactory.

Future developments

In the future it is likely that more and more non-operative methods of haemostasis will be developed. Previous experience in many centres suggests that these techniques will be applied enthusiastically before there is any scientific evidence of their benefit to patients. Laser and electrocoagulation therapy are becoming more widely used despite their potential drawbacks and cost. Although trials indicate that rebleeding can be reduced by laser therapy, a great deal of specialized expertise must be generated to emulate these results. Other endoscopic techniques seem unlikely to contribute much to patient management in the next decade, and despite encouraging reports of their effectiveness have yet to prove themselves in controlled trials, although it is possible that injection sclerotherapy with submucosal adrenalin or sclerosants may find a place in the therapy of bleeding peptic ulcer disease.

Effective medical therapy which would reduce rebleeding would obviously be the greatest advance, as it would not require any great expertise to apply and would avoid the need for expensive equipment. It seems unlikely that newer H2 receptor antagonists will have any advantage over current medication, and neither tranexamic acid nor prostaglandin analogues seem likely to make a major impact, despite the recent successful trial of tranexamic acid. Of the currently available agents only somatostatin holds much promise (Dykes & Wheatley 1987), but again this is an expensive drug with difficulties associated with its administration.

The answer may come from research into why ulcers bleed in the first instance, and why only a percentage of them rebleed. This problem has received comparatively little attention in the past, particularly the question of whether any reversible factors are associated with rebleeding. At the cost of being accused of 'riding a hobby-horse', we would maintain that rebleeding may be associated with increased tryptic activity in gastric juice, a phenomenon that seems to be more common in bleeding ulcers than non-bleeding ulcers (Wheatley et al 1989). Prophylactic antitrypsin therapy with aprotinin may provide a pharmacological method of reducing rebleeding.

However, it still seems unlikely that any drug can substantially affect the chronically inflamed artery sitting in an ulcer base. Thus surgery is destined to remain the principle method of controlling massive or recurrent bleeding. We need to establish more precisely which patients require surgery and which can be safely managed conservatively, and which operations are the most effective at controlling bleeding with the lowest overall mortality rate and the lowest short- and long-term morbidity. Multicentre studies will be needed to achieve these aims, as single centres do not manage sufficient numbers of patients to allow comparisons of mortality with different therapeutic approaches. Young (1982), in a *BMJ* editorial, summed up the current situation very succinctly: 'The ordinary clinician managing persisting haemorrhage must pin his hopes not on modern technological advances but on efficient and prompt replacement of blood loss, early feeding, and skill in judging the appropriate moment for surgical intervention.

REFERENCES

Allan R N, Dykes P W 1976 A study of the factors influencing mortality rates from gastrointestinal haemorrhage. Quarterly Journal of Medicine 45: 533–550

Allum W H, Brearley S, Wheatley K E, Dykes P W, Keighley M R B 1989 Acute haemorrhage from gastric malignancy. In press

Barer D, Ogilvie A, Henry D et al 1983 Cimetidine and tranexamic acid in the treatment of acute upper-gastrointestinal-tract bleeding. New England Journal of Medicine 308: 1571–1575

Beckly D E, Casebow M P 1986 Prediction of rebleeding from peptic ulcer experience with an endoscopic Doppler device. Gut 27: 96–99

Bergqvist D, Dahlgren S, Hessman Y 1980 Local inhibition of the fibrinolytic system in patients with massive upper gastrointestinal haemorrhage. Upsala Journal of Medical Science 85: 173–178

Biggs J C, Hugh T B, Dodds A J 1976 Tranexamic acid and upper gastrointestinal haemorrhage — a double blind trial. Gut 17: 729–734

Blair S D, Janvrin S B, McCollum C N, Greenhalgh R M 1986 Effect of early blood transfusion on gastrointestinal haemorrhage. British Journal of Surgery 73: 783–785

Bown S G, Salmon P R, Brown P, Read A E 1981 Upper gastrointestinal haemorrhage. Journal of the Royal College of Physicians of London 15: 265–268

Brearley S, Hawker P C, Dykes P W, Keighley M R B 1987a Per-endoscopic bipolar diathermy coagulation of visible vessels using a 3.2 mm probe — a randomised clinical trial. Endoscope 19: 160–163

Brearley S, Hawker P C, Morris D L, Dykes P W D, Keighley M R B 1987b Selection of patients for surgery following peptic ulcer haemorrhage. British Journal of Surgery 74: 893–896

Bulmer E 1927 The mortality from haematemesis. Lancet ii: 168–171

Bulmer E 1932 Mortality from haematemesis. Lancet ii: 720–722

Christiansen J, Yotis A 1986 The role of somatostatin and a long-acting analogue, SMS 201–995, in acute bleeding due to peptic ulceration. Scandinavian Journal of Gastroenterology 21 (Suppl 119): 109–113

Clason A E, Macleod D A D, Elton R A 1986 Clinical factors in the prediction of further haemorrhage or mortality in acute upper gastrointestinal haemorrhage. British Journal of Surgery 73: 985–987

Collins R, Langman M 1985 Treatment with histamine H2 antagonists in acute upper gastrointestinal haemorrhage. New England Journal of Medicine 313: 660–666

Cormack F, Chakrabarti R R, Jouhar A J, Fearnley G R 1973 Tranexamic acid in upper gastrointestinal haemorrhage. Lancet i: 1207–1208

Cotton P B, Russell R C G 1977 Diseases of the alimentary system — haematemesis and melaena. British Medical Journal i: 37–39

Cotton P B, Rosenberg M T, Waldram R P L, Axon A T R 1973 Early endoscopy of oesophagus, stomach, and duodenal bulb in patients with haematemesis and melaena. British Medical Journal ii: 505–509

Devitt J E, Brown F N, Beattie W G 1966 Fatal bleeding ulcer. Annals of Surgery 164: 840–844

Dronfield M W 1987 Special units for acute upper gastrointestinal bleeding. British Medical Journal 294: 1308–1309

Dronfield M W, Atkinson M, Langman M J S 1979 Effect of different operation policies on mortality from bleeding peptic ulcer. Lancet i: 1126–1128

Dronfield M W, Langman M J S, Atkinson M et al 1982 Outcome of endoscopy and barium radiography for acute upper gastrointestinal bleeding: controlled trial in 1037 patients. British Medical Journal 284: 545–548

Duggan J M 1986 Ten year follow-up of gastrointestinal hemorrhage patients. Australia and New Zealand Journal of Medicine 16: 33–38

Dykes P W, Wheatley K E 1987 Acute gastrointestinal haemorrhage. Current Opinion in Gastroenterology 3: 1006–1014

Engqvist A, Bostrom O, Feilitzen F et al 1979 Tranexamic acid in massive haemorrhage from the upper gastrointestinal tract: a double blind study. Scandinavian Journal of Gastroenterology 14: 839–844

Fleischer D 1986 Endoscopic therapy of upper gastrointestinal bleeding in humans. Gastroenterology 90: 217–234

Foster D N, Miloszewski K J A, Losowsky M S 1978 Stigmata of recent haemorrhage in diagnosis and prognosis of upper gastrointestinal bleeding. British Medical Journal i: 1173–1177

Gatehouse D, Dimock F, Burdon D W, Alexander-Williams J, Keighley M R B 1978 Prediction of wound sepsis following gastric operations. British Journal of Surgery 65: 551–554

Gilbert D A, Silverstein F E, Tedesco F J 1981 National ASGE survey on upper gastrointestinal bleeding: complications of endoscopy. Digestive Diseases and Sciences 26 (July suppl): pp 55s–59s

Hajiro K, Matsui H, Tsujimura D 1986 Endoscopic hemostasis with hemoclips, local injection and other new techniques: The Japanese experience. Endoscopy 18: 62–67 (suppl 2)

Herrington J L, Davidson J R, III 1987 Bleeding gastroduodenal ulcers: choice of operations. World Journal of Surgery 11: 304–314

Hoffman J, Devantier A, Koelle T, Jensen H-E 1987 Parietal cell vagotomy as an emergency procedure for bleeding peptic ulcer. Annals of Surgery 206: 583–585

Hunt P S 1985 Surgical management of bleeding chronic peptic ulcer. In: Hunt P S (ed) Gastrointestinal Haemorrhage (Clinical Surgery International 11). Churchill Livingstone, Edinburgh, pp 37–46

Hunt P S 1987 Bleeding gastroduodenal ulcers: selection of patients for surgery. World Journal of Surgery 11: 289–294

Hunt P S, Hansky J, Korman M G 1979 Mortality in patients with haematemesis and melaena: a prospective study. British Medical Journal i: 1238–1240

Hunt P S, Hansky J, Korman M G 1982 Bleeding carcinomatous ulcer of the stomach. Medical Journal of Australia i: 494

Hunt P S, Francis J K, Hansky J et al 1983 Reduction in mortality from upper gastrointestinal haemorrhage. Medical Journal of Australia 2: 552–555

Johnston D, Lyndon P J, Smith R B, Humphrey C S 1973 Highly selective vagotomy without a drainage procedure in the treatment of haemorrhage, perforation and pyloric

stenosis due to peptic ulcer. British Journal of Surgery 60: 790–797

Jones F A 1956 Hematemesis and melena with special reference to causation and to the factors influencing the mortality from bleeding peptic ulcers. Gastroenterology 30: 166–190

Kernohan R M, Anderson J R, McKelvey S T D, Kennedy T L 1984 A controlled trial of bipolar electrocoagulation in patients with upper gastrointestinal bleeding. 1984 British Journal of Surgery 71: 889–891

Kiefhaber P, Kiefhaber K, Huber F, Nath G 1986 Endoscopic neodymium: YAG laser coagulation in gastrointestinal hemorrhage. Endoscopy 18: 46–51 (suppl 2)

Laine L 1987 Multipolar electrocoagulation in the treatment of active upper gastrointestinal haemorrhage. New England Journal of Medicine 316: 1613–1617

Lauritsen K, Laursen L S, Havelund T, Bytzer P, Rask-Madsen J 1985 Controlled trial of arbaprostil in bleeding peptic ulcer. British Medical Journal 291: 1093

Levine B A, Sirinek K R, Gaskill H V 1985 Topical prostaglandin E2 in the treatment of acute upper gastrointestinal hemorrhage. Archives of Surgery 120: 600–604

Lewin D C, Truelove S 1949 Haematemesis with special reference to chronic peptic ulcer. British Medical Journal i: 383–386

Madden M V, Griffith G H 1986 Management of upper gastrointestinal bleeding in a district general hospital. Journal of the Royal College of Physicians 20: 212–215

Mailer C, Goldberg A, Harden R M, Grey-Thomas I, Burnett W 1965 Diagnosis of upper gastrointestinal bleeding. British Medical Journal ii: 784–789

Matthewson K, Swain C P, Bland M et al 1987 A randomised comparison of Nd-YAG laser, heater probe and no endoscopic therapy for bleeding peptic ulcers. Gut 10: A1342

Morris D L 1983 Early or delayed surgery for gastrointestinal ulcer. M D thesis, University of Birmingham, p 43–45

Morris D L, Hawker P C, Brearley S, Simms M, Dykes P W, Keighley M R B 1984 Optimal timing of operation for bleeding peptic ulcer: prospective randomised trial. British Medical Journal 288: 1277–1280

Murray W R 1986 Surgical management of haemorrhage from peptic ulceration. British Journal of Surgery 73: 947–948

Murray W R, Laferla G, Cooper G, Archibald M 1986 Duodenal ulcer healing after presentation with haemorrhage. Gut 27: 1387–1389

Nilsson F, Wahlberg J 1981 Survival and emergency surgery in upper gastrointestinal bleeding. Acta Chirurgica Scandinavica 147: 555–559

Northfield T C 1971 Factors Predisposing to recurrent haemorrhage after acute gastrointestinal bleeding. British Medical Journal i: 26–28

O'Brien J D, Day S J, Burnham W R 1986 Controlled trial of small bipolar probe in bleeding peptic ulcers. Lancet i: 464–467

Panes J, Viver J, Forne M, Garcia-Olivares E, Marco C, Garau J 1987 Controlled trial of endoscopic sclerosis in bleeding peptic ulcers. Lancet ii: 1292–1294

Peterson W L, Barnett C, Smith H J, Allen M H, Corbett D 1981 Routine early endoscopy in upper-gastrointestinal-tract bleeding. New England Journal of Medicine 304: 925–929

Pingleton S K 1987 Recognition and management of upper

gastrointestinal hemorrhage. American Journal of Medicine 83 (Suppl 6a): 41–45

Raimes S A, Venables C W 1987 Acute upper gastrointestinal bleeding. Hospital Update 13: 669–684

Rofe S B, Duggan J M, Smith E R, Thursby C J 1985 Conservative treatment of gastrointestinal haemorrhage. Gut 26: 481–484

Rogers P N, Murray W R, Shaw R, Brar S 1988 Surgical management of bleeding gastric ulceration. British Journal of Surgery 75: 16–17

Salmon P R 1986 In: Lancaster Smith M J (ed) Peptic ulcer. Update-Sibert, London p 29–32

Schiller K F R, Truelove S C, Williams D G 1970 Haematemesis and melaena with special reference to factors influencing the outcome. British Medical Journal ii: 7–14

Smart H L, Langman M J S 1986 Late outcome of bleeding gastric ulcers. Gut 27: 926–928

Snook J A, Holdstock G E, Bamforth J 1986 Value of a simple biochemical ratio in distinguishing upper and lower sites of gastrointestinal haemorrhage. Lancet i: 1064–1065

Somerville K, Faulkner G, Langman M J S 1986 Non-steroidal anti-inflammatory drugs and bleeding peptic ulcer. Lancet i: 462–464

Stael von Holstein C C S, Eriksson S B S, Kallen R 1987 Tranexamic acid as an aid to reducing blood transfusion requirements in gastric and duodenal bleeding. British Medical Journal 294: 7–10

Steger A C, Galland R B, Spencer J 1987 Remaining indications for vagotomy with drainage or antrectomy in duodenal ulcer. Annals of the Royal College of Surgeons of England 68: 24–26

Stephan R N, Kupper T S, Geha A S, Baue A E, Chaudry I H 1987 Hemorrhage without tissue trauma produces immunosupression and enhances susceptibility to sepsis. Archives of Surgery 122: 62–68

Stevenson G W, Cox R R, Roberts C J C 1976 Prospective comparison of double-contrast barium meal examination and fibreoptic endoscopy in acute upper gastrointestinal haemorrhage. British Medical Journal ii: 723–724

Storey D W, Bown S G, Swain C P, Salmon P R, Kirkham J S, Northfield T C 1981 Endoscopic prediction of recurrent bleeding in peptic ulcers. New England Journal of Medicine 305: 915–916

Swain C P, Kirkham J S, Salmon P R, Bown S G, Northfield T C 1986 Controlled trial of Nd-YAG laser photocoagulation in bleeding peptic ulcers. Lancet i: 1113–1117

Taylor D E M, Whamond J S, Penhallow J E 1987 Effect of haemorrhage on wound strength and fibroblast function. British Journal of Surgery 74: 316–319

Torres A J, Landa I, Hernandez F et al 1986 Somatostatin in the treatment of severe upper gastrointestinal bleeding: a multicentre controlled trial. Britsih Journal of Surgery 73: 786–789

Vellacott K D, Dronfield M W, Atkinson M, Langman M J S 1982 Comparison of surgical and medical management of bleeding peptic ulcers. British Medical Journal 284: 548–550

Venables C W 1981 Gastroduodenal surgery In: Dykes P W, Keighley M R B (eds) Gastrointestinal haemorrhage. Wright-PSG, Bristol, p 337–356

Wara P 1985 Endoscopic prediction of major rebleeding — prospective study of stigmata of hemorrhage in bleeding ulcer. Gastroenterology 88: 1209–1214

Wheatley K E, Poxon V, Dykes P W, Keighley M R B. 1989 Intragastric fibrinolysis in bleeding peptic ulcer disease. In press

Young A E 1982 Stopping the haemorrhage from peptic ulcers. British Medical Journal 284: 530

Zambertas C, Cregreen R J, Forrest J A H, Finlayson N D C 1982 Accuracy of early endoscopy in acute upper gastrointestinal bleeding. British Medical Journal 285: 1540

7 Acute cholecystitis, calculous and acalculous

R. C. N. WILLIAMSON

Incidence

Definitions

Acute biliary pain has become the third commonest cause for admission to a surgical ward in Britain (Jones 1982). The actual frequency of acute cholecystitis depends upon definitions. Many patients with gallstones have episodic attacks of pain, which typically radiates from the right hypochondrium to the back. When examined during an acute attack they are likely to be tender in the right upper quadrant and the gallbladder may be palpable. The cause of the acute attack is impaction of a calculus in the neck of the gallbladder or cystic duct, and as the stone slips back into the gallbladder or is passed, so the pain subsides. There is no good term for this transient syndrome. It is often called biliary colic, though the pain seldom fluctuates as sharply as the true colic of intestinal or ureteric obstruction. Doubtless there is some degree of acute inflammatory change in the wall of such an obstructed gallbladder, but the term acute cholecystitis is generally reserved for those with clearcut evidence of constitutional upset: tenderness and guarding in the hypochondrium, symptoms of greater duration than 24 h and especially pyrexia ($> 37.5°C$) (Mitchell & Morris 1982).

Calculous cholecystitis

About 90% of acute cholecystitis is associated with gallstones. It should therefore be a disease of middle-aged and elderly women. Several series report a female preponderance of 62–71% (Essenhigh 1966, Glenn 1976, Stryker & Beal 1983, Addison & Finan 1988), but others suggest a more even distribution (Huber et al 1983, Jenkinson et al 1985). There is general agreement that the disease is commoner (and the prognosis worse) in the elderly. Acute cholecystitis is the indication for 10–15% of cholecystectomies (Crumplin et al 1985, Ganey et al 1986), and the disease seems to be getting commoner (Mitchell & Morris 1982).

Acalculous cholecystitis

The remaining 10% of acute cholecystitis is acalculous, i.e. the gallbladder is devoid of stones. Different series report an actual incidence of between 6% and 17% (Williamson 1988), and the proportion may be increasing (Glenn & Becker 1982). Up to half these patients with acute acalculous cholecystitis have idiopathic disease (Glenn 1979): there is no obvious predisposing cause for the attack. Many of the others are seriously ill before the development of an acutely inflamed gallbladder. Acute acalculous cholecystitis is increasingly encountered among patients treated in an intensive therapy unit (Fabian et al 1986). When it follows trauma, sepsis or major surgical operations it is a serious event that can be difficult to recognize and may cause death (Williamson 1988).

Acute cholecystitis can develop in the absence of gallstones as a complication of certain specific infections (e.g. typhoid fever, leptospirosis) and autoimmune diseases (e.g. Sjögren's disease, polyarteritis nodosa) (Williamson 1988). Occasionally it is the presenting feature of carcinoma of the gallbladder (Payne 1969). One important variant is acute emphysematous cholecystitis, in which the gallbladder is invaded by gas-forming bacteria. Another unusual condition, xanthogranulomatous cholecystitis, seldom presents acutely though microscopic foci of haemorrhage and necrosis can often be seen in the resected gallbladder (Reyes et al 1981).

This chapter will consider the pathogenesis of the various forms of acute cholecystitis. Since the presentation and principles of management are broadly similar irrespective of aetiological type, the features of a typical case of calculous cholecystitis will be discussed, followed by the salient differences to be seen among the rarer variants. The frequency of complications, and thus the worse prognosis of acute acalculous cholecystitis and its emphysematous form merit detailed attention.

Pathogenesis

Calculous obstruction

Most cases of acute cholecystitis develop when a gallstone suddenly obstructs the neck of the gallbladder or the cystic duct (Pellegrini & Way 1987). Acute mucosal inflammation is not the inevitable sequel of this event; in experimental animals, for example, either simple dilatation of the gallbladder (hydrops) or shrinkage follow ligature of the cystic duct (Morris et al 1952) and ductal occlusion by tissue glue (Salomonowitz et al 1984).

Bacterial infection of the stagnant bile is an obvious mechanism by which obstruction of the gallbladder could lead to the clinical syndrome of acute cholecystitis. Organisms can be cultured from the bile in 65% of patients, the exact proportion depending upon the urgency of operative intervention (Claesson et al 1986). Among patients operated upon within two days of the onset of symptoms of acute cholecystitis, 81% had positive gallbladder cultures, but the figure fell to 50% when there was further delay. These results do not support the prevailing opinion (Pellegrini & Way 1987, Jivegard et al 1987) that bacterial infection is secondary in acute calculous cholecystitis. Intes-

tinal organisms predominate, some 20% being anaerobes (Claesson et al 1986). Experimental injection of various bacteria into the gallbladder lumen will produce suppurative cholecystitis, but only in the presence of an obstructed cystic duct (Pellegrini & Way 1987). Simultaneous culture of the same organism from blood and bile in several cases of acute acalculous cholecystitis (Lindberg et al 1970, Orlando et al 1983) shows that bloodborne infection is a plausible concept, but whether organisms normally reach the gallbladder via blood, bile or lymph is unknown.

Although bacteria can often be isolated from the bile in acute cholecystitis, it is most unlikely that they are the sole miscreants. The normal chemical constituents of the bile may themselves be injurious. Thus bile acids can damage the mucosal barrier of rabbit gallbladder wall, an effect that is counteracted by lecithin (Heuman et al 1980). It may be relevant that patients with cholelithiasis have more deoxycholic acid and less lecithin than normal in bile (Heuman et al 1980). *Lysolecithin* is normally present in small amounts, but in acute cholecystitis the lysolecithin:lecithin ratio is increased 25-fold (Sjödahl & Wetterfors 1974). Since lysolecithin can readily induce experimental cholecystitis, this metabolic disorder may be of crucial importance (Sjödahl & Tagesson 1983). Conversion of lecithin to lysolecithin could be brought about by phospholipase-A, released perhaps by epithelial trauma, or B-glucuronidase derived from luminal bacteria (Pellegrini & Way 1987). Moreover, phospholipase-A acts on lecithin to release arachidonic acid, a prostaglandin precursor, and prostaglandins could also mediate the inflammatory response (Sjödahl & Tagesson 1983, Jivegard et al 1987). It seems likely, therefore, that the trauma accompanying gallstone impaction triggers the formation of an abnormal bile, which leads to mucosal damage with or without the assistance of enteric bacteria.

Acalculous disease

As already mentioned, acute cholecystitis is an occasional complication of *septicaemia*, for example in typhoid fever (Glenn 1979). With or without such an acute episode, typhoid patients may subsequently develop chronic acalculous cholecystitis, secreting salmonellae into the bile (and thence the faeces) for the rest of their lives. Carcinoma of the gallbladder has occasionally been reported as a complication of long-standing typhoid cholecystitis (Axelrod et al 1971). Acute hydrops of the gallbladder can occur in children with typhoid, leptospiral, streptococcal and other systemic infections; in one such patient the dilatation settled with nonsurgical treatment (Cohen et al 1986). Thomas and colleagues (1981) described one case of staphylococcal septicaemia in a young man, who subsequently developed acute abdominal pain and was found to have a necrotic gallbladder with a sealed perforation. In this patient, as in others with acute acalculous cholecystitis, the causative organism was cultured from the bile as well as the blood. Nevertheless, in a third or more of patients with acalculous inflammation the bile is sterile on culture, and many of those with proven bactobilia have concomitant aetiological features to explain the attack (Lindberg et al 1970, Ottinger 1976, Orlando et al 1983, Devine et al 1984).

Acute acalculous cholecystitis can be classified as follows, and tends to develop in patients who are seriously ill or stressed.

Primary, i.e. idiopathic, acute acalculous cholecystitis

Secondary acute acalculous cholecystitis
  Surgical operations
  Multiple trauma
  Burns
  Severe sepsis
  Recent childbirth

Rare varieties of acute acalculous cholecystitis
  Torsion
  Trauma
  Arterial injuries
  Endoprosthesis
  Collagen diseases

Thus it can follow major operations remote from the biliary tract or multiple injuries including burns. Possibly the first such case was reported by Duncan in 1844 and followed an operation for femoral hernia; gangrenous cholecystitis was found

at autopsy, but there were no gallstones. An attack of calculus cholecystitis could just be coincidental in such circumstances, but 33–47% of the *post-operative* cases and no less than 87–92% of the *post-traumatic* cases are acalculous (Jönsson & Andersson 1976, Du Priest et al 1979, Devine et al 1984). The difference probably reflects the age of the two groups. Several of the trauma patients reported have been young soldiers injured in battle, (Lindberg et al 1970, Weeder et al 1970), whereas three-quarters of the postoperative patients have been over 50 years old and thus more likely to have gallstones (Jönsson & Andersson 1976). Likewise, males outnumbered females by 7:1 in a review of 35 series of postoperative attacks and by 21:1 in a review of 20 series of post-traumatic attacks (Jönsson & Andersson 1976); when calculous cholecystitis followed operation or trauma the sex distribution was equal.

Several aetiological mechanisms have been implicated in acute acalculous cholecystitis, viz:

Increased bile viscosity:
  Blood transfusion
  Dehydration
Bile stasis:
  Parenteral nutrition
  Assisted ventilation
  Vagotomy
Papillary obstruction:
  Opiates
  Papillitis
Cystic duct obstruction:
  Abnormal cystic duct
  Enlarged cystic lymph node
Ischaemia:
  Sympathetic tone
  Atherosclerosis
  Vasculitis
Infection:
  Septicaemia
  Cystic duct obstruction

Bile viscosity. In 1970 Lindberg and colleagues reported 12 cases among 2400 American soldiers wounded in Vietnam and evacuated to Clark Air Base in the Philippines. Gallbladder symptoms developed 10–35 days after the battle injury, and two patients died. A consistent feature among these casualties was the need for multiple blood transfusions; all but one received in excess of 10 units of blood to replace losses associated with fractures and amputations. Although none of the patients developed jaundice, it was suggested that haemolysis of the transfused blood could have increased the pigment load and thus the *viscosity of the bile*, causing chemical irritation of the gallbladder mucosa. Clearly dehydration could have similar effects (Glenn & Wantz 1956). It is notewothy that these soldiers had received between 2 and 11 operations before developing cholecystitis, so that several other aetiological mechanisms could have been involved (see below); indeed, transfusion alone seems of relatively minor importance (Flancbaum et al 1985).

Bile stasis. Acalculous cholecystitis has been reported as a complication of prolonged parenteral nutrition, both in adults (Long et al 1978, Petersen & Sheldon 1979) and premature infants (Thurston et al 1986). The mechanism may be one of decreased gallbladder contractility, because circulating levels of cholecystokinin are low in the absence of food from the gut (Glenn & Wantz 1956, Gullick 1960). Thus bile stasis develops together with an increase in bile viscosity; inspissation of the gallbladder contents occurs as the organ continues to absorb water. Glenn and Wantz (1956) noted that postoperative cholecystitis often followed resumption of oral feeding after a fast. They suggested that forceful contraction of the gallbladder to try and expel the stagnant, viscid bile was the crucial factor in pathogenesis. In support, serial cholecystograms have shown that postoperative evacuation of the gallbladder is delayed until the resumption of food by mouth (Gullick 1960). However, the temporal association between oral re-feeding and onset of cholecystitis has not been confirmed in subsequent reports.

Serial use of ultrasonography confirms distension of the gallbladder and sludge formation in patients fed intravenously (Peterson & Sheldon 1979). In neonates total parenteral nutrition causes intrahepatic cholestasis and can lead to the rapid development of gallstones (Whitington & Black 1980). Again, ultrasound scans may show acute dilatation of the gallbladder in hyperalimented infants (Bowen 1984). However, sonography cannot readily distinguish between hydrops (mucocoele) of the gallbladder and acalculous cholecystitis in children (Bowen 1984). Another factor leading to biliary stasis in critically ill patients is the use of ventilatory support for concomitant respiratory failure (Orlando et al 1983). In one series (Flancbaum et al 1985), 16 of 18 patients (89%) who developed acalculous cholecystitis after major trauma had received positive end-expiratory pressure (PEEP) of 50–200 mm H_2O; interestingly, all 18 patients had also received more than 20 units of blood. In dogs, continuous positive-pressure ventilation causes increased pressure and decreased flow in the bile duct (Johnson & Hedley-Whyte 1975).

Obstruction. Stasis may be compounded by physical obstruction of the biliary tree. Large doses of opiates are often administered to patients in an intensive therapy unit, and these could clearly cause prolonged spasm of the sphincter of Oddi (Flancbaum et al 1985). Biliary scintigraphy shows delayed appearance of the radionuclide in the intestine (but not the gallbladder) among healthy volunteers given narcotic drugs (Joehl et al 1984). Obstructive causes loomed large in a series of Greek patients with acalculous cholecystitis, 80 with acute disease and 50 with chronic disease (Lygidakis 1981). Primary papillitis, tortuosity of the cystic duct and recent vagotomy (presumably causing biliary stasis) were remarkably common in each group. In children, where 30% of gallbladder disease is acalculous, cystic duct obstruction could result from congenital narrowing, local inflammation or compression by enlarged lymph nodes (Ternberg & Keating 1975, Traynelis & Hrabovsky 1985). One child was actually born with a mass in the right upper quadrant; laparotomy at 3 days revealed acute acalculous cholecystitis with complete occlusion of the cystic duct (Washburn & Barcia 1980).

Ischaemia. The advanced age of many patients with acute acalculous cholecystitis (Fox et al 1984, Johnson 1987) raises the possibility that ischaemia plays a part in its pathogenesis. Vascular occlusion doubtless accounts for the acute cholecystitis sometimes seen in polyarteritis nodosa (Li Volsi et al 1973). Besides atheroma of the cystic artery, increased sympathetic tone in injured or postoperative patients might critically reduce the blood supply to the gallbladder mucosa (Orlando et al 1983); sympathectomy protects against experimental acute cholecystitis in dogs (Howard et al 1952). Vasoconstrictor drugs such as adrenaline or dopamine might contribute to vascular damage in the gallbladder of a shocked patient (Du Priest et al 1979). In one series, 3 of 8 patients with postoperative cholecystitis were shocked before the onset of the disease (Ziv et al 1987). A prolonged increase in intraluminal pressure, resulting e.g. from narcotic therapy, could further reduce perfusion of the organ. It has also been suggested that trauma and sepsis might lead to activation of Factor XII, with consequent damage to the gallbladder vasculature (Glenn & Becker 1982). Thus the pathogenesis of acute acalculous cholecystitis is probably multifactorial, as tissue hypoxia renders the mucosa susceptible both to irritants in an abnormally concentrated bile and to circulating micro-organisms.

Presentation and diagnosis

Clinical features

Most patients who develop acute (calculous) cholecystitis have a previous history of biliary colic or flatulent dyspepsia, but for some 25% this is the first clinical manifestation of gallstones (Pellegrini & Way 1987). Not uncommonly the attack follows a rich or heavy meal. The pain starts in the right hypochondrium and may radiate to the epigastrium or back. Nausea and vomiting are common. With increasing inflammation of the gallbladder the pain settles in the right subcostal area. There is localized tenderness with rebound tenderness and a positive Murphy's sign: a 'catch' just before the zenith of deep inspiration during palpation over the gallbladder. The distended gallbladder can sometimes be felt as a tender mass. Mild jaundice may be detected in 10–15% of cases (Essenhigh 1966, Pellegrini & Way 1987). Jaundice may reflect common duct stones, cholangitis affecting the liver or partial obstruction of the bile duct by inflammatory oedema caused by impaction of a stone in Hartmann's pouch (Mirizzi's syndrome) (Stryker & Beal 1983, Witte 1984). Pyrexia is variable, ranging from a mild elevation to a high swinging fever, when concomitant cholangitis or Gram-negative septicaemia should be suspected.

Laboratory tests

There is generally a neutrophil leucocytosis ($>10 \times 10^9$/l) accompanied by some abnormality in liver function tests. Even in the absence of clinically apparent jaundice the serum bilirubin, together with one or more transaminase enzymes, may be elevated (Stryker & Beal 1983). The presence of bile in the urine on testing is a useful pointer to disease of the biliary tract and helps to differentiate acute cholecystitis from mimicking conditions such as peptic ulcer, retrocaecal appendicitis, renal colic, pyelitis, angina and the Curtis-FitzHugh syndrome of gonococcal perihepatitis (Pellegrini & Way 1987). A substantial increase in bilirubin and alkaline phosphatase levels indicates obstruction of the common duct. Mild elevation in serum amylase is consistent with uncomplicated cholecystitis, but higher values (> 1000 iu/l) suggest acute pancreatitis. Biliary sepsis is one of the commonest causes of Gram-negative septicaemia, especially in the elderly, so blood cultures should be obtained if pyrexia and toxicity are marked (Glenn 1976). Blood urea may be raised in such patients, who are at risk of developing renal failure.

Radiological diagnosis

Plain abdominal radiographs will reveal calcified gallstones in 10–20% of patients (Watts & Toouli 1984, Pellegrini & Way 1987), but appearances are otherwise nonspecific except in emphysematous cholecystitis (see below). Oral cholecystography is too cumbersome in the acute context. Endoscopic retrograde cholangiography is contraindicated in gallbladder sepsis and CT scanning is unhelpful. Intravenous cholangiography, formerly popular, has been supplanted by *ultrasonography* and cholescintigraphy as the mainstays of diagnosis (Gill et al 1985). In particular, ultrasound scanning is readily available and non-invasive (Dillon & Parkin 1980, Stryker & Beal 1983). Besides gallstones, it will show gallbladder distension and

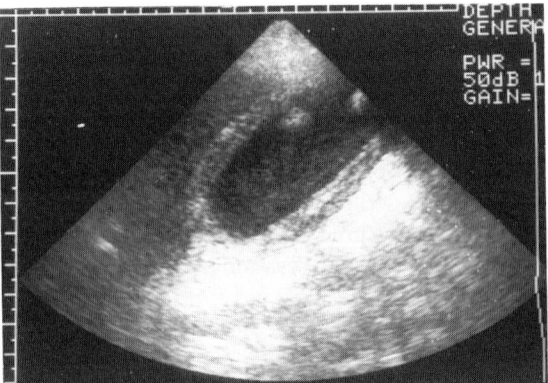

Fig. 7.1 Acute cholecystitis in a woman aged 62. Ultrasound scan shows distension of the gallbladder with diffuse thickening of the wall and echogenic calculi in the lumen.

mural thickening (Fig. 7.1). Scans can be obtained at the bedside using a portable real-time scanner.

Cholescintigraphy involves the intravenous injection of a derivative of iminodiacetic acid, such as HIDA or PIPIDA, labelled with the radionuclide technetium (^{99m}Tc). Non-visualization of the gallbladder despite good hepatic uptake and entry of isotope into the duodenum (Fig. 7.2) indicates cystic duct obstruction, and in appropriate clinical circumstances is virtually diagnostic of acute cholecystitis (Cabellon et al 1984). This statement holds true for both the calculous and the acalculous varieties (Swayne 1986). Radionuclide scans may also show increased pericholecystic activity (the 'rim' sign) in the presence of gangrene (Bushnell et al 1986), and free peritoneal spill of the radionuclide will diagnose perforation of the gallbladder (Swayne 1986, Siskind et al 1987). An indium-labelled leucocyte scan is another way of diagnosing an acutely inflamed gallbladder (Datz 1986).

Management of acute calculous disease

Preoperative management

Cholecystectomy is the treatment of choice for acute cholecystitis in all but those who are very frail or unfit. In many patients the acute attack will settle with medical therapy, but the risk of complications and the strong likelihood of recurrence are clear indications for an early operation. Just how early that should be is discussed below.

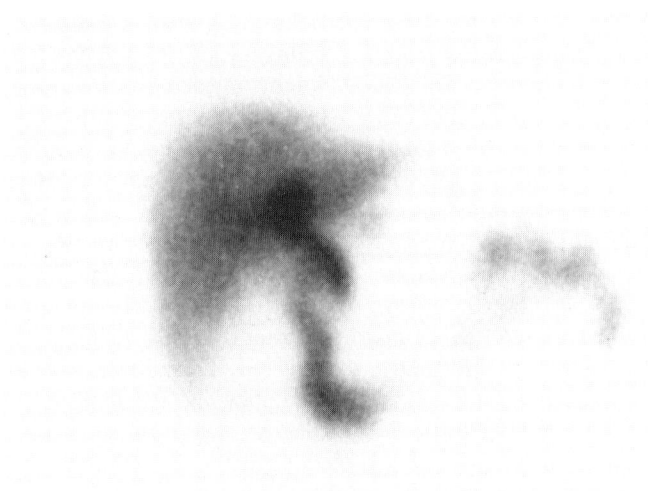

Fig. 7.2 Acute cholecystitis in a man aged 56. Cholescintigram (15-min scan) shows prompt excretion of radionuclide by the liver with filling of the bile duct and upper small bower but not the gallbladder.

The principles of non-operative treatment are as follows: intravenous fluid replacement, nasogastric suction if vomiting persists, adequate analgesia (usually pethidine by injection at first), antibiotics and vigilant observation for evidence of increasing tenderness, which demands urgent operation. Although antibiotics are of unproven benefit in controlled trials (Pellegrini & Way 1987), their routine use is justified in acute cholecystitis because of the risks of ascending cholangitis (and septicaemia) and empyema of the gallbladder. Most attacks will respond to a single agent, such as a cephalosporin, but in patients with severe constitutional upset combination therapy including metronidazole, gentamicin and/or penicillin should be considered. During this initial period of management an early attempt should be made to clinch the diagnosis by means of ultrasonography, supplemented if necessary by cholescintigraphy (see above).

Optimal timing of operation

A small proportion of patients admitted with acute cholecystitis have such severe symptoms and signs, both local and general, that urgent operation is mandatory. There were 21 such cases (7%) among 304 patients retrospectively reviewed at Oxford between 1974–1978 (Mitchell & Morris 1982); another 16 (5%) were deemed unfit for operation, making medical treatment obligatory. For the remaining 88% there was a clear choice between early or later cholecystectomy.

Traditional management for acute cholecystitis has been to assist the acute attack to settle, to confirm the diagnosis at leisure and to discharge the patient from hospital to await cholecystectomy after a minimum of 4 weeks. The rationale for this policy is that inflammatory oedema and adhesions make early cholecystectomy hazardous and that in most cases the delay is not associated with serious problems (Paterson-Brown & Chan 1987). Before the advent of effective antibiotics that could achieve adequate concentrations in bile, there may have been an additional concern about the risk of developing septicaemia during operation in the presence of acute infection. Lastly, the delay al-

lows plenty of time for an unequivocal diagnosis to be established.

Among the 267 Oxford patients whose clinical condition did not dictate initial management, three-quarters (198) were treated conservatively (Mitchell & Morris 1982). The relative safety of this course of action is highlighted by the fact that there were only three deaths in the group and that subsequent elective operations (performed in the majority) were mostly uneventful. However, in 23% the response to medical therapy was considered unsatisfactory and these patients came to operation during the initial admission. Moreover, half the group (54%) developed further symptoms while languishing on the waiting list for operation, and a third of these (18%) required emergency readmission. Overall, one quarter of the patients (69) were selected for early operation from the outset, and there was only one death in this group. Thus the mortality rates of the two treatment arms were very similar (1.4% vs. 1.5%), and the only clear difference to emerge from this retrospective survey was a saving of 5.4 hospital days in favour of the early operation policy. The avoidance of recurrent symptoms is an additional benefit that is difficult to quantitate.

The question of early or delayed operation for acute cholecystitis has been put to the test in four controlled prospective trials carried out during the last 20 years (der Linden & Sunzel 1970, McArthur et al 1975, Lahtinen et al 1978, Jarvinen & Hastbacka 1980). There were approximately 200 patients in each group in total, and the results have conveniently been summarized by Pellegrini & Way (1987). The policy of early operation was attended by a shorter total hospital stay (c. 9 days), fewer deaths (0 vs. 5) and a lower incidence of failure, i.e. cholecystectomy was not performed as planned. No particular risks were encountered in those receiving early operation, and sometimes an important missed diagnosis (e.g. appendicitis) was corrected. Experience has shown that an aggressive policy is particularly justified in men, in diabetics and in the elderly, all of whom appear to be at greater risk of complications (Jenkinson et al 1985, Pellegrini & Way 1987). There is much to commend the advice of Jenkinson and colleagues (1985) that when elderly men develop symptoms of gallstones they should have an early elective operation before acute cholecystitis supervenes.

My own policy for managing acute cholecystitis is therefore as follows. All patients are admitted to hospital and treated expectantly at first (as outlined in the previous section) unless there is evidence of generalized peritonitis, in which case emergency laparotomy is undertaken. For those with marked local tenderness and/or a mass and with constitutional symptoms that fail to settle promptly, laparotomy is performed after 24–48 h because of the risk of gangrene and incipient perforation; ultrasonography is performed during the interim. The majority of patients who respond to medical treatment are kept in hospital while the diagnosis is being confirmed, and the gallbladder is removed on the next convenient operating list. In practice, prior knowledge of the gallstones can be anticipated in about a third of patients admitted with acute cholecystitis (Mitchell & Morris 1982). If the attack settles but the diagnosis remains in doubt and/or the patient is unfit or reluctant for operation, surgery is postponed for 1–2 months to resolve these problems.

Operative procedures

1. Cholecystectomy Complete removal of the gallbladder is desirable in acute cholecystitis and nearly always feasible, though less severe alternatives are discussed below. The operation is generally straightforward (Lahtinen et al 1978), but sometimes (and unpredictably) it can be a difficult technical challenge. A more difficult and bloody dissection can be anticipated during urgent cholecystectomy (for incipient or established gangrene) (Mitchell & Morris 1982), though sometimes gross oedema actually assists enucleation of the gallbladder from its bed. A few days later resolving oedema may obscure the important anatomical landmarks, yet fibrosis can have the same effect at interval cholecystectomy after a delay of 1–2 months. Although there were no bile duct injuries among the Oxford patients or the four prospective trials described above, this remains an ever-present threat, particularly if the surgeon forgets the frequency and the various types of congenital anomalies in biliary anatomy.

The technique of cholecystectomy for acute cholecystitis is described elsewhere (Williamson 1987, Pellegrini & Way 1987), but certain principles merit repetition. It helps to decompress a distended gallbladder at the outset, and the Ochsner suction trocar is a convenient means for performing this step. Generally blunt dissection is adequate to separate the gallbladder from the liver after incising the peritoneum, and the fundus-first technique is particularly appropriate. Subsequently the cystic duct can safely be followed to its junction with the common hepatic duct. Since bile duct stones are present in 15–20% of patients with acute cholecystitis (Jones 1982), an operative cholangiogram should be obtained unless the patient is very sick or there is severe local inflammation. If the cystic duct is grossly inflamed and friable it should be ligated with care or transfixed. Bile cultures should always be obtained, and adequate drainage should be provided to the subhepatic space at the end of the operation. Irrespective of preoperative treatment, an acute cholecystectomy should always be 'covered' with appropriate antibiotics. Wound infection can be anticipated in about 5% of cholecystectomies for acute cholecystitis and subhepatic abscess in about 2% (Payne 1969, Claesson et al 1986).

2. Choledochotomy In one series of 256 patients with acute cholecystitis, stones were encountered in the common bile duct in 32 cases (12.5%) (Stryker & Beal 1983). If stones are felt or visualized radiologically within the bile duct, they should be removed to relieve or prevent cholangitis and obstructive jaundice. Unless there is a good deal of inflammation in the vicinity, exploration of the bile duct can proceed routinely. Clearance of the stones should be checked by means of choledochoscopy and/or a postexploratory cholangiogram (Williamson 1987). T-tube drainage of the bile duct should be employed. Judgement is required if ductal stones are associated with suppurative cholangitis and/or severe periductal sepsis, e.g. in the presence of a perforated gallbladder. Under such circumstances it is usually wise to limit the procedure to incision and irrigation of the bile duct with removal of as many calculi as possible. Decompression of the duct in this fashion and T-tube drainage will arrest the process of ascending cholangitis, liver abscess and septicaemia. Once life has been saved, retained calculi can be dealt with later by dissolution or extraction via the T-tube or endoscopic papillotomy. To carry out a biliary bypass, whether choledochoduodenostomy or transduodenal sphincteroplasty, in the presence of suppurative cholangitis is to risk anastomotic dehiscence. It should be emphasized that it is unusual for acute cholecystitis to coexist with suppurative cholangitis, however.

3. Cholecystostomy In 1881 Halsted carried out a cholecystostomy on his own mother (Jones 1982). Nowadays there is probably only one indication for a formal operative cholecystostomy: an elderly patient who is seriously ill and has a palpable gallbladder mass (like Mrs Halsted). Under these circumstances the gallbladder can be decompressed under local or light general anaes-

thesia and death averted thereby. In the Oxford series of patients with acute cholecystitis, 2 of 21 patients requiring urgent operation received cholecystostomy and 6 of the 46 who had an early operation after failed medical treatment (Mitchell & Morris 1982). By contrast only 1 cholecystostomy was required for 163 patients with a histological diagnosis of acute cholecystitis undergoing operation in a Florida district general hospital (Ganey et al 1986). This proportion (0.6%) is indeed low in view of the fact that the participating surgeons adopted a policy of very early operation for this disease and had no bile duct injuries.

Cholecystostomy used to be advised much more readily in acute cholecystitis (Glenn 1976), with rates as high as 35% (Gingrich et al 1968). One series from Sydney (1963–70) included 25 patients

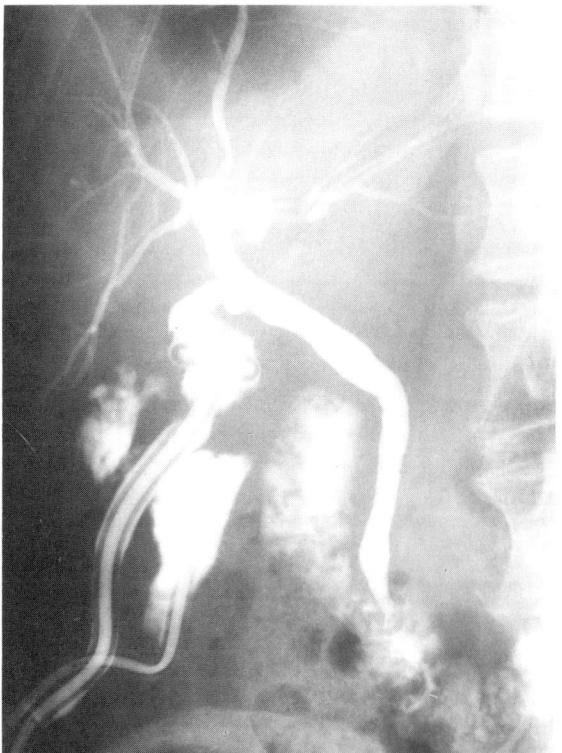

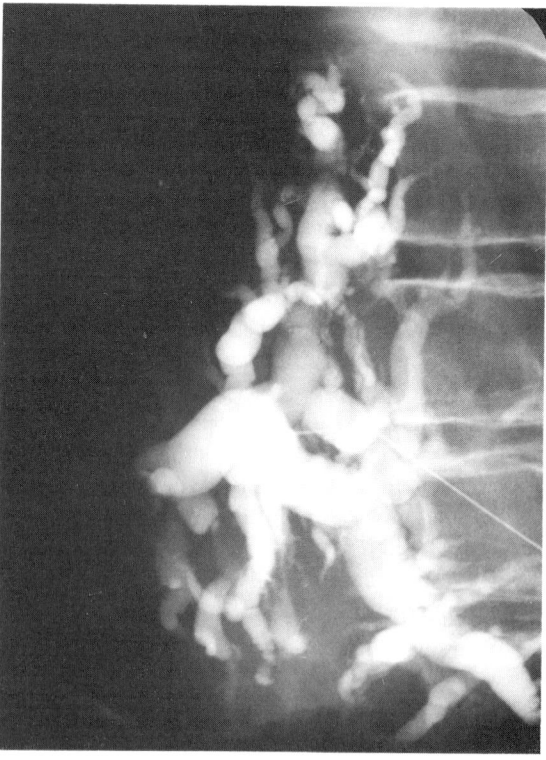

A   B

Fig. 7.3A,B Carcinoma of the gallbladder presenting as an empyema in a man aged 78. The patient developed pain, fever and a mass, and a distended gallbladder was drained of pus by cholecystostomy. Postoperative cholecystography via the Malecot drainage catheter (A) shows an otherwise normal biliary tree with some extravasation from the gallbladder. Recovery was uneventful, but 9 months later the patient became jaundiced. A percutaneous transhepatic cholangiogram (B: oblique view) confirms complete obstruction of the common hepatic duct by a carcinoma of the gallbladder that had been previously overlooked.

(Pheils & Duraiappah 1975) and another contemporaneous series from Boston no less than 77 patients (Welch & Malt 1972); it is doubtful if many hospitals could match these figures today. The mortality rates in these two series (8–25%) confirm that the operation was being undertaken in seriously ill patients. Although potentially life-saving under such circumstances, residual problems were common: retained stones, recurrent cholecystitis, extrusion of the tube, persistent fistula. Several patients require a subsequent cholecystectomy to render the biliary tract free of disease. In one such patient, illustrated in Fig. 7.3, cholecystostomy carried out for empyema of the gallbladder failed to diagnose the underlying carcinoma. Acute cholecystitis is an established (though rare) complication of gallbladder cancer (Payne 1969).

Percutaneous cholecystostomy offers an attractive alternative means of decompressing the gallbladder and relieving toxicity in these patients. Klimberg and colleagues (1987) report 15 high-risk patients with acute cholecystitis treated by this means, 10 with calculous disease and 5 with acalculous disease. Under ultrasound control a fine needle was inserted through the liver and into the gallbladder, to be followed by a 6.5 French accordion catheter. In all but one case there was resolution of symptoms and signs within 24 h; indeed, pain could resolve almost immediately. The remaining patient died of overwhelming sepsis. Other reports confirm the promise of this new technique (Van Sonnenberg et al 1986), though hypotension may occur as a result of a vasovagal reaction and there is a theoretical risk of biliary peritonitis. Moreover, subsequent cholecystectomy will still be required in many of the survivors unless the gallbladder can safely be ablated by injection of sclerosant down the tube (Salomonowitz et al 1984), a procedure that remains experimental at the present time.

4. Subtotal cholecystectomy In many ways this is a better option than formal cholecystostomy when gross inflammation is encountered at operation, making it very difficult to identify the junction between cystic duct and bile duct (Pellegrini & Way 1987). The body of the gallbladder is opened and all stones are removed under direct vision. The neck of the gallbladder, which may be firmly ad-herent to the bile duct in such cases, is left in situ and is oversewn. It is sometimes possible to insert a catheter and obtain a cholangiogram before closing off the stump of the gallbladder. The body and fundus of the gallbladder are peeled off the liver and removed unless they too are very adherent, in which case the back wall is also left in situ; its mucosa is then destroyed by the use of diathermy. A running suture will control bleeding from the edge of the gallbladder remaining in situ (Bornman & Terblanche 1985). Unless stones have been left behind in the bile duct, further biliary surgery should not be required after subtotal cholecystectomy.

Atypical attacks and their management

Acute acalculous cholecystitis

Symptoms and signs are essentially the same as in the calculous variety, except that there is obviously no previous history of cholelithiasis and the early clinical features may be overshadowed by the concomitant illness. Thus the classical signs of fever, tenderness and a mass are often not detected until gangrene and even perforation of the gallbladder has occurred (Williamson 1988). The diagnosis of acute acalculous cholecystitis in seriously ill patients requires a high index of clinical suspicion. Leucocytosis may be accompanied by hyper-bilirubinaemia and elevations in liver enzymes and amylase (Fabian et al 1986). In the presence of peritonitis, perforated stress ulcer is an alternative possibility (Shields 1973). Ultrasonography may show distension of the gallbladder, thickening of its wall, intraluminal sludge and a halo denoting subserosal oedema (Beckman et al 1985). Scintigraphy using ^{99m}Tc HIDA may be more sensitive in confirming the diagnosis and showing complications (Fox et al 1984, Swayne 1986).

Delayed diagnosis undoubtedly contributes to the high mortality rate of this disease. In a recent study, perforation of the gallbladder was five times as likely to occur if operation was not performed within 48 h of the onset of symptoms (Johnson 1987). The post-traumatic and postoperative types are particularly dangerous, with at least a 60% incidence of gangrene and perforation of the gallbladder (Ottinger 1976, Du Priest et al 1979, Devine et al 1984). Thus the diagnosis of acute acalculous cholecystitis is a clear indication for emergency laparotomy, and there is no case for a trial of conservative therapy. Because gangrene is so common, cholecystectomy (total or subtotal) is a much better option than cholecystostomy. In children, however, where gangrene is uncommon, this statement may not hold true (Ternberg & Keating 1975). Similarly children who develop acute hydrops of the gallbladder secondary to a systemic infection may settle with percutaneous aspiration of the gallbladder or even with conservative treatment (Cohen et al 1986).

Acute emphysematous cholecystitis

May and Strong (1971) collected 115 cases of this unusual disease since the original description by Stolz in 1901. Although Stolz believed that the gas had developed from postmortem decomposition of the tissues, it is now known that gas-forming anaerobes are to blame, notably clostridia but also coliforms and streptococci (Rosoff & Meyers 1966). Gas bubbles are to be seen in the wall of

the gallbladder, but also in its lumen and occasionally throughout the biliary tree. The appearance of the gas-filled gallbladder on plain abdominal radiographs and on ultrasound scan (Fig. 7.4) is classical. A fistula between the gallbladder and the intestine can give a similar radiological picture but without the striking clinical features of emphysematous cholecystitis. Rarely patients present with a pneumoperitoneum following perforation (Radin & Halls 1987).

Many more men than women present with acute emphysematous cholecystitis (at least three times), with a peak incidence in the sixth and seventh decades. Between 20% and 30% of patients are diabetic (Rosoff & Meyers 1966). This fact, together with evidence of endarteritis obliterans in the cystic artery, raises the possibility that the primary lesion is a vascular occlusion (May & Strong 1971). Alternatively, cystic duct obstruction might allow tension and ischaemia in the gallbladder wall, again with secondary infection by intestinal bacteria in susceptible individuals. Whatever the aetiology, affected patients have a sudden onset of pain with a palpable mass and marked toxicity. Urgent treatment is required with intravenous fluids and antibiotics (penicillin, metronidazole) and control of associated diabetes. Cholecystectomy should be performed once the

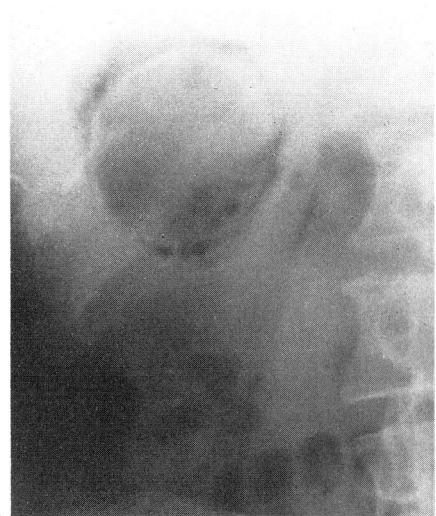
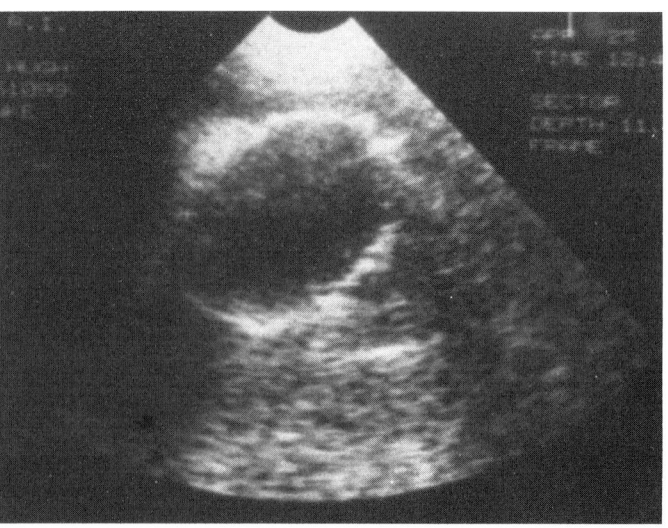

Fig. 7.4A,B Acute emphysematous cholecystitis in a 65-year-old diabetic man. Plain abdominal X-ray (A) shows the tell-tale ring of gas in the wall of a distended gallbladder. Ultrasonogram (B) shows bright echoes in the gallbladder wall and no calculi.

patients respond or as a matter of urgency in the absence of any improvement. Gangrene is common; gallstones are often absent. Although recent data are scarce, the mortality rate is probably higher than for other forms of acute cholecystitis (Pellegrini & Way 1987).

Torsion of the gallbladder

This is a rare cause of acute necrotizing cholecystitis. Unlike emphysematous cholecystitis, patients are typically elderly women with visceroptosis (Ashby 1965), though young adults and children can also be affected (Greenwood 1963). However, the presentation is similar, with a sudden onset of pain and vomiting, leucocytosis and a tender mass that may be palpable in the right subcostal or lumbar regions. The underlying aetiology is an excessively mobile gallbladder with a long cystic duct, but there are two varieties of this pattern (Schlinkert et al 1984). In the first (presumably congenital) the gallbladder floats free on the cystic duct and artery with no attachment to the liver. In the second (probably acquired) it is suspended from the liver on a long mesentery. Exceptionally torsion can be confined to part of the gallbladder (the fundus) (Schlinkert et al 1984) or affect one half of a double gallbladder (Recht 1952), or the entire organ 'floats' into an epigastric hernia and becomes incarcerated (Goldman et al 1985).

Torsion of the gallbladder presents like a case of severe acute cholecystitis, and the diagnosis is hardly ever suspected preoperatively. Sonographic and CT appearances are nonspecific: mural thickening, luminal distension and absence of calculi (Quinn et al 1987). Krabbel did achieve a correct preoperative diagnosis in 1920, but he had encountered a similar case only 18 days beforehand. His unusually rich experience of the condition was insufficient to prevent him from overlooking the diagnosis in a third case seen 9 months later. Occasionally patients have recurrent attacks of pain and swelling owing to subacute torsion with spontaneous resolution (Ashby 1965). Otherwise prompt laparotomy is required to remove the strangulated organ. Cholecystectomy is easy to perform, but the gallbladder should be untwisted before excision to free the adjacent common hepatic duct (Butsch & Luchette 1985).

Iatrogenic cholecystitis

This variant is becoming commoner. Acute cholecystitis can result from infusion of chemotherapeutic agents into the hepatic artery (Carrasco et al 1983). The indication is usually colorectal carcinoma metastatic to the liver. Implantable pumps allow the delivery of several courses of drugs such as 5-fluorouracil and adriamycin over weeks and months. Inflammation can proceed to gangrene and perforation or develop into chronic cholecystitis with recurrent episodes of pain (Pietrafitta et al 1986).

Traumatic cholecystitis occasionally results from abdominal injuries causing intraluminal haemorrhage (Penn 1962), and percutaneous aspiration of the gallbladder for diagnostic or therapeutic procedures could clearly have the same effect. Gangrenous cholecystitis with intraluminal haemorrhage has been reported in a patient with renal failure undergoing haemodialysis (McFadden & Smith 1987). We have recently encountered a case of acalculous cholecystitis with patchy mucosal necrosis associated with an indwelling endoprosthesis placed through a benign bile-duct stricture.

There are two aspects to management of this type of problem. In the first place clinicians must be aware of the possibility of cholecystitis and gallbladder infarction when treating patients in this manner. If symptoms and signs develop, ultrasonography should be performed as a prelude to cholecystectomy. In the second place it is a sensible precaution to remove the gallbladder when carrying out ligation and/or cannulation of the hepatic artery for secondary malignant disease (Pietrafitta et al 1986).

Complications

Gangrene

Ischaemic necrosis of the gallbladder wall can develop, sometimes rapidly, in association with severe acute cholecystitis. It is generally believed that necrosis is not so much the consequence of cystic artery occlusion as of increasing pressure within the gallbladder lumen following cystic duct obstruction (Pellegrini & Way 1987). However, the occurrence of gangrene and perforation in diabetics with cholecystitis or patients with hepatic artery ligation suggests that vascular occlusion can certainly play a part. It is difficult to estimate the incidence of gangrene in acute cholecystitis. If the gallbladder resected during the first few days of an attack is carefully inspected, patches of necrosis are quite commonly seen. Some 10–15% of patients with acute calculous cholecystitis show evidence of peritonitis and require emergency laparotomy for gangrene with or without perforation (Jones 1982). In acute acalculous cholecystitis the figure is undoubtedly higher, and in post-operative and post-traumatic cases it may reach 60% (Williamson 1988). Diffuse gangrene (gallbladder infarction) may give rise to bizarre complications such as bleeding into the colon (Brady & Welch 1985) or pulmonary bile embolism (Proia et al 1986).

Empyema

By definition the gallbladder is inflamed and contains pus. Empyema or suppurative cholecystitis is an uncommon but potentially lethal complication which particularly affects the elderly. The gallbladder is usually obstructed by stones, but empyema can develop in acute acalculous cholecystitis (Ottinger 1976, Devine et al 1984). Thornton and colleagues (1983) reported 32 patients with empyema of the gallbladder among 1327 cases of gallbladder disease seen at the Bristol Royal Infirmary between 1976 and 1981 (an incidence of 2.4%). The mean age was 71 years and there was a 25% mortality rate, mostly from septicaemia. Although most patients developed empyema as a consequence of acute cholecystitis requiring emergency admission, 6 of the 32 (19%) had little or no antecedent history; perhaps these cases represented infection of a pre-existing mucocele. Tenderness was nearly always present in the right hypochondrium and was accompanied by leucocytosis and deranged liver function tests, but fever and a mass were found in barely half the group.

Thus empyema of the gallbladder is a dangerous condition that may present with a relative paucity of physical signs. Although it is an unusual event in acute cholecystitis (comprising 6% of patients in one large series — Essenhigh 1966), the possible development of empyema is another reason to support an aggressive policy of early operation in this disease.

Perforation

Like the appendix, the gallbladder is a blind-ended sac which can perforate if intraluminal tension becomes high enough. Perforation complicates 3–15% of attacks of acute calculous cholecystitis (Essenigh 1968, Lahtinen et al 1978, Jarvinen & Hastbacka 1980, Ranson 1987) and 11–28% of attacks of acute acalculous cholecystitis (Ottinger 1976, Du Priest et al 1979, Orlando et al 1983, Devine et al 1984, Johnson 1987). Reasons for the discrepancy include the insidious onset of acalculous disease and the thickening of the wall associated with chronic cholecystitis in patients with stones. Perforation is common in the elderly, in diabetics and those with acute typhoid cholecystitis (Ranson 1987). Half the patients in one recent report had serious intercurrent medical problems, including carcinoma, diabetes and cirrhosis (Roslyn et al 1987). Perforation of the gallbladder can be classified as follows (Niemeier 1934): 1. acute, leading to generalized biliary peritonitis; 2. subacute, leading to a pericholecystic abscess walled off by inflammatory adhesions; 3. chronic, leading to a cholecystenteric fistula. Free perforation is diagnosed on the basis of diffuse tenderness and marked toxicity with or without jaundice; however, the diagnosis is often not made until laparotomy or even autopsy (Roslyn et al 1987). Pericholecystic abscess mimics empyema of the gallbladder, with a mass and leucocytosis. In the third type the fistula is usually not discovered until after the acute attack has settled. Ultrasound and CT scanning can detect fluid collections outside the gallbladder, and cholescintigraphy may show extravasation of radionuclide (Siskind et al 1987).

Contamination of the general peritoneal cavity with infected bile produces a severe constitutional upset, and these patients require vigorous resuscitation with intravenous fluids and antibiotics before emergency cholecystectomy is performed. Reviewing six series of perforated gallbladders reported since 1961, Ranson (1987) collected 100 patients with free perforation and 39 with localized perforation. The overall mortality rate of free perforation was 31%, falling to 22% with surgical treatment. The overall mortality rate of localized perforation was 18%, falling to 6% with surgical treatment. The lessons are clear.

Outcome

Overall mortality

From the United States, Glenn (1976) reported 2021 patients undergoing surgical treatment for acute cholecystitis between 1932 and 1974, among whom there were 68 deaths, giving a mortality rate of 3.4%. It seems likely that there were at least as many deaths in patients treated nonoperatively during this period, including perhaps a few cases undiagnosed during life. From the United Kingdom, Essenhigh (1966) reported 429 patients with acute cholecystitis between 1953–1962. His overall mortality rate of 7.7% is probably in the same league as that of the American series therefore.

Mitchell & Morris (1982) compared Essenhigh's earlier Oxford data with those from a more recent period (1974–1978) in the same city. They found a sharp drop in mortality rate to 1.6% and attributed this improvement to the increased proportion of patients receiving operation during the initial admission (45% vs. 27%). Elsewhere in Britain, Payne (1969) reported a 1.9% mortality rate for acute cholecystitis during a similar period (1952–1966) to Essenhigh. His policy of early operation was endorsed by the fact that no deaths occurred among 133 patients in this group. Likewise Pickleman and Gonzalez (1986) had only 2 deaths in a personal series of 120 cholecystectomies for acute cholecystitis in the USA. Thus although an overall death rate of 5% may be given for acute cholecystitis (Pellegrini & Way 1987), better figures can certainly be achieved by an aggressive approach.

The effect of age

Nowadays death from acute cholecystitis is distinctly uncommon below the age of 65 years. In Glenn's enormous series (1976) the mortality rate of patients over 65 years old (9.3%) was much higher than that of their juniors (1.4%); others report the same trend (Mitchell & Morris 1982, Huber et al 1983, Pickleman & Gonzalez 1986, Addison & Finan 1988). Moreover, the proportion of elderly patients is increasing (Glenn 1976). Elderly and even aged patients tolerate elective cholecystectomy reasonably well but may succumb to cardiorespiratory complications when hospitalized with acute inflammatory disease (Houghton et al 1985). They are also more susceptible to empyema and perforation, developments that clearly jeopardize the chance of survival.

Diabetics with acute cholecystitis are often thought to fare worse than non-diabetics with the disease (Pellegrini & Way 1987), though one recent survey found no such difference (Pickleman & Gonzalez 1986). During the 1960s prophylactic cholecystectomy was commonly recommended for diabetics with silent gallstones. A recent study from Cleveland has challenged this policy (Ransohoff et al 1987). Although the mortality rate among diabetics with acute cholecystitis was twice that of non-diabetics (6.5% vs. 2.7%), the difference was not statistically significant. A trend towards a higher complication rate among diabetics undergoing emergency biliary surgery in another survey was attributed to their greater age and higher incidence of cardiovascular and renal disease (Sandler et al 1986).

The effect of biliary disease on pregnancy has been reviewed by Hiatt and colleagues (1986) in a series of 26 patients. Nine of the patients required operation for acute cholecystitis during the pregnancy, and 5 of these patients lost the fetus (including 2 by intent). However, two cholecystectomies were safely undertaken during the third trimester. Ultrasonography is the diagnostic investigation of choice. Operative cholangiography should be carried out using a lead shield to protect the lower abdomen.

Acalculous cholecystitis

The outlook is much more serious for the minority of patients (about 10%) with acute acalculous disease. Many of them are elderly, when gangrene and perforation are particularly likely to supervene. Glenn and Becker (1982) reported an overall mortality rate of 9.6% for acute acalculous cholecystitis compared with 4.3% for the calculous variety. The postoperative and post-traumatic forms of acute cholecystitis include a high proportion of acalculous cases and are particularly lethal, with mortality rates of 32–47% (Ottinger 1976, Du Priest et al 1979, Devine et al 1984). Thus the development of necrotising cholecystitis is often the terminal event in patients who are critically ill in an intensive therapy unit.

Prophylaxis

The risk of acute cholecystitis and the safety of elective cholecystectomy justify a policy of early operation in patients with symptomatic gallstones irrespective of age. This maxim is particularly apposite for elderly men (Jenkinson et al 1985). As for acalculous cholecystitis, it has been suggested that periodic administration of oral fat or intravenous cholecystokinin (CCK) might overcome the biliary stasis that predisposes to its development in susceptible patients. Although there is no evidence to support such a regime, prophylactic CCK could therefore be of benefit for patients undergoing major operation, those with multiple trauma and those maintained on total parenteral nutrition (Petersen & Sheldon 1979, Flancbaum et al 1985).

Conclusions

Gallstones are common and are responsible for 90% of attacks of acute cholecystitis. Most affected patients will have had previous symptoms before developing the acute attack. Sudden obstruction of the cystic duct by a stone leads to changes within the lumen of the gallbladder (increased tension, increased lysolecithin content) that can trigger the inflammatory process with or without the assistance of bacteria derived from the gut. Acalculous acute cholecystitis may develop spontaneously, especially in patients recovering from major surgery or multiple trauma. Aetiological features include biliary obstruction and stasis, increased bile viscosity and mucosal ischaemia. Acalculous cholecystitis is a rare complication of septicaemia, torsion and therapeutic manoeuvres such as ligation and cannulation of the hepatic artery.

Fever, local tenderness and leucocytosis are sometimes accompanied by a mass and mild jaundice. Ultrasonography and cholescintigraphy are clearly established as the best means of confirming the diagnosis. Patients with peritonitis or severe constitutional upset need emergency laparotomy after a short period of vigorous resuscitation. Gangrene, empyema or perforation will often be found at operation, especially in acalculous disease. For the majority who respond to initial conservative management, there is much to commend a routine policy of early operation during the next few days. Cholecystectomy is nearly always the procedure of choice, but occasionally partial cholecystectomy or percutaneous cholecystostomy may be appropriate.

An overall mortality rate of 2–5% can be anticipated in acute cholecystitis. For the ordinary calculous variety, death is virtually confined to the elderly, in whom both local complications and intercurrent disease are common. Acute acalculous disease has a mortality rate of about 10%. When cholecystitis complicates major surgery or multiple injuries, at least a third of patients die.

REFERENCES

Addison N V, Finan P J 1988 Urgent and early cholecystectomy for acute gallbladder disease. British Journal of Surgery 75: 141–143
Ashby B S 1965 Acute and recurrent torsion of the gall-bladder. British Journal of Surgery 52: 182–184
Axelrod L, Munster A M, O'Brien T F 1971 Typhoid cholecystitis and gallbladder carcinoma after interval of 67 years. Journal of the American Medical Association 217: 83

Beckman I, Dash N, Sefczek R J et al 1985 Ultrasonographic findings in acute acalculous cholecystitis. Gastrointestinal Radiology 10: 387–389
Bornman P C, Terblanche J 1985 Subtotal cholecystectomy: For the difficult gallbladder in portal hypertension and cholecystitis. Surgery 98: 1–6
Bowen A 1984 Acute gallbladder dilatation in a neonate: emphasis on ultrasonography. Journal of Pediatric Gastroenterology and Nutrition 3: 304–308

Brady E, Welch J P 1985 Acute hemorrhagic cholecystitis causing hemobilia and colonic necrosis. Diseases of the Colon and Rectum 28: 185–187

Bushnell D L, Perlman S B, Wilson M A, Polcyn R E 1986 The rim sign: association with acute cholecystitis. Journal of Nuclear Medicine 27: 353–356

Butsch J L, Luchette F 1985 Torsion of the gallbladder. Archives of Surgery 120: 1323

Cabellon S, Brown J M, Cavanaugh D G 1984 Accuracy of the hepatobiliary scan in acute cholecystitis. American Journal of Surgery 148: 607–608

Carrasco C H, Freeny P C, Chuang V P, Wallace S 1983 Chemical cholecystitis associated with hepatic artery infusion chemotherapy. American Journal of Roentgenology 141: 703–706

Claesson B E B, Holmlund D E W, Matzsch T W 1986 Microflora of the gallbladder related to duration of acute cholecystitis. Surgery Gynecology and Obstetrics 162: 531–535

Cohen E K, Stringer D A, Smith C R, Daneman T W 1986 Hydrops of the gallbladder in typhoid fever as demonstrated by sonography. Journal of Clinical Ultrasound 14: 633–635

Crumplin M K H, Jenkinson L R, Kassab J Y, Whitaker C M Al-Boutiahi F H 1985 Management of gallstones in a district general hospital. British Journal of Surgery 72: 428–432

Datz F L 1986 Utility of indium[111]-labeled leukocyte imaging in acute acalculous cholecystitis. American Journal of Roentgenology 147: 813–814

der Linden W van, Sunzel H 1970 Early versus delayed operation for acute cholecystitis. A controlled clinical trial. American Journal of Surgery 120: 7–13

Devine R M, Farnell M B, Mucha P Jr 1984 Acute cholecystitis as a complication in surgical patients. Archives of Surgery 119: 1389–1393

Dillon E, Parkin G J S 1980 The role of upper abdominal ultrasonography in suspected acute cholecystitis. Clinical Radiology 31: 175–179

Duncan J 1844 Femoral hernia: gangrene of the gallbladder; extravasation of bile; peritonitis; death. Northern Journal of Medicine 2: 151–153. Cited by Johnson L B 1987

Du Priest R W Jr, Khaneja S C, Cowley R A 1979 Acute cholecystitis complicating trauma. Annals of Surgery 189: 84–89

Essenhigh D M 1966 Management of acute cholecystitis. British Journal of Surgery 53: 1032–1038

Essenhigh D M 1968 Perforation of the gall-bladder. British Journal of Surgery 55: 175–178

Fabian T C, Hickerson W L, Mangiante E C 1986 Posttraumatic and postoperative acute cholecystitis. American Surgeon 52: 188–192

Flancbaum L, Majerus T C, Cox E F 1985 Acute posttraumatic acalculous cholecystitis. American Journal of Surgery 150: 252–256

Fox M S, Wilk P J, Weissmann H S, Freeman L M, Gliedman M L 1984 Acute acalculous cholecystitis. Surgery, Gynecology and Obstetrics 159: 13–16

Ganey J B, Johnson P A Jr, Prillaman P E, McSwain G R 1986 Cholecystectomy: clinical experience with a large series. American Journal of Surgery 151: 352–357

Gill T, Dillon E, Leahy L, Reeder A, Peel A L G 1985 Ultrasonography, HIDA scintigraphy or both in the diagnosis of acute cholecystitis. British Journal of Surgery 72: 267–268

Gingrich R A, Awe W C, Boyden A M, Peterson C G 1968 Cholecystostomy in acute cholecystitis. Factors influencing morbidity and mortality. American Journal of Surgery 116: 310–315

Glenn F 1976 Acute cholecystitis. Surgery, Gynecology and Obstetrics 143: 56–58

Glenn F 1979 Acute acalculous cholecystitis. Annals of Surgery 189: 458–465

Glenn F, Becker C G 1982 Acute acalculous cholecystitis. Annals of Surgery 195: 131–136

Glenn F, Wantz G E 1956 Acute cholecystitis following the surgical treatment of unrelated disease. Surgery Gynecology and Obstetrics 102: 145–153

Goldman G, Rafael A J, Hanoch K 1985 Acute acalculous cholecystitis due to an incarcerated epigastric hernia. Postgraduate Medical Journal 61: 1017–1018

Greenwood R K 1963 Torsion of the gallbladder. Gut 4: 27–29

Gullick H D 1960 A roentgenologic study of gallbladder evacuation following nonbiliary tract surgery. Annals of Surgery 151: 403–408

Heuman R, Norrby S, Sjödahl R, Tiselius H-G, Tagesson C 1980 Altered gallbladder bile composition in gallstone disease. Relation to gallbladder wall permeability. Scandinavian Journal of Gastroenterology 15: 581–586

Hiatt J R, Hiatt J C G, Wiliams R A, Klein S R 1986 Biliary disease in pregnancy: strategy for surgical management. American Journal of Surgery 151: 263–265

Houghton P W J, Jenkinson L R, Donaldson L A 1985 Cholecystectomy in the elderly: a prospective study. British Journal of Surgery 72: 220–222

Howard J M, Milford M T, De Bakey M E 1952 The significance of the sympathetic nervous system in acute cholecystitis. Surgery 32: 251–258

Huber D F, Martin E W, Cooperman M 1983 Cholecystectomy in elderly patients. American Journal of Surgery 146: 719–722

Jarvinen H J, Hastbacka J 1980 Early cholecystectomy for acute cholecystitis: a prospective randomized study. Annals of Surgery 191: 501–505

Jenkinson L R, Crumplin M K H, Kassab J Y, Whitaker C J 1985 Early elective cholecystectomy — an alternative to early cholecystectomy in acute cholecystitis. Annals of the Royal College of Surgeons of England 67: 162–163

Jivegard L, Thornell E, Svanvik J 1987 Pathophysiology of acute obstructive cholecystitis: implications for non-operative management. British Journal of Surgery 74: 1081–1084

Joehl R, Koch K L, Nahrwold D L 1984 Opioid drugs cause bile duct obstruction during hepatobiliary scans. American Journal of Surgery 147: 134–138

Johnson E E, Hedley-Whyte J 1975 Continuous positive-pressure ventilation and choledochoduodenal flow resistance. Journal of Applied Physiology 39: 937–942

Johnson L B 1987 The importance of early diagnosis of acute acalculous cholecystitis. Surgery, Gynecology and Obstetrics 164: 197–203

Jones P F 1982 Acute cholecystitis: a case for early surgery? British Medical Journal 285: 1376–1377

Jönsson P-E, Andersson A 1976 Postoperative acute acalculous cholecystitis. Archives of Surgery 111: 1097–1100

Klimberg S, Hawkins I, Vogel S B 1987 Percutaneous cholecystostomy for acute cholecystitis in high-risk patients. American Journal of Surgery 153: 125–129

Krabbel M 1920 Die Stieltorsion der Gallenblase. Deutsche
Zeitschriftfür Chirurgie 154: 76–86

Lahtinen I, Alhava E M, Auke S 1978 Acute cholecystitis
treated by early and delayed surgery. A controlled clinical
trial. Scandinavian Journal of Gastroenterology
13: 673–678

Lindberg E F, Grinnan G L B, Smith L 1970 Acalculous
cholecystitis in Viet Nam casualties. Annals of Surgery
171: 152–157

Li Volsi V A, Perzin K H, Porter M 1973 Polyarteritis
nodosa of the gallbladder presenting as acute cholecystitis.
Gastroenterology 65: 115–123

Long T N, Helmbach D M, Carrico C J 1978 Acalculous
cholecystitis in critically ill patients. American Journal of
Surgery 136: 31–36

Lygidakis N J 1981 Surgery for acalculous cholecystitis. An
organic and not a functional disease. American Journal of
Gastroenterology 76: 27–31

McArthur P, Cuschieri A, Sells R A, Shields R 1975
Controlled clinical trial comparing early with interval
cholecystectomy for acute cholecystitis. British Journal of
Surgery 62: 850–852

McFadden D W, Smith G W 1987 Hemodialysis-associated
hemorrhagic cholecystitis. American Journal of
Gastroenterology 82: 1081–1083

May R E, Strong R 1971 Acute emphysematous
cholecystitis. British Journal of Surgery 58: 453–458

Mitchell A, Morris P J 1982 Trends in management of acute
cholecystitis. British Medical Journal 284: 27–30

Morris C R, Hohf R P, Ivy A C 1952. An experimental
study of the role of stasis in the etiology of cholecystitis.
Surgery 32: 673–685

Niemeier O W 1934 Acute free perforation of the
gallbladder. Annals of Surgery 99: 922–924

Orlando R, III, Gleason E, Drezner A D 1983 Acute
acalculous cholecystitis in the crtically ill patient.
American Journal of Surgery 145: 472–476

Ottinger L W 1976 Acute cholecystitis as a postoperative
complication. Annals of Surgery 184: 162–165

Paterson-Brown S, Chan S T F 1987 Early versus delayed
cholecystectomy for acute cholecystitis. British Journal of
Hospital Medicine 37: 546–548

Payne R A 1969 Evaluation of the management of acute
cholecystitis. British Journal of Surgery 56: 200–202

Pellegrini C A, Way L W 1987 Acute cholecystitis. In: Way
L W, Pellegrini C A (eds) Surgery of the gallbladder and
bile ducts. Saunders, Philadelphia, pp 251–264

Penn I 1962 Injuries of the gall-bladder. British Journal of
Surgery 49: 636–641

Petersen S R, Sheldon G F 1979 Acute acalculous
cholecystitis: a complication of hyperalimentation.
American Journal of Surgery 138: 814–817

Pheils M T, Duraiappah B 1975 Cholecystostomy for acute
cholecystitis. Medical Journal of Australia 1: 418–419

Pickleman J, Gonzalez R P 1986 The improving results of
cholecystectomy. Archives of Surgery 121: 930–934

Pietrafitta J J, Anderson B G, O'Brien M J, Deckers P J
1986 Cholecystitis secondary to infusion chemotherapy.
Journal of Surgical Oncology 31: 287–293

Proia A D, Fetter B F, Woodard B H, Stickel D L, Meyers
W C 1986 Fatal pulmonary bile embolism following acute
acalculous cholecystitis. Archives of Surgery
121: 1206–1208

Quinn S F, Fazzio F, Jones E 1987 Torsion of the
gallbladder: findings on CT and sonography and role of

percutaneous cholecystostomy. American Journal of
Roentgenology 148: 881–882

Radin D R, Halls J M 1987 Emphysematous cholecystitis
presenting with pneumoperitoneum. American Journal of
Roentgenology 149: 1175–1176

Ransohoff D F, Miller G L, Forsythe S B, Hermann R E
1987 Outcome of acute cholecystitis in patients with
diabetes mellitus. Annals of Internal Medicine
106: 829–832

Ranson J H C 1987 Perforation of the gallbladder. In: Way
L W, Pellegrini C A (eds) Surgery of the gallbladder and
bile ducts. Saunders, Philadelphia pp 265–273

Recht W 1952 Torsion of a double gallbladder. A report of
a case and a review of the literature. British Journal of
Surgery 39: 342–344

Reyes C V, Jablokow V R, Reid R 1981
Xanthogranulomatous cholecystitis: report of seven cases.
American Surgeon 47: 322–325

Roslyn J J, Thompson J E Jr, Davies H, DenBesten L 1987
Risk factors for gallbladder perforation. American Journal
of Gastroenterology 82: 636–640

Rosoff L, Meyers H 1966 Acute emphysematous
cholecystitis. An analysis of ten cases. American Journal
of Surgery 111: 410–423

Salomonowitz E, Frick M P, Simmons R L et al 1984
Obliteration of the gallbladder without formal
cholecystectomy. Archives of Surgery 119: 725–729

Sandler R S, Maule W F, Baltus M E 1986 Factors
associated with postoperative complications in diabetics
after biliary tract surgery. Gastroenterology 91: 157–162

Schlinkert R T, Mucha P Jr, Farnell M B 1984 Torsion of
the gallbladder. Mayo Clinic Proceedings 59: 490–492

Shields M A 1973 Acute acalculous cholecystitis: an
important complication of trauma. Journal of the Royal
College of Surgeons of Edinburgh 18: 83–86

Siskind B N, Hawkins H B, Cinti D C, Zeman R K,
Burrell M I 1987 Gallbladder perforation. An imaging
analysis. Journal of Clinical Gastroenterology 9: 670–678

Sjödahl R, Wetterfors J 1974 Lysolecithin and lecithin in
the gallbladder wall and bile; their possible roles in the
pathogenesis of acute cholecystitis. Scandinavian Journal
of Gastroenterology 9: 519–525

Sjödahl R, Tagesson C 1983 On the development of primary
acute cholecystitis. Scandinavian Journal of
Gastroenterology 18: 577–579

Stolz A 1901 Ueber Gasbildung in den Gallenwegen. Archiv
der pathologischer Anatomie 165: 90–123

Stryker S J, Beal J M 1983 Acute cholecystitis and
common-duct calculi. Archives of Surgery 118: 1063–1064

Swayne L C 1986 Acute acalculous cholecystitis: sensitivity
in detection using technetium-99m iminodiacetic acid
cholescintigraphy. Radiology 160: 33–38

Ternberg J L, Keating J P 1975 Acute acalculous
cholecystitis. Complication of other illnesses in childhood.
Archives of Surgery 110: 543–547

Thomas W E G, Thornton J R, Thompson M H 1981
Staphylococcal acalculous cholecystitis. British Journal of
Surgery 68: 136

Thornton J R, Heaton K W, Espiner H J, Eltringham W K
1983 Empyema of the gallbladder — reappraisal of a
neglected disease. Gut 24: 1183–1185

Thurston W A, Kelly E N, Silver M M 1986 Acute
acalculous cholecystitis in a premature infant treated with
parenteral nutrition. Canadian Medical Association Journal
135: 332–334

Traynelis V C, Hrabovsky E E 1985 Acalculous cholecystitis in the neonate. American Journal of Diseases of Children 139: 893–895

Van Sonnenberg E, Wittich G R, Casola G et al 1986 Diagnostic and therapeutic percutaneous gallbladder procedures. Radiology 160: 23–26

Washburn M E, Barcia P J 1980 Uncommon cause of a right upper quadrant abdominal mass in the newborn: acute cholecystitis. American Journal of Surgery 140: 704–705

Watts J McK, Toouli J 1984 Cholecystitis and choledocholithiasis. In: Bouchier I A D, Allan R N, Hodgson, H J F, Keighley M R B (eds) Textbook of gastroenterology. Baillière Tindall, London p 1416

Weeder R S, Bashant G H, Muir R W 1970 Acute non-calculous cholecystitis ascciated with severe injury. American Journal of Surgery 119: 729–732

Welch J P, Malt R A 1972 Outcome of cholecystostomy. Surgery, Gynecology and Obstetrics 135: 717–720

Whitington P F, Black D D 1980 Cholelithiasis in premature infants treated with parenteral nutrition and furosemide. Journal of Pediatrics 97: 647–649

Williamson R C N 1987 Surgery of the biliary tract and pancreas. In: Kirk R M, Williamson R C N (eds) General surgical operations.Churchill Livingstone, Edinburgh pp 171–195

Williamson R C N 1988 Acalculous disease of the gallbladder. Gut 29: 860–872

Witte C L 1984 Choledochal obstruction by cystic duct stone. Annals of Surgery 50: 241–243

Ziv Y, Feigerberg Z, Zer M, Dintsman M 1987 Acute cholecystitis complicating unrelated disease: etiological considerations. American Journal of Gastroenterology 82: 1165–1168

8 *Early management of acute gallstone pancreatitis*

M. J. McMAHON

Acute pancreatitis is becoming an increasingly common disease in many westernized countries, including the UK. Gallstones and alcohol abuse are the commonest causes of attacks of acute pancreatitis. Although alcohol is responsible for much of the increase in prevalence, gallstones remain the principal cause of pancreatitis in many parts of the world. Statistically, patients who develop pancreatitis secondary to gallstones are more likely to be women and over 60 years of age. Superficially, attacks of pancreatitis due to gallstones are similar to those associated with alcohol abuse, but the relatively older age of many of the patients and the coexistence of other diseases associated with the 'westernized' lifestyle,

such as hypertension and congestive cardiac failure, probably contribute to a higher mortality rate; also the presence of obstruction and infection within the biliary tract lead to complications such as cholangitis. Patients who develop pancreatitis secondary to gallstones, like those whose attacks are secondary to alcohol abuse, are subject to complications such as pancreatic abscess, necrosis and pseudocyst, but it is probably uncommon for chronic pancreatitis to be a consequence.

The exact mechanism whereby a gallstone causes acute pancreatitis is unknown but many suggestions have been made (Fig. 8.1). There is no clear consensus concerning the optimal diagnosis of gallstones in patients with pancreatitis, and there are a variety of management options, some of which are controversial and unproven.

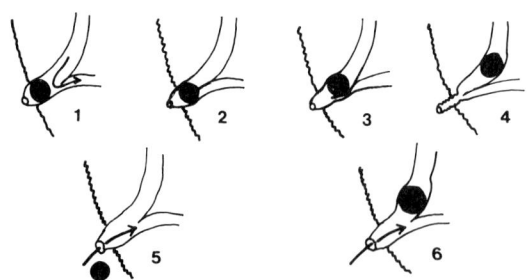

Fig. 8.1 Suggested mechanisms for the induction of acute pancreatitis by gallstones. 1. The classic 'common channel' theory in which bile refluxes into the pancreatic duct behind a stone obstructing the common channel formed by the junction of biliary and pancreatic ducts. 2. Obstruction of both ducts by a stone in the common channel without the opportunity for reflux. 3. Obstruction of the pancreatic duct by a stone lodged in the adjacent portion of the distal common bile duct. 4. Obstruction of the distal bile duct by a stone with spasm of the ampulla. 5. Duodenopancreatic reflux after the passage of a stone from the bile duct into the duodenum. 6. Duodenopancreatic reflux resulting from the presence of a stone in the lower bile duct.

Pathogenesis of gallstone-related pancreatitis

The relationship between acute pancreatitis and gallstones was recognised by Opie (1901) and Halsted (1901). These authors suggested possible mechanisms, including the 'retrojection' of bile into the pancreas caused by the blockage of the ampullary outlet by a stone in a 'common channel' of sufficient length to allow free communication between the bile duct and the pancreatic duct above the stone. Almost half a century was to pass before the association between acute pancreatitis and gallstones was proven. Molander & Bell (1946), in a study of a large number of autopsies, found gallstones to be six times more common in patients with pancreatitis than in the general population. Attacks of pancreatitis due to gallstones are frequently recurrent if the gallstones remain untreated, and both Raker & Bartlett (1953) and Howard (1960) showed that cholecystectomy was highly successful as a measure for the prevention of further attacks of pancreatitis.

Widespread acceptance of the Opie and Halsted 'common channel' theory was prevented by the frequent observation that only about 5% of patients who had suffered an attack of acute pancreatitis due to gallstones could be shown to have a stone lodged at the ampulla. Moreover, neither the pancreas nor the pancreatic duct is usually stained with bile when laparotomy is carried out in the early stages of acute pancreatitis due to gallstones (the duct was stained bright green in Opie and Halsted's case). The reason for the low frequency of impacted gallstones became apparent from studies carried out by Acosta & Ledesma (1974) and Kelly (1976). By sieving the faeces of patients, they showed that it was possible to recover gallstones from the faecal matter in a high proportion of patients after an attack of acute pancreatitis but not when the patient was admitted to hospital with other clinical manifestations of gallstone disease. The inference from these studies — that gallstones were causing pancreatitis by their presence in the lower part of the common duct, but that most of them pass spontaneously into the duodenum — was confirmed by Acosta et al (1978), who reported on the findings of a policy of operative intervention within the first 48 hours in a series of patients with acute pancreatitis due to gallstones, and in 72% found that a stone was lodged at the lower end of the common duct. Subsequently, it has been shown that patients with pancreatitis are most likely to have small and perhaps irregularly shaped gallstones and a functioning gallbladder (McMahon & Shefta 1980, Houssin et al 1983, Farinon et al 1987, Taylor & Armstrong, 1987). There now seems little doubt, therefore, that most cases of acute pancreatitis due to gallstones are caused by the migration of a stone from the gallbladder into the duodenum with transient obstruction in the ampullary region. Exactly how the migrating stone triggers the attack has been the subject of much controversy and remains an enigma.

Some of the mechanisms that have been suggested to explain the relationship between gallstones and the induction of acute pancreatitis are shown in Figure 8.1. Reflux of bile into the pancreatic duct behind a gallstone occluding the 'common channel' was the mechanism suggested by Opie and Halsted. From animal experiments it is quite clear that the injection of bile into the pancreatic duct can cause severe pancreatitis, especially when it is injected under pressure or if the bile contains micro-organisms, activated pancreatic proteases or duodenal enterokinase. However, in the absence of pressure or activated enzymes it is probable that bile is not particularly toxic to the pancreas. Moreover, in experimental animals, the pressure of secretion is such that it is more likely that pancreatic juice will flow into the bile than bile into the pancreatic duct (Elmslie et al 1966). There has been a great deal of controversy concerning the frequency of the 'common channel'. Although careful studies of autopsy material suggest that a common channel of sufficient length to allow intercommunication of biliary and pancreatic secretions behind a stone is a minority finding (Sterling 1954, Berman et al 1960), there seems little doubt that reflux of contrast medium into the pancreatic duct during the performance of an intraoperative cholangiogram is considerably more common in patients who have had gallstone-related pancreatitis than in patients who have alternative symptom complexes due to gallstones (Taylor & Rimmer 1980, McMahon et al 1981). The induction of hyperamylasaemia when the pancreatic duct opacifies during cholangiography (Howell & Bergh 1950) and the frequently dilated nature of the pancreatic duct in which reflux occurs during cholangiography (Cuschieri & Hughes 1973) can be interpreted as evidence to support the hypothesis that the anatomical arrangement of the lower end of the common bile duct predisposes to reflux into the pancreatic duct and hence to pancreatitis. It is equally possible that the changes are a consequence rather than a cause of pancreatitis. Recently, Schmitz-Moorman et al (1986) have suggested that the 'common channel' is less frequent in patients who develop gallstone-related acute pancreatitis, and the cholangiographic findings of Acosta et al (1980) only showed reflux of contrast

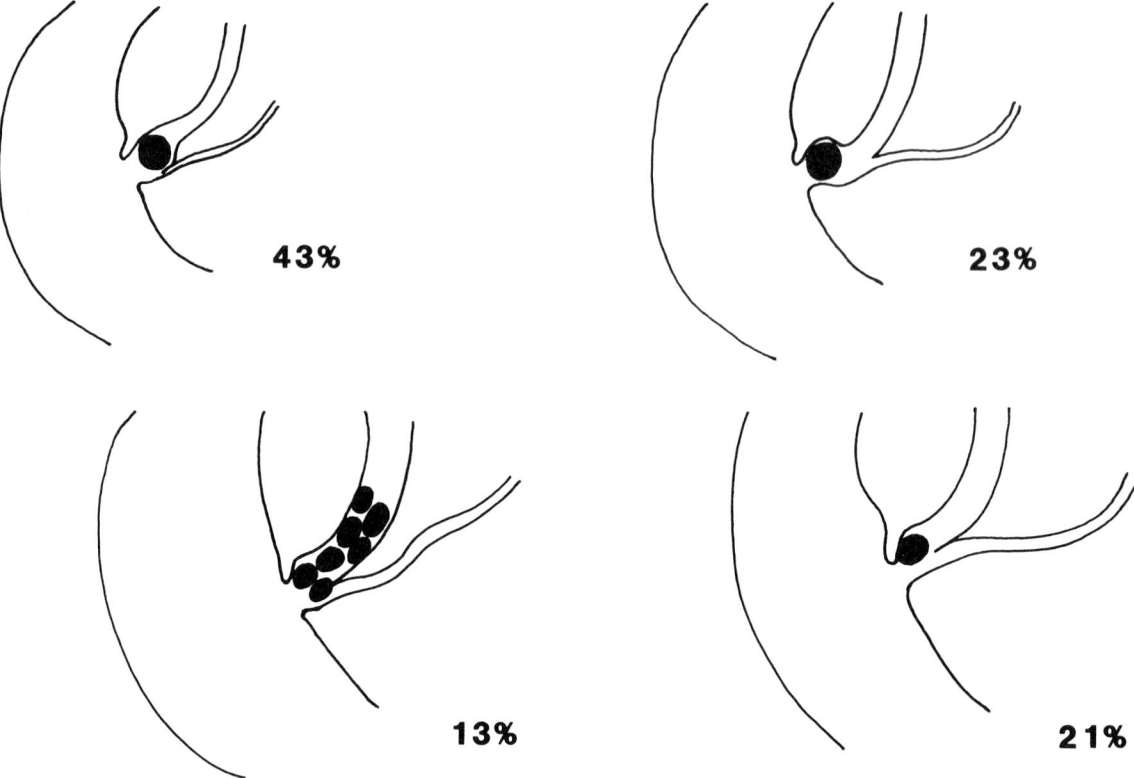

Fig. 8.2 Types of ampullary obstruction in 47 patients with acute pancreatitis due to gallstones based upon the findings of operative cholangiography. (From Acosta et al 1980)

medium into the pancreatic duct in only 23% of patients who underwent surgical intervention early in the course of the disease (Fig. 8.2). Despite the theories, there is no evidence that a common channel is a necessary prerequisite for pancreatitis, and there is no evidence that reflux of bile into the pancreatic duct occurs in patients who develop gallstone-related pancreatitis.

It is probable that during migration, gallstones occlude the pancreatic duct by their presence in the common channel, or in the lower part of the bile duct where it lies closely adjacent to the pancreatic duct. There are no convincing experimental models of gallstone-related pancreatitis, but perhaps the best is in the opossum, where there is a considerable length of common channel. In this animal, obstruction of the pancreatic duct alone causes mild pancreatitis but the disease becomes more severe if the pancreatic and bile ducts

are ligated independently, or if the common channel itself is ligated (Senninger et al 1986).

Reflux of duodenal contents into the pancreas through a patulous ampulla was advocated as a cause by McCutcheon (1968) and recent editorial comments have argued in its favour (*Lancet* 1988, Barry 1988). However, in my opinion there is little evidence to favour this mechanism and much to oppose it. There is some evidence for sphincter dysfunction in patients who have had pancreatitis associated with gallstones. Cuschieri et al (1984) showed that in patients undergoing cholecystectomy, who had previously had an attack of acute pancreatitis, the sphincter of Oddi complex exhibited a hypotonic response to an infusion of saline which was uninfluenced by a cerulein analogue in contrast to the increased manometric pressure in response to saline, infusion and marked relaxation in response to the cerulein analogue, found in patients who had previously had an attack of cholecystitis or biliary colic. The significance of these findings is unclear, and it is arguable whether the patulous sphincter was a predisposing factor for pancreatitis, or a consequence of the migration of a gallstone.

In summary, it is known that acute pancreatitis results from the migration of gallstones from the bile duct into the duodenum and their temporary lodgement at the lower end of the common duct. Certain anatomical and functional features of the biliary tract appear to be associated with pancreatitis, but their significance is unclear and a causal relationship to pancreatitis has not been established. From a practical point of view it seems reasonable to assume that it is the presence of the stone in the lower common duct or ampulla that gives rise to the pancreatitis, but in many patients the stone passes onwards rapidly and may have done so by the time the patient arrives in hospital. Two important issues arise. Firstly, is there therapeutic advantage to be gained from extracting the stone from the lower common duct during the early stages of the attack? Secondly, how can patients in the early stage of the hospital admission who not only have gallstones, but still have a stone in the lower common bile duct be detected?

Some patients with gallstone-associated pancreatitis have a very mild attack, so mild perhaps that an ultrasound scan shows no abnormality is evident within the pancreas, and little abnormality is seen at laparotomy a few days after admission to hospital. This has prompted the suggestion that gallstones and hyperamylasaemia may be a separate entity from gallstone-related acute pancreatitis (Roth 1974, Lesser & Warshaw 1975). If such a separate entity does exist, then the source of the amylase remains obscure, although a possible explanation is the reflux of pancreatic juice from the pancreatic duct into the biliary tract from whence it passes into the plasma (the 'common channel theory' in reverse). Certainly, there do appear to be rare occasions when amylase-rich bile can be detected (Bradley et al 1981), but until the existence of alternative mechanisms for the production of hyperamylasaemia in patients with gallstones is firmly established it is probably acceptable to argue that in some patients the degree of pancreatitis is so mild that morphological evidence of its presence is difficult to establish. The situation may be analogous to ligation of the pancreatic duct in experimental animals, which may produce little more than slight oedema of the gland but a measurable rise in plasma amylase. For the clinician, it is probably safest to assume that hyperamylasaemia in a patient with the symptoms of biliary colic represents mild acute pancreatitis, but it should be remembered that the stone that causes the pancreatitis may lead to coexistent pathology in the biliary tract such as cholecystitis (Mackie et al 1985).

The diagnosis of gallstones in patients with acute pancreatitis

Patients with gallstone-related acute pancreatitis are usually elderly (mean age about 65 years) and frequently female. Thus, in an elderly woman with symptoms of biliary colic and a raised plasma amylase level, the diagnosis of acute pancreatitis due to gallstones can be predicted with confidence upon the basis of clinical features and a single enzyme assay. In other patients the relationship between pancreatitis and gallstones may not be as clear. With increasing emphasis upon the urgent or emergency management of gallstone-related pancreatitis, precise recognition of the presence of associated gallstones has become important.

In addition to clinical features, the magnitude of the amylase rise in patients with acute pancreatitis can be a guide to the cause of the attack, higher levels being usual in patients with gallstone-related attacks compared to those with attacks due to alcohol (Paloyan & Simonowitz 1976). Moreover, amylase levels tend to fall more rapidly in patients with gallstone-related attacks (McMahon & Mayer 1984). Unfortunately, amylase levels are not sufficiently specific to be of great diagnostic value. Computer analysis of clinical data and the results of routine laboratory investigations available on the day of admission was shown to predict the presence of gallstones in patients with acute pancreatitis with an accuracy of 92% (Graham & Wyllie 1979), but the facility is not widely available, and it is possible that the programme might require modification for the spectra of acute pancreatitis found in different hospitals.

The diagnosis of gallstones in patients with acute pancreatitis during the early stages of the attack is most helped by radiological or biochemical investigations.

Radiological detection of gallstones during the early stages of acute pancreatitis

Traditional radiological contrast techniques are of little value for the urgent diagnosis of gallstones in patients with acute pancreatitis. Kaden et al (1955) showed that 65% of apparently normal gallbladders failed to fill, or filled abnormally, when an oral cholecystogram was performed during the first week of relatively mild acute pancreatitis. Intravenous cholangiography performed a little better, but the biliary tract was still not visualized in 35% of patients (Johnson et al 1959).

Radionuclide scans

Radionuclide imaging using ^{99m}Tc-HIDA was shown by Fonseca et al (1979) to be able to differentiate acute cholecystitis from acute pancreatitis. In cholecystitis the gallbladder characteristically failed to take up the isotope, but 13 of 15 patients with pancreatitis appeared to have a functioning gallbladder; the cause of pancreatitis in these patients was not stated. If acute pancreatitis results from the migration of gallstones from the gallbladder into the duodenum, ^{99}Tc-HIDA would be expected to enter the gallbladder, particularly as the cystic duct tends to be somewhat dilated in these patients (McMahon & Shefta 1980). The findings of Glazer at al (1981) were accordingly unexpected. Thirty-six patients with acute pancreatitis underwent a ^{99m}Tc-HIDA scan within three days of admission. Twenty of the patients were shown to have pancreatitis due to gallstones and in none of them was the gallbladder visualized. The remaining patients, whose pancreatitis was not due to gallstones, showed evidence of gallbladder filling with ^{99m}Tc-HIDA. Because the lack of gallbladder function appeared to be a temporary phenomenon in some patients, the data might be interpreted to suggest that there was temporary occlusion of the cystic

duct in patients with pancreatitis, perhaps by oedema or spasm, or by the migration of further stones. This possibility was supported by Zeman (1981), who also observed that in patients with acute pancreatitis there was non-visualization of the gallbladder when a radionuclide scan was carried out in the early stages. The specificity of the finding in gallstone-related pancreatitis was questioned, however, because it was observed in patients subsequently shown to have a normal gallbladder.

Neoptolemos et al (1983) studied 50 patients with acute pancreatitis and carried out radionuclide biliary scanning with ^{99m}Tc-HIDA within the first 72 h of onset of symptoms. Thirty-four of the patients had pancreatitis shown to be due to gallstones, but in only 53% of them was the scan positive, i.e. the gallbladder did not fill. Sixteen patients had pancreatitis not due to gallstones and 31% of them had a positive scan. The results were compared with those from 51 patients with acute cholecystitis, in all of whom the scan was positive, as it was in 82% of a further 51 patients with biliary colic. The authors concluded that radionuclide scanning was of little value for the identification of gallstones as a cause of acute pancreatitis. Consistent with their findings were those of Stone et al (1981), who found that a radionuclide scan showed non-filling of the gallbladder in only 38% of 26 patients with gallstone-related pancreatitis.

Ultrasonography for the detection of gallstones

Although clearly inferior to CT for visualization of the pancreas during the early stages of acute pancreatitis, ultrasound can visualize the gallbladder in 70–95% of patients, with a greater than 90% accuracy for the detection of gallstones (Stone et al 1981, McKay et al 1982). The technique is dependent upon the expertise of the operator as well as the quality of the equipment. It is probable that published series, most of which come from large university hospitals with enthusiastic clinicians and radiologists, represent the best that can be expected of ultrasound. When an ultrasound scan was performed six weeks after the attack of pancreatitis in 99 patients, it had a sensitivity of 86% and a specificity of 93% for the detection of gallstones (Goodman et al 1985). However, in the same centre ultrasound carried out during the first 72 h after admission only visualized 80% of gallbladders, and although 92% of gallstones in the visualized gallbladders were detected, the overall detection rate was only 67% (Neoptolemos et al 1984). It is important to remember that stones detected by ultrasound early in the course of acute pancreatitis are usually in the gallbladder and do not indicate that gallstones have caused the attack, merely that they are present. Other features such as dilatation of the extrahepatic biliary tree or visualization of a stone in the bile duct may be present, and visualization of the lower bile duct is usually poor during the early stages of acute pancreatitis, especially when the attack is severe.

The use of CT for the early evaluation of severe acute pancreatitis is becoming more routine. Gallstones can be visualized (Fig. 8.3), but there is no evidence that the diagnostic accuracy of CT in the presence of gallstones is greater than that of ultrasound.

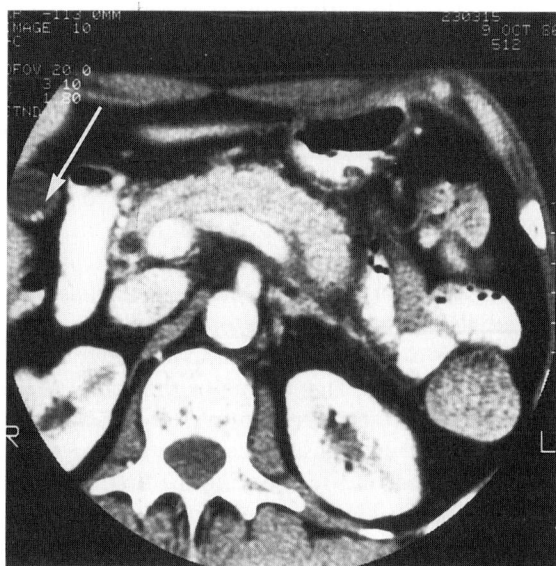

Fig. 8.3 Demonstration of small stones in the gallbladder by CT in a patient who had suffered an attack of acute pancreatitis. (Reproduced by kind permission of Dr A. G. Chalmers)

Biochemical techniques for the detection of gallstones during acute pancreatitis

When jaundice occurs in a patient with acute pancreatitis who has no history of alcohol abuse, there is a high probability of a common duct stone (Frieden 1965). In Leeds, liver function tests were studied during the early stages of acute pancreatitis in order to evaluate their role in the detection of gallstones. Surprisingly, AST (aspartate transaminase, glutamic oxaloacetic transaminase) appeared to discriminate between gallstone and non-gallstone related attacks better than bilirubin or alkaline phosphatase (McMahon & Pickford 1979). A plasma AST level greater than 60 iu/l was found in 88% of attacks associated with gallstones but in none of the attacks due to other causes. Inclusion of the bilirubin or alkaline phosphatase level did not appear to enhance the predictive value of transaminase. It was interesting that 24 h later, the predictive value of transaminase was considerably lower.

These findings were controversial and disputed by some, probably because the inclusion of transaminase levels in blood samples collected at a later stage in the attack reduced the diagnostic value. Further experience in Leeds confirmed the diagnostic value of AST (Fig. 8.4) (Mayer & McMahon 1985). We were also able to demonstrate the transient nature of the rise in transaminase in a fortuitous study of a patient who developed acute pancreatitis related to gallstones whilst in hospital. Transaminase had risen from a previously normal value to 210 iu/l within 2 h of the onset of abdominal pain and hyperamylasaemia, but had fallen back to 56 iu/l 12 h later. In our larger experience 12 (14.5%) of 83 patients with acute pancreatitis not associated with gallstones were found to have a transaminase level above 60 iu/l on the day of admission. One of the 12 was subsequently found to have an ampullary tumour, another developed pancreatitis as a consequence of ERCP examination and a third had undergone mobilization of the duodenal loop and palpation of the common duct at diagnostic laparotomy. The AST was elevated above 60 iu/l in 84% of the 132 attacks of pancreatitis associated with gallstones.

The high predictive value of transaminase early

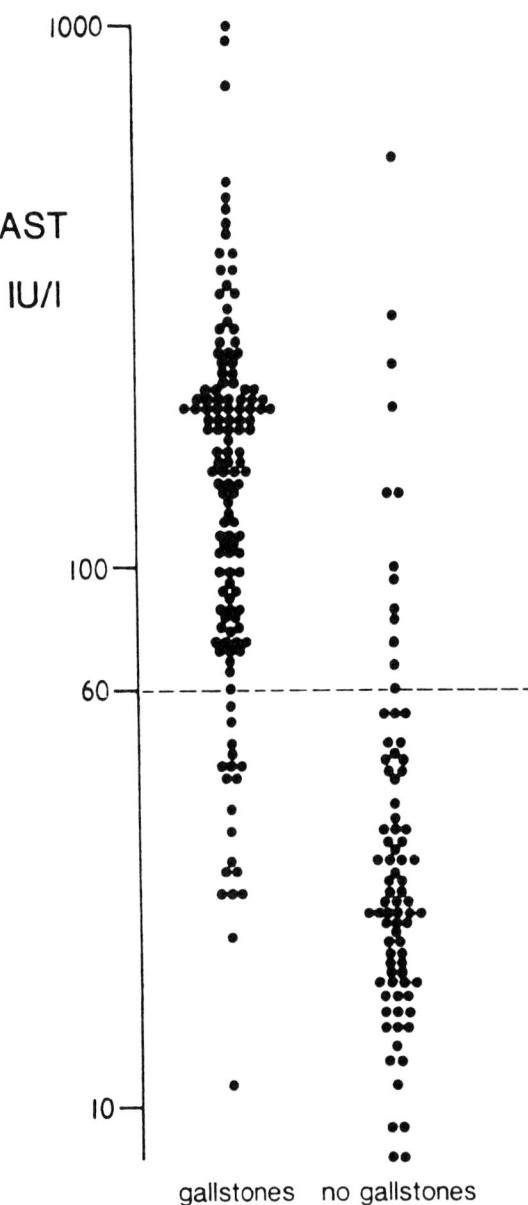

Fig. 8.4 Plasma AST levels on the day of admission to hospital in 132 attacks of acute pancreatitis associated with gallstones and 83 attacks in which no stone could be detected. (Reproduced from Mayer & McMahon 1985, with permission)

in the course of pancreatitis was confirmed by Van Gossum et al (1984), who suggested ALT (alanine transaminase) was slightly better than AST. Neop-

tolemos et al (1984) found that an ALT level above 60 iu/l detected 67% of patients with acute pancreatitis related to gallstones, with a 12% false positive rate when the blood sample was drawn during the first 72 h of the attack. The majority of blood samples were collected on the day of admission. When used in combination with ultrasound, biochemical techniques detected 81% of gallstone-related attacks.

In Leeds, we have been unable to enhance the predictive power of transaminase by the inclusion of data from other biochemical investigations. Blamey et al (1983) did not find ALT or AST as useful, although each had independent predictive value. In addition, they considered alkaline phosphatase, age, gender and amylase to be of value. The differences between their findings and ours might be related to the fact that they considered plasma samples obtained during the initial 48 h after admission rather than the day of admission only.

Diagnosis of gallstones early in the course of acute pancreatitis — what is the best buy?

If it is considered important to know the cause of acute pancreatitis early in the course of the attack, two diagnostic techniques are appropriate. The simplest is the routine measurement of plasma transaminase (AST or ALT) as early as possible in the course of the attack. We routinely send a plasma sample to the laboratory for transaminase measurement at the time of admission, requesting that the plasma be separated and saved in order that the assay can be performed as a routine during normal laboratory hours. Detection of gallstones by radiological techniques after an attack of acute pancreatitis can be difficult, and knowledge of the transaminase level at the time of the acute attack provides important corroborative information. As well as measuring transaminase, it is routine to request an ultrasound scan during the first few days of the attack. This examination is usually performed when the patient is well enough to travel to the radiology department. It is not my practice at the present time to undertake urgent surgical or endoscopic intervention for gallstones in patients with acute pancreatitis, and the routine management of the attack is rarely contingent upon a knowledge of the cause. Nevertheless, this is a controversial topic and current attitudes may have changed by the time this volume is published, creating a greater imperative for the urgent diagnosis of gallstones.

Urgent surgery for the patient with gallstone-related pancreatitis

The traditional approach to gallstones in patients with acute pancreatitis was to treat the attack conservatively, send the patient home, carry out appropriate investigations and then re-admit for cholecystectomy. The objective was to remove the gallbladder and its contained stones and hence the source of further attacks of pancreatitis. The major disadvantage of this plan of action is that it exposes the patient to the risk of another attack of acute pancreatitis whilst cholecystectomy is awaited. This risk is real rather than hypothetical and can lead to the death of the patient (Mayer et al 1984). There is now a large body of opinion that the best policy for prophylactic surgery in patients with gallstone-related acute pancreatitis is to remove the gallbladder during the same admission, but allow sufficient time for the patient to become convalescent from the attack of acute pancreatitis. In some patients, who are elderly or infirm or who have a severe attack of acute pancreatitis, it might be advisable to wait longer. This chapter is concerned with early management of gallstones in patients with acute pancreatitis and will therefore address the problem of the stone that has caused the present attack rather than consider stones in the gallbladder which might cause future attacks.

The case for urgent intervention by operation or endoscopic techniques in patients with gallstone-related pancreatitis depends upon the demonstration that clearance of the duct, and more specifically the ampullary region, reduces morbidity and mortality rates. Acosta et al (1978) related the severity of pancreatitis to the duration of ampullary obstruction by a stone in 49 patients who underwent surgical exploration within 48 hours of the onset of symptoms (Fig. 8.5). They concluded that 'rapid remission occurs if patency of the ampulla is restored before 48 h'. This find-

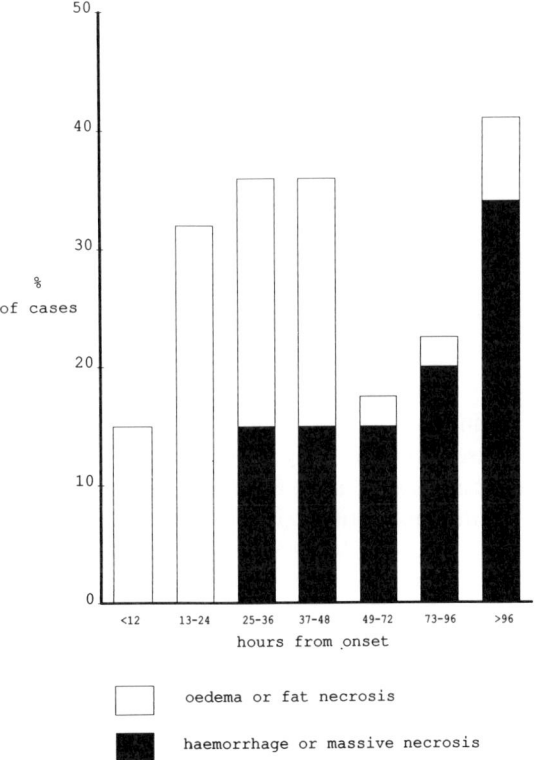

Fig. 8.5 The relationship between the severity of acute pancreatitis and the time elapsed between the onset of symptoms and laparotomy. (From the data of Acosta et al 1980)

ing is consistent with a previous publication in which they had compared results for patients who receive conventional medical treatment, usually accompanied by elective cholecystectomy at a later date, with those for a series of patients operated on to remove the gallbladder and explore the bile duct between 6 and 48 h after the onset of symptoms (Acosta et al 1978). Sixteen percent of the conventionally treated patients died, compared to 2% of those who underwent the urgent biliary exploration. It is important to note, however, that this was not a randomized study. Conventionally treated patients were admitted between 1964 and 1972 and those who underwent urgent exploration between 1972 and 1975. It is possible, therefore, that many other factors such as improvements in fluid and electrolyte management, anaesthesia and intensive care, together with the prophylactic use of antibiotics etc., may have been responsible for the difference in mortality rates. A contrary conclusion was drawn from the experience of Tondelli et al in Basel (1982). Urgent surgical intervention was carried out in 16 patients with gallstone-related pancreatitis, 5 of whom died. However, the indication for surgical intervention was to confirm the diagnosis of pancreatitis, or because another condition such as cholecystitis or cholangitis was suspected.

Mercer et al (1984) recorded their experience of urgent intervention (within 48 h) in 34 patients with 'biliary pancreatitis', who had symptoms or signs compatible with biliary colic or cholecystitis and an increase in serum amylase. The mean amylase level was only 621 iu/l, so that many of the patients would not fulfil the diagnostic criteria of acute pancreatitis related to gallstones that we use in Leeds. Cholecystectomy was carried out together with operative cholangiography and, when appropriate, exploration of the common bile duct. Despite the fact that 20 of the patients were operated on within 24 hours of admission, only 12 of them (35%) were found to have a common duct stone. None of the patients had haemorrhagic pancreatitis. All patients made steady progress after operation, and there were no deaths. The authors concluded that their findings were generally applicable to patients with acute pancreatitis due to gallstones and thus recommended urgent evaluation and treatment. They felt that this would reduce the morbidity and mortality rates resulting from operation at a later stage in the disease. From the data presented, it is unlikely that the patients in this series are representative of gallstone pancreatitis as a whole, and one must doubt the general applicability of the conclusions.

Kelly (1980) recorded his experience of 24 patients with gallstone-related pancreatitis who were operated on within 48 h. In contrast to the patients recorded by Mercer et al, an impacted ampullary stone was found in 63% of the patients. A quarter of them developed complications of the operation and three died. This mortality rate is to be compared to no deaths and a 7% incidence of complications in 146 patients operated on between 5 and 8 days after admission, but of importance is the indication used by Kelly for urgent operation. If the patients failed to show improvement with normal conservative management, exploration was undertaken, so that this group of patients were probably those with the most severe pancreatitis. Nevertheless, only four of them were considered to have haemorrhagic pancreatitis on the evidence available at laparotomy.

The only controlled trial of urgent surgical intervention in patients with gallstone-related pancreatitis was reported by Stone et al in 1981. Patients were randomly assigned to operation within 72 h of admission, or to conservative management with elective operation three months later. 'Urgent intervention' was cholecystectomy combined with transduodenal sphincteroplasty and pancreatic ductal septotomy. Stones were cleared from the common bile duct using a Fogarty catheter. Ductal stones were found in 75% of the 36 patients who underwent emergency surgery compared to 28% of the 29 who received an elective operation. In addition, stones were found in the duodenum in 31% of the emergency surgery group. One patient died at early operation, but none of the patients treated conservatively died during the course of the attack of pancreatitis, although two of them died after elective operation.

The published experience does not, in my opinion, confirm the view of Acosta et al that urgent surgical intervention reduces the morbidity and mortality of acute gallstone-related pancreatitis. Moreover, the data suggest that morbidity and mortality are increased rather than reduced by early surgical intervention. A possible explanation might be the fact that Acosta's original reasoning, that the duration of ampullary obstruction was causally related to the severity of pancreatitis, is incorrect.

Experimental work in the pig by Farias et al (1986) suggests that the duration of ductal obstruction may not be critical. Haemorrhagic pancreatitis was created by injecting a bile salt trypsin solution retrogradely into the pancreatic duct. The duct was ligated for 24 h after the injection, in half the animals and in the other half for 2 h only. There was no difference in mortality rate or in severity of acute pancreatitis. The extent to which this model parallels human pancreatitis is unclear, but the results do question the importance of the duration of ductal obstruction to the severity of the attack.

An alternative explanation for the disappointing results of urgent surgical intervention is that patients during the acute stage of pancreatitis are ill-equipped to withstand laparotomy and surgical exploration of the biliary tract. If this is so, it suggests that the advantages of duct clearance are likely to emerge if it can be achieved by non-operative methods. Therefore, there is great interest in endoscopic sphincterotomy as a means to this end.

If laparotomy is undertaken during the early stages of acute pancreatitis due to gallstones, what action should be taken as far as the biliary tract is concerned? This is not an easy question to answer on the basis of established fact. It is likely that the patient will have relatively severe pancreatitis because it is not usually necessary to undertake diagnostic laparotomy in patients with mild attacks. It is usually the fear that a lesion such as perforated peptic ulcer or mesenteric infarction may be present that prompts the laparotomy. My advice is to leave the biliary tract alone unless there is evidence of cholangitis or cholecystitis. To avoid trauma to the pancreas, the decision to explore the common duct should be made after performing an operative cholangiogram, because the external appearance of the duct, which may be oedematous and inflamed, is probably a poor guide to the presence of stones in patients with a recent attack of pancreatitis. In my view, the duct should only be explored if a stone is present. There is no evidence that decompression of the biliary tract influences the progress of acute pancreatitis, but the healing of wounds in patients with acute pancreatitis appears to be poor and even the insertion of a T-tube into the common duct may expose the patient to the risk of a subphrenic abscess or a biliary fistula.

If it is necessary to explore the duct, the procedure should be undertaken with extreme care to avoid unnecessary damage to the pancreas. Few of the stones that cause acute pancreatitis become truly impacted and most can be adequately removed or eased through into the duodenum via a supraduodenal choledochotomy. Despite the experience of Stone et al (1981), I would be reluctant to advocate transduodenal sphincterotomy because of the potential risk of a leak from the duodenum.

The role of endoscopic sphincterotomy in management

Safrany and Cotton (1981) showed that ERCP with endoscopic sphincterotomy was both feasible and safe during the early stages of acute pancreatitis due to gallstones. Eleven patients were studied: 6 of them had stones impacted at the ampulla and the remainder stones in the bile duct. Interestingly, one patient had a gallstone in the pancreatic duct. The authors claimed prompt and persistent improvement following sphincterotomy. A further report confirming the safety, and also claiming the benefit, of early sphincterotomy came from Scandinavia (Rosseland & Solhaug 1984). The issue has become very controversial in the wake of a series of publications from Leicester (UK). ERCP was performed within 72 h of admission in 68 patients with pancreatitis related to gallstones (Neoptolemos et al 1988). Patients were predicted as 'mild' or 'severe' according to the modified Glasgow Prognostic Scoring System (Imrie et al 1978). Common duct stones were found in 61% of cholangiograms from patients with a predicted severe attack compared to only 35% of those with a predicted mild attack. Furthermore, the common bile duct diameter was greatest in patients with predicted severe attacks and a stone in the common duct. Complications of pancreatitis occurred most commonly in patients with predicted severe attacks and common duct stones.

Many of the patients were incorporated into a randomized trial of ERCP and endoscopic sphincterotomy (Neoptolemos et al 1988). Fifty-nine patients were randomized to receive ERCP plus endoscopic sphincterotomy (if appropriate) within 72 hours admission and 62 patients were treated conventionally. Conventional treatment included cholecystectomy during the same admission in only two patients. A diagnosis of pancreatitis was based upon consistent clinical features and a plasma amylase level >1000 iu/l. Gallstones were identified by a combination of ultrasound and biochemical methods. ERCP and endoscopy sphincterotomy were performed by a single highly skilled and experienced endoscopist, and sphincterotomy was only undertaken if a stone was identified in the common duct. After sphincterotomy stones in the duct were extracted. There was no difference in outcome between the predicted 'mild' patients who underwent sphincterotomy and the predicted 'mild' patients who were managed conventionally. However, there was a highly significant reduction in the complications that occurred in the predicted 'severe' patients who were managed by ERCP and sphincterotomy. Six out of 25 patients in this group developed complications and 1 patient died, compared to 17 out of 28 patients, including 5 deaths, in the conventionally managed group. Twelve of the patients who were predicted 'severe' received sphincterotomy in addition to ERCP. As the ERCP alone has no clear therapeutic influence, the benefit of the procedure was presumably confined to the sub-group of 20% of the total number randomized to urgent ERCP who also received a sphincterotomy. About half the patients could be eliminated on the basis of the fact that they were predicted 'mild' by the Glasgow criteria. If the results of this study are supported by others, the workload imposed by a routine policy of urgent ERCP in patients with severe pancreatitis associated with gallstones should not be excessive, particularly if it leads to a reduction of expensive complications and reduced time in hospital. Nevertheless, it is possible that few hospitals possess an endoscopist who is sufficiently skilled or experienced to enable these results to be reproduced, and it remains to be seen whether the policy is more universally applicable.

Cholangitis in patients with gallstone-related pancreatitis

A proportion of patients who are admitted to hospital with a clinical diagnosis of acute pancreatitis develop evidence of cholangitis. In a prospective study of acute pancreatitis in Bristol, Glasgow and Leeds, 7 out of 439 patients (1.5%) developed evidence of acute cholangitis and 3 died (McMahon et al 1985). Most of the patients were elderly (mean age 73 years), and in each case the pancreatitis was judged to be mild at the time of admission. Clinical deterioration was characterized by pyrexia, jaundice, rigors and hypertension and occurred 2 to 8 days after ad-

mission. Three of the 4 patients who were treated conservatively died, while all 3 patients treated by operative intervention survived. At laparotomy or autopsy, the pancreas showed evidence of oedema only. Neoptolemos et al (1987) recorded evidence of coexistent cholangitis and pancreatitis in 32 patients over a 10-year period, which amounted to 14% of all cases of gallstone-related acute pancreatitis. Again, most patients were elderly and predominantly female. In contrast to the Bristol, Glasgow, and Leeds experience, 63% of the patients had a predicted severe attack of pancreatitis. Twenty-three patients had a successful ERCP, and common bile duct stones were identified in 15 of them. Treatment included endoscopic sphincterotomy and surgery, and one patient died. Nine patients did not undergo cholangiography, although 4 received surgery, and 3 of them died.

The difference in the prevalence and severity of the associated pancreatitis in these two studies is considerable and probably reflects the criteria used to make a diagnosis of cholangitis. Both studies indicate that cholangitis can be an important cause of death in patients with pancreatitis and gallstones, particularly in the elderly. They suggest that active intervention by surgery, or preferably endoscopy, may reduce the risk of death.

Summary

In summary, gallstones cause acute pancreatitis during transient obstruction of the pancreatic or bile ducts, and in so doing they can also cause cholangitis or cholecystitis. The causative role of gallstones in a patient with pancreatitis may be suspected from the clinical features of the attack and may be confirmed in 80–90% of patients on the day of admission by measurement of plasma transaminase (ALT or AST >60 iu/l) combined with ultrasound examination. There is no established role for urgent surgery in most patients with gallstone-related pancreatitis, but cholecystectomy during the convalescent stages of the attack (during the same admission) is becoming routine. The possibility that morbidity and mortality rates can be reduced in severe attacks by urgent endoscopic sphincterotomy is intriguing and exciting, but its role has not yet been established despite a positive result from the single controlled trial that has been completed. Elderly patients with pancreatitis related to gallstones can develop acute cholangitis. Surgical exploration or preferably endoscopic sphincterotomy appears to be indicated.

REFERENCES

Acosta J M, Ledesma C L 1974 Gallstone migration as a cause of acute pancreatitis. New England Journal of Medicine 290: 484–487

Acosta J M, Rossi R, Galli O M R, Pellegrini C A, Skinner D B 1978 Early surgery for acute gallstone pancreatitis: Evaluation of a systemic approach. Surgery 83: 367–370

Acosta J M, Pellegrini C A, Skinner D B 1980 Etiology and pathogenesis of acute biliary pancreatitis. Surgery 88: 118–125

Barry R E 1988 The pathogenesis of acute pancreatitis. British Medical Journal 296: 589

Berman L G, Prior J T, Abramow S M, Ziegler D D 1960 A study of the pancreatic duct system in man by the use of vinyl acetate casts of postmortem preparations. Surgery Gynecology and Obstetrics 110: 391–403

Blamey S L, Osborne D H, Gilmour W H, O'Neill J, Carter D C, Imrie C W 1983 The early identification of patients with gallstone associated pancreatitis using clinical and biochemical factors only. Annals of Surgery 198: 574–578

Bradley J A, Bradley P, McMahon M J 1981 Diagnostic peritoneal lavage in acute pancreatitis — the value of microscopy of the lavage fluid. British Journal of Surgery 68: 245–246

Cuschieri A, Hughes J H 1973 Pancreatic reflux during operative choledochography. British Journal of Surgery 60: 933–936

Cuschieri A, Cumming J G R, Wood R A B, Baker P R 1984 Evidence for sphincter dysfunction in patients with gallstone associated pancreatitis: effect of ceruletide in patients undergoing cholecystectomy for gallbladder disease and gallstone associated pancreatitis. British Journal of Surgery 71: 885–888

Elmslie R, White T T, Magee D F 1966 The significance of reflux of trypsin and bile in the pathogenesis of human pancreatitis. British Journal of Surgery 53: 809–816

Farias L R, Frey C F, French S, Gunther R 1986 The role of ductal obstruction on the course of hemorrhagic pancreatitis in the pig. International Journal of Pancreatology 1: 51–59

Farinon A M, Ricci G L, Sianesi M, Percudani M, Zanella E 1987 Pathophysiologic role of microlithiasis in gallstone pancreatitis. Surgery Gynecology and Obstetrics 164: 252–256

Fonseca C, Greenberg D, Rosenthall L, Arzoumanian A, Lisbona R 1979 ^{99m}Tc-IDA imaging in the differential diagnosis of acute cholecystitis and acute pancreatitis. Radiology 130: 525–527

Frieden J H 1965 The significance of jaundice in acute pancreatitis. Archives of Surgery 90: 422–425

Glazer G, Murphy F, Clayden G S, Lawrence R G, Craig O 1981 Radionuclide biliary scanning in acute pancreatitis. British Journal of Surgery 68: 766–770

Goodman A J, Neoptolemos J P, Carr-Locke D L, Finlay D B L, Fossard D P 1985 Detection of gallstones after acute pancreatitis. Gut 26: 125–132

Graham D F, Wyllie F J 1979 Prediction of gallstone pancreatitis by computer. British Medical Journal i: 515–517

Halsted W S 1901 Retrojection of bile into the pancreas, a cause of acute haemorrhagic pancreatitis. Bulletin of the Johns Hopkins Hospital 12: 179–182

Houssin D, Castaing D, Lemoine J, Bismuth H 1983 Microlithiasis of the gallbladder. Surgery Gynecology and Obstetrics 157: 20–24

Howard J M 1960 In: Howard J M, Jordan G L (eds) Surgical Diseases of the Pancreas. Pitman Medical. London pp 169–189

Howell C W, Bergh G S 1950 Pancreatic duct filling during cholangiography: its effect upon serum amylase levels. Gastroenterology 16: 309–316

Imrie C W, Benjamin I S, Ferguson J C et al 1978 A single centre double blind trial of trasylol therapy in primary acute pancreatitis. British Journal of Surgery 65: 337–341

Johnson H C, Minor B D, Thompson J A, Weens H S 1959 Diagnostic value of intravenous cholangiography during acute cholecystitis and acute pancreatitis. New England Journal of Medicine 260: 158–160

Kaden V G, Howard J M, Doubleday L C 1955 Cholecystographic studies during and immediately following acute pancreatitis. Surgery 38: 1082–1086

Kelly T R 1976 Gallstone pancreatitis: pathophysiology. Surgery 80: 488–492

Kelly T R 1980 Gallstone pancreatitis: the timing of surgery. Surgery 88: 345–350

Kelly T R 1984 Gallstone pancreatitis. Local predisposing factors. Annals of Surgery 200: 479–485

Lancet 1988 Obstruction or reflux in gallstone-associated acute pancreatitis (Editorial). Lancet i: 915–917

Lesser P B, Warshaw A L 1975 Differentiation of pancreatitis from common bile duct obstruction with hyperamylasaemia. Gastroenterology 68: 636–641

McCutcheon A D 1968 A fresh approach to the pathogenesis of pancreatitis. Gut 9: 296–310

McKay A J, Imrie C W, O'Neill J, Duncan J G 1982 Is an early ultrasound scan of value in acute pancreatitis? British Journal of Surgery 69: 369–371

Mackie C R, Wood R A B, Preece P E, Cuschieri A 1985 Surgical pathology at early elective operation for suspected acute gallstone pancreatitis: preliminary report of a prospective trial. British Journal of Surgery 72: 179–181

McMahon M J, Mayer A D 1984 Comparison of the clinical features of acute pancreatitis due to gallstones and alcohol. In: Gyr K E, Singer M V, Sarles H (eds) Pancreatitis — concepts and classification. Elsevier. Amsterdam, pp 379–388

McMahon M J, Pickford I R 1979 Biochemical prediction of gallstones early in an attack of acute pancreatitis. Lancet ii: 541–543

McMahon M J, Shefta J R 1980 Physical characteristics of gallstones and the calibre of the cystic duct in patients with acute pancreatitis. British Journal of Surgery 67: 6–9

McMahon M J, Playforth M J, Booth E W 1981 Identification of risk factors for acute pancreatitis from routine radiological investigation of the biliary tract. British Journal of Surgery 68: 465–467

McMahon M J, Mayer A D, Shearer M G et al 1985 Cholangitis and acute pancreatitis. Gut 26: A648

Mayer A D, McMahon M J 1985 Biochemical identification of patients with gallstones associated with acute pancreatitis on the day of admission to hospital. Annals of Surgery 210: 68–75

Mayer A D, McMahon M J, Benson E A, Axon A T R 1984 Operations upon the biliary tract in patients with acute pancreatitis: aims, indications and timing. Annals of the Royal College of Surgeons of England 66: 179–183

Mercer L C, Saltzstein E C, Peacock J B, Dougherty S H 1984 Early surgery for biliary pancreatitis. American Journal of Surgery 148: 749–753

Molander D W, Bell E T 1946 Relation of cholelithiasis to acute haemorrhagic pancreatitis. Archives of Pathology 41: 17–18

Neoptolemos J P, Fossard D P, Berry J M 1983 A prospective study of radionuclide biliary scanning in acute pancreatitis. Annals of the Royal College of Surgeons of England 65: 180–182

Neoptolemos J P, Hall A W, Finlay D F, Berry J M, Carr-Locke D L, Fossard D P 1984 The urgent diagnosis of gallstones in acute pancreatitis: a prospective study of three methods. British Journal of Surgery 71: 230–233

Neoptolemos J P, Carr-Locke D L, Leese T, James D 1987 Acute cholangitis in association with acute pancreatitis: incidence, clinical features and outcome in relation to ERCP and endoscopic sphincterotomy. British Journal of Surgery 74: 1103–1106

Neoptolemos J P, Carr-Locke D L, London N, Bailey I, Fossard D P 1988 ERCP findings and the role of endoscopic sphincterotomy in acute gallstone pancreatitis. British Journal of Surgery 75: 954–960

Neoptolemos J P, Carr-Locke D L, London N J, Bailey I A, James D, Fossard D P 1988 Results of a controlled trial of urgent ERCP and endoscopic sphincterotomy in patients with pancreatitis due to gallstones. Lancet 2: 979–983

Opie E L 1901 The aetiology of acute haemorrhagic pancreatitis. Bulletin of the Johns Hopkins Hospital 12: 182–188

Paloyan D, Simonowitz D 1976 Diagnostic considerations in acute alcoholic and gallstone pancreatitis. American Journal of Surgery 132: 327–331

Raker J W, Bartlett M K 1953 Acute pancreatitis; the fate of the patient surviving one or more acute attacks. New England Journal of Medicine 249: 751–757

Rosseland A R, Solhaug J H 1984 Early or delayed endoscopic papillotomy in gallstone pancreatitis. Annals of Surgery 199: 165–167

Roth J A 1974 Patients with hyperbilirubinaemia and hyperamylasaemia: is the diagnosis pancreatitis or biliary lithiasis? American Surgeon 40: 321–325

Safrany L, Cotton P B 1981 A preliminary report: Urgent sphincterotomy for acute gallstone pancreatitis. Surgery 189: 424–428

Schmitz-Moorman P, Schwerk W, Sinn P 1986 Histological alterations of the pre-ampullary comon bile and pancreatic duct in acute biliary and nonbiliary pancreatitis. Digestion 34: 93–100

Senninger N, Moody F G, Coelho J C V, Van Burren D L 1986 The role of biliary obstruction in the pathogenesis of acute pancreatitis in the opossum. Surgery 99: 688–693

Sterling J A 1954 The common channel for bile and pancreatic ducts. Surgery Gynecology and Obstetrics 98: 420–424

Stone H H, Fabian T C, Dunlop W E 1981 Gallstone pancreatitis. Biliary tract pathology in relation to time of operation. Annals of Surgery 194: 305–312

Taylor T V, Rimmer S 1980 Pancreatic-duct reflux in patients with gallstone pancreatitis. Lancet i: 848–850

Taylor T V, Armstrong C P 1987 Migration on gallstones. British Medical Journal 294: 1320–1322

Tondelli P, Stutz K, Harder F, Schupisser J-P, Allgower M 1982 Acute gallstone pancreatitis: best timing for biliary surgery. British Journal of Surgery 69: 709–710

Van Gossum A, Seferian V, Rodzynek J J, Wettendorff P, Cremer M, Delcourt A 1984 Early detection of biliary pancreatitis. Digestive Disease and Science 29: 97–101

Zeman R K 1981 Diagnostic analysis of cholecystigraphy and ultrasonography in acute cholecystitis. American Journal of Surgery 141: 446–451

9

Surgical complications of acute pancreatitis

E. L. BRADLEY III

Today, spontaneous uncomplicated recovery from acute pancreatitis with supportive treatment is the rule, and the overwhelming number of people who develop acute pancreatitis merely find the experience uncomfortable. With the widespread appreciation of the magnitude of plasma volume sequestration in acute pancreatitis, few people now expire from the ravages of untreated hypovolaemia, as was common in the past. Currently, it is the development of a *complication* of acute pancreatitis that accounts for most morbidity and mortality from this disease. Significant complications are estimated to occur in 30% of cases of acute pancreatitis, which ultimately prove to be fatal in one-third to one-half of these patients (Bradley 1982a).

It has often been stated that acute pancreatitis is a disease of seven days (known as Gliedman's Law). The experience of most physicians is that the vast majority of patients will have recovered and been discharged within a week of the onset of symptoms. The important clinical corollary to this law is that patients who *continue* to show signs of active disease after one week of supportive treatment should be suspected of having developed some complication of the disease. In the presence of persistent inflammation, specific complications should be sought to account for the prolonged course. Waiting until potentially serious complications become clinically obvious can no longer be accepted as good medical practice; anticipation is the key.

Systemic complications of acute pancreatitis, such as pancreatic psychosis, acute respiratory distress syndrome, renal insufficiency or various coagulopathies rarely result in the necessity for surgical intervention by themselves. However, when these systemic complications exist together in configuration, multiple organ system failure exists, and a source of pancreatic sepsis should always be sought.

Rather than systemic complications, it is the local or regional complications of acute pancreatitis that constitute most cases of surgical interest. A glance at the following table will reveal the breadth of the possible surgical complications of the acute form of the disease. While this list of complications is not necessarily synonymous with a list of indications for surgery, it does represent a number of conditions for which surgery is often necessary. Each will be discussed in turn.

Surgical complications of acute pancreatitis

1. Necrosis
   a. Pancreatic necrosis
   b. Acute pseudocyst
   c. Intestinal necrosis
2. Infection
   a. Infected pancreatic necrosis
   b. Pancreatic abscess
   c. Infected pseudocyst
3. Haemorrhage
   a. Stress ulceration
   b. Vascular necrosis
4. Obstruction
   a. Acute cholangiopathy
   b. Intestinal obstruction

Pancreatic 'sepsis'

Considerable confusion continues to surround the clinical management of patients with acute pancreatitis and systemic signs of toxicity: i.e. elevated temperature, tachycardia, abdominal pain, ileus, guarding, and increased white blood cell count (often with a left shift). The source of this confusion is twofold.

First, it is not possible to distinguish between acute oedematous pancreatitis, pancreatic necrosis, infected pancreatic necrosis, pancreatic abscess, acute pseudocyst and infected pseudocyst on clinical grounds alone (Mendez et al 1980). Others have also concluded that the clinical courses of each of these diverse conditions are remarkably similar and that they cannot be differentiated on a clinical basis (Sostre et al 1985; Hunter et al 1982). Unfortunately, accurate differentiation is mandatory for effective therapy, which might range among these conditions from persistent observation all the way to widespread exploration and extensive debridement. Recognition of the similarity of the clinical courses of these varied conditions is a critical first step toward differentiation by more sophisticated methodology.

Secondly, no generally accepted definitions of these conditions exist. International conferences on pancreatitis have been held in Marseilles in 1963 (Sarles 1965), Cambridge in 1983, (Sarner & Cotton 1984) and again in Marseilles in 1984 (Singer et al 1985). However, the focus of these conferences was primarily upon chronic pancreatitis, and clear-cut definitions of those conditions clinically expressed as pancreatic 'sepsis' did not emerge. As a consequence, the confusion in definitions of acute pancreatitis and its complications is widespread in the medical and surgical communities. In a recent search of 112 English-language articles in the past 10 years dealing with 'pancreatic abscess', we found that only 10 had even bothered to define the condition (Bradley 1987). To make matters even worse, no two definitions were the same! Another case in point is the word 'phlegmon'. Originally used by Kune to describe a persistent sterile inflammatory mass of oedematous pancreatic and peripancreatic tissues (Kune & King 1973), other authors subsequently extended the original definition to include necrosis and infection (Warshaw 1974). As a consequence, we now have a term which refers to a mass which is composed of oedema or necrosis and is either sterile or infected, depending upon who is using the term. Iatrogenic incompatibility may represent one of the largest impediments to progress in the management of inflammatory diseases of the pancreas! Currently, one man's 'abscess' is another's 'infected pseudocyst' or perhaps even 'infected pancreatic necrosis.' Because the natural history of these conditions varies widely (from 90% recovery to 100% mortality), such confusion in terminology has generally invalidated comparison of data between institutions.

Without accurate and specific definitions for those conditions presenting as pancreatic sepsis, comparison of diagnostic and treatment regimens is hazardous. Such limitations assume particular importance when mortality rates from differing surgical approaches are to be compared. The suggested list of definitions in Table 9.1 will be used throughout this chapter.

Pancreatic necrosis

Evidence is rapidly accumulating that the development of necrosis is the primary determinant of whether an individual episode of acute pancreatitis becomes morbid. In extensive series of pancreatic resections for clinically 'severe' pancreatitis, both Léger et al (1981) and Beger and his co-workers (1985) found evidence of pancreatic or peripancreatic necrosis in the overwhelming majority of patients. For the first time, these observations have provided a firm histological and pathogenetic basis for why some episodes of acute pancreatitis are more severe than others.

In 1974 Ranson and his co-workers introduced a clinical grading system for the express purpose of grading the severity of an individual episode of acute pancreatitis. Using retrospective computer analysis, they were able to identify 11 clinical and biochemical variables that could be significantly correlated with morbidity and mortality in acute pancreatitis. A number of other investigators have subsequently proposed clinical grading systems for stratifying the severity of an episode of pancreatitis (Jacobs et al 1977; Banks et al 1983; Agarwal &

Table 9.1 Definitions of conditions presenting as pancreatic sepsis

1. **Acute interstitial pancreatitis** Sterile inflammation and oedema of the pancreas; fat necrosis may be present.

   a. Occasionally, peripancreatic tissue may become involved in a prolonged inflammatory process referred to as 'phlegmon', an ambiguous term which could be discontinued.
   b. CT findings: uniform enhancement of pancreatic tissue with an intravenous bolus of contrast material.
   c. Needle aspiration (rarely required): no bacteria.

2. **Necrotizing pancreatitis** Inflammation with devitalized pancreatic on peripancreatic tissue; necrosis may be local or diffuse and may result in loss of integrity of the major pancreatic duct, and/or thrombosis of the splenic vein.

   a. Necrosis may be restricted to the pancreas (pancreatic necrosis), or involve peripancreatic tissues (peripancreatic necrosis) or both.
   b. CT findings: local or diffuse non-enhancement of involved tissue with an intravenous bolus of contrast material.
   c. Needle aspiration: no bacteria

3. **Infected pancreatic or peripancreatic necrosis** As above but with infection

   a. Necrosis may be restricted to the pancreas or involve peripancreatic tissues or both.
   b. CT scan with vascular enhancement shows areas of non-perfusion.
   c. CT scan or ultrasound guided needle aspiration: gram stain and culture positive.

4. **Pancreatic abscess** A collection of classically purulent material in the region of the pancreas, enclosed by inflammatory walls. May have resulted from liquefaction of areas of necrosis which became secondarily infected, or from a pseudocyst which has become secondarily infected.

   a. Objective evidence of antecedent pancreatitis is necessary to eliminate other causes of lesser sac abscess. May or may not communicate with the major duct.
   b. CT findings: enhancement of pancreas with intravenous contrast; decreased intensity in region of abscess.
   c. Needle aspiration: classically purulent material; positive for bacteria.

5. **Acute pseudocyst** An effusion of pancreatic juice enclosed by fibrous walls in a patient with acute pancreatitis.

   a. Communicates with the pancreatic ductal system.
   b. CT findings: low tissue density and absence of enhancement in the region of the pseudocyst with an intravenous bolus of contrast material.
   c. needle aspiration: thin fluid, high in amylase which does not contain bacteria.

6. **Loculated fat necrosis** A collection of liquefied fat enclosed by inflammatory walls, often mistakenly called a pseudocyst.

   a. Does not communicate with the pancreatic ductal system.
   b. CT findings: core tissue density and absence of enhancement in the region of the loculation with intravenous bolus of contrast material.
   c. Needle aspiration: yellow-hued liquid or semi-solid material, low in amylase, which does not contain bacteria.

Table 9.2 Similarities in clinical grading systems for acute pancreatitis

	Ranson et al 1974	Jacobs et al 1977	Banks et al 1983	Agarwal & Pitchumoni 1986
Cardiac	(−)	BP<90,HR >130	BP<90,HR> 130	BP<90,HR>130
Pulmonary	PO$_2$<60	Intubation	PO$_2$<60 ARDS	PO$_2$<60
Renal	BUN, CR	BUN, CR	BUN, CR	UO<50 ml/h
Metabolic	Ca<2 (−) ↓ HCT	CA<2 (−) ↓ HCT	CA<2 Alb<3.2 ↓ HCT	CA<2 CA<3.2 ↓ HCT
No. of cases	100	514	75	76
Mortality rate	n.a.	n.a.	56%	41%
Others	wbc>16	wbc>20	n.s.	n.s.

(−), not evaluated; n.a., not applicable; n.s., not significant; ARDS, Acute respiratory distress syndrome; UO, urinary output; BUN, blood urea nitrogen; CR, creatinine; CA, serum calcium (mmol/l); HCT, haematocrit; PO$_2$, partial pressure of oxygen in arterial blood (mm Hg); alb, albumin (g/l); wbc, white blood count ($\times 10^9$/l).

Pitchumoni 1986). Superficially, these grading systems appear to be quite dissimilar. However, if the systems are arranged by organ systems as shown in Table 9.2, marked similarities begin to appear. These similarities serve to reinforce the basic validity of the concept of clinical grading for acute pancreatitis. However, the essential similarity of these systems raises another important question. Why should these various clinical and biochemical parameters correlate with morbidity and mortality in acute pancreatitis?

When the Ranson criteria were introduced, they represented the first objective data system for studying acute pancreatitis. Accordingly, they were widely accepted as a method for the stratification and comparison of data from different institutions. Almost no one questioned *why* they were valid. Because of the marked similarities between the grading systems, and because clinical severity can be correlated with the presence of pancreatic or peripancreatic necrosis, it now seems clear that tissue necrosis has become the most important determinant of the severity of an episode of acute pancreatitis. Furthermore, a direct correlation between the extent of necrosis and mortality risk has now been demonstrated (Gebhart & Gall 1981, Beger et al 1985). Accordingly, rather than attempting to continue to differentiate the various causes of pancreatic sepsis by nonspecific means, a search for indicators of the presence of pancreatic necrosis should now become the focus of our diagnostic efforts.

Despite earlier claims, neither methaemoglobin (Geokas et al 1974) nor RNAse (Warshaw & Lee 1979) has proved to be sufficiently specific or sensitive for identifying patients with pancreatic necrosis. More recently, however, other serum tests for the identification of pancreatic necrosis have received considerable attention (McMahon et al 1984). Buchler and his co-workers (1986) have now accumulated a considerable experience with C-reactive protein as an indicator of pancreatic or peripancreatic necrosis. In a prospective study of 35 patients, the overall accuracy rate for C-reactive protein in predicting pancreatic necrosis was 95% when values of C-reactive protein exceeded 100 mg%. Recent limited experience in our institution corroborates these observations. Furthermore, serum levels of alpha-1-protease in-

hibitor (>3.5 g/l) and alpha-2-macroglobulin (<2 g/l) are also highly correlated (85% accuracy) with the presence of tissue necrosis (Buchler et al 1986). Reproduction of these claims in other institutions and patient populations would greatly facilitate the clinical management of these patients.

A second approach to identifying pancreatic necrosis has been through contrast-enhanced CT scanning (dynamic pancreatography). Since neither conventional CT scanning nor ultrasonography has proved to be consistently useful in detecting pancreatic necrosis (Crass et al 1985, Rotman et al 1986), other approaches should be sought. Dynamic pancreatography appears to offer considerable promise in identifying these patients (Block et al 1984). Following a large intravenous bolus of contrast material (200 ml), the pancreas will enhance in normal patients, or in those with acute interstitial (oedematous) pancreatitis. Areas of non-enhancement (patchy or diffuse) are seen in patients with pancreatic or peripancreatic necrosis (Figs 9.1, 9.2). Animal experiments have shown that pancreatic enhancement is dependent upon an intact microcirculation (Nuutinen et al 1986). Presumably, ischaemic pancreatic necrosis is the reason for diminished or absent contrast-medium perfusion in patients with pancreatic necrosis. Originally proposed by Kivisarri et al in 1980, others are now also accumulating favourable experiences with this technique (Schroder et al 1980, Maier 1987). Dynamic pancreatography has been accurate in predicting necrosis in the six patients in whom it was used in our institution.

Once pancreatic or peripancreatic necrosis has been identified, a question arises as to whether all patients with demonstrated necrosis require surgery. Widespread necrosis probably requires surgical debridement. However, in the absence of secondary infection (see below), many workers now feel that a policy of observation only is safe in cases of patchy or limited necrosis. The validity of these approaches remains to be determined. Clinical studies are in progress.

Infected pancreatic necrosis

In the past, marked plasma sequestration accounted for the vast majority of deaths from acute

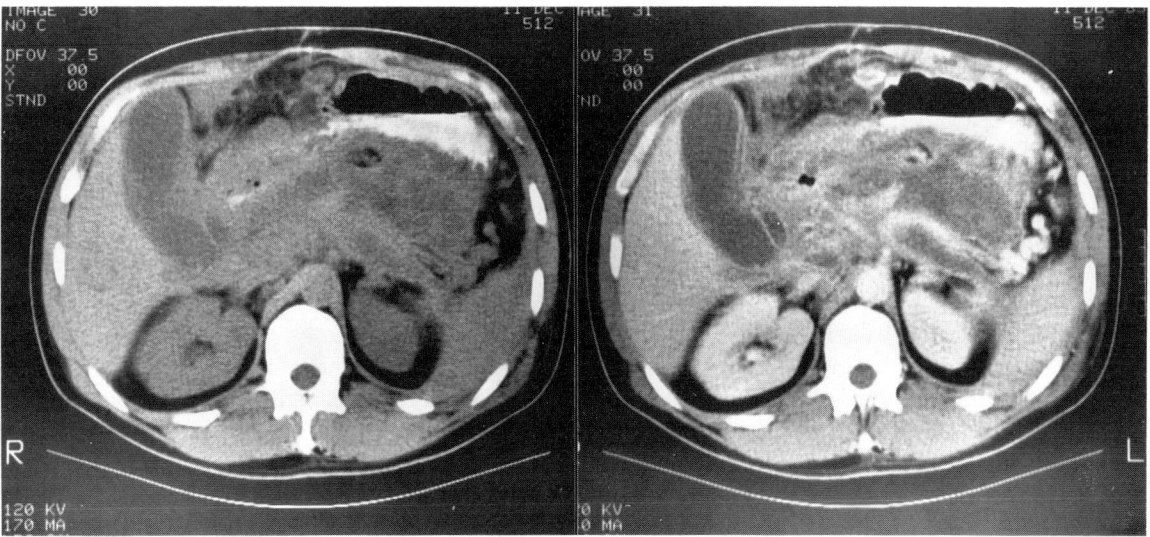

Fig. 9.1 Conventional CT scan on left. Note large indiscriminate mass in region of pancreas. Dynamic pancreatogram on right fails to opacify pancreatic tissue. Note absence of contrast material anterior to splenic vein. Extensive *pancreatic* necrosis was found at surgery.

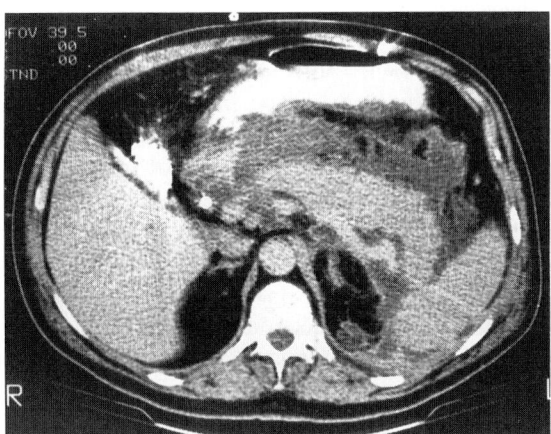

Fig. 9.2 Dynamic pancreatogram showing extensive *peripancreatic* necrosis. Note contrast in splenic vein, as well as the body and tail of the pancreas. At exploration, marked necrosis of peripancreatic tissues with preservation of pancreatic parenchyma was found.

pancreatitis. Today, with the advent of invasive monitoring, deaths from hypovolaemia are rare. More than 80% of the current deaths from acute pancreatitis are due to some form of secondary infection (Buggy & Nostrant 1983, Renner et al 1985). It therefore appears that we are keeping people alive longer through the initial period of hypovolaemia, only to expose them to the later,

often fatal, consequences of the disease. This concept springs from the observation that the overall mortality rate in acute pancreatitis has not changed in the past 40 years (Bradley 1982a, Ranson et al 1985) despite marked advances in intensive care. It seems clear that if we are to make any inroads in the morbidity and mortality of acute pancreatitis, we must shift our attention to the management of infection in these patients.

Infection of pancreatic necrosis probably occurs as a secondary phenomenon. Sterile necrosis is commonly observed in resected pancreatic specimens (Léger et al 1981, Beger et al 1985). Non-bacterial necrosis has been identified by needle aspiration in a patient with severe pancreatitis and subsequently confirmed by surgical exploration (Sostre et al 1985). Even in severe acute pancreatitis bacteria are not commonly found either by needle aspiration (Gerzof et al 1987) or from tissue cultures of resected glands (Beger et al 1986) in the first week after the onset of pancreatitis. After the second week, however, the incidence of bacteria in the necrotic tissue rises sharply to as high as 40–50% of cases (Beger et al 1986). These findings are consistent with secondary infection of pancreatic necrosis.

Perhaps because the vast majority of bacteria found in these patients are gram-negative, (*E. coli*,

Klebsiella and *Aerobacter* account for 70% of infections; Beger et al 1986, Bradley 1987), transcolonic 'migration' of bacteria from the colon to the adjacent pancreas has been suggested as the source of secondary infection (Onderdonk et al 1974). The pathophysiology of such putative migration remains obscure, but it might involve loss of a normal mucosal barrier. Recently, animal experiments have suggested another possible mechanism. It has been observed that monocytes are capable of transporting viable bacteria which have been phagocytosed but not destroyed. In the presence of active inflammation, these impaired monocytes can aggregate at the site of the inflammation and can release the viable bacteria to the inflamed tissues when they themselves are destroyed (Wells et al 1986).

Regardless of the mechanism involved, secondary infection of pancreatic or peripancreatic necrosis is an ominous development. Beger and his co-workers have shown that the morbidity and mortality of infected necrosis is significantly higher (32%) than that of non-infected necrosis (9.8%) (Beger et al 1985).

The choice of a particular antibiotic for patients with infected necrosis is made difficult by a lack of basic information. Studies purporting to show no advantage for antibiotics in acute pancreatitis have been flawed by poor choice of agent (ampicillin does not enter pancreatic tissue or juice) and by limited stratification (only mild to moderate pancreatitis has been studied). No studies as to the efficacy of antibiotics in severe (necrotic) pancreatitis have as yet been performed. Until such time as reliable antibiotic studies are available, limited clinical studies suggest that metronidazole, chloramphenicol and trimethoprim — sulphamethoxozole reach therapeutic levels in the pancreas (Wallace et al 1986). Water-soluble antibiotics (such as the beta-lactams) were not found in pancreatic juice in anti-microbial concentrations (Gregg et al 1985).

Diagnosis

Recognition of infected necrosis can still be difficult. Even though contrast-enhanced CT scanning and serum monitoring of C-reactive protein may indicate that necrosis is present, neither test will establish whether secondary infection of the necrosis has occurred. Furthermore, since many workers feel that limited non-infected necrosis does not need surgery, one can easily appreciate the importance of determining whether secondary infection has developed. To obviate this problem, Gerzof et al (1987) have advocated transcutaneous needle aspiration bacteriology whenever pancreatic necrosis has been demonstrated. Under CT guidance, a thin needle is advanced into the area of non-perfusion seen on the dynamic pancreatogram, and an aspirate is taken for Gram stain and culture. If the Gram stain is positive for bacteria in an area of poor perfusion, infected necrosis is presumed to be present. Hill et al (1984), Hiatt et al (1987) and the present author have all had favourable experiences with this technique.

Management

Even though some controversy exists regarding the management of limited, non-infected necrosis, few people would advocate wait-and-see policy toward infected necrosis. Since non-surgical treatment of infected pancreatic necrosis is uniformly fatal (Kune 1968, Frey et al 1979), the only pertinent question is the type of drainage to be used.

Although guided transcutaneous catheter drainage of these collections of infected necrosis has been advocated (Karlson et al 1982), this technique has not been particularly successful due to the particulate nature of the necrotic material and the propensity of the small calibre transcutaneous catheters to occlude. Persistent sepsis and recurrent abscesses are the rule in patients with transcutaneous catheter drainage (Bolooki et al 1968, Ranson et al 1985, Pemberton et al 1986, Bradley 1987), and for these reasons this technique cannot be recommended for such patients.

Currently, infected pancreatic necrosis is most often approached by abdominal exploration, debridement and closed drainage. However, in the 25 years that surgeons have followed these recommendations since they were proposed by Altemeier and Alexander in 1963, mortality rates of 30–60% have been common (Miller et al 1974, Camer et al

1975, Holden et al 1976, Ranson & Spencer 1977, Donohue et al 1980, Aranha et al 1982, Becker et al 1984). Perhaps as a reflection of dissatisfaction with such results, surgical controversy has previously centred on the number and types of drains to be used (Holden et al 1976, Owens & Hamit 1977, Aranha et al 1982). However, in three of the largest series, neither the number nor the types of drains could be correlated with results from surgery (Miller et al 1974, Camer et al 1975, Frey et al 1979).

In reviewing the stated causes of death in patients with pancreatic sepsis undergoing conventional surgical exploration over the past 10 years, we found that 76% of deaths were due to persistent or recurrent sepsis! (Bradley 1987). This observation suggested to us that the conventional closed surgical approach was not doing the job for which it was designed. Furthermore, questions as to why conventional surgical drainage was not sucessful in patients with infected pancreatic necrosis assumed increasing importance.

In 1976, we began to treat patients with infected pancreatic necrosis by anterior laparotomy, finger debridement of necrotic tissues, placement of Adaptic® non-adherent gauze (Johnson & Johnson) over exposed blood vessels and intestine, and packing the abdomen open with moist laparotomy pads (open drainage) (Davidson & Bradley 1981), (Fig. 9.3).

Because of the propensity for infected pancreatic necrosis to track widely in the relatively defence-less retroperitoneum, widespread unroofing of the retroperitoneum is necessary to prevent overlooked extensions. This is accomplished by taking down both colic flexures, performing a Kocher manoeuvre and opening the retroperitoneum above and behind the pancreas for additional necrosis. Dressings are changed in the operating room every 2–3 days under light anaesthesia and further debridement is carried out as necessary. When intestinal adhesion has occurred, dressing changes are carried out on the ward. Patients are hyperalimented and wounds are permitted to heal by secondary intention (Fig. 9.4). As our experience grew (Bradley & Fulenwider 1984, Bradley 1987) we found that the average length of hospitalization decreased from 58 days to 33 days.

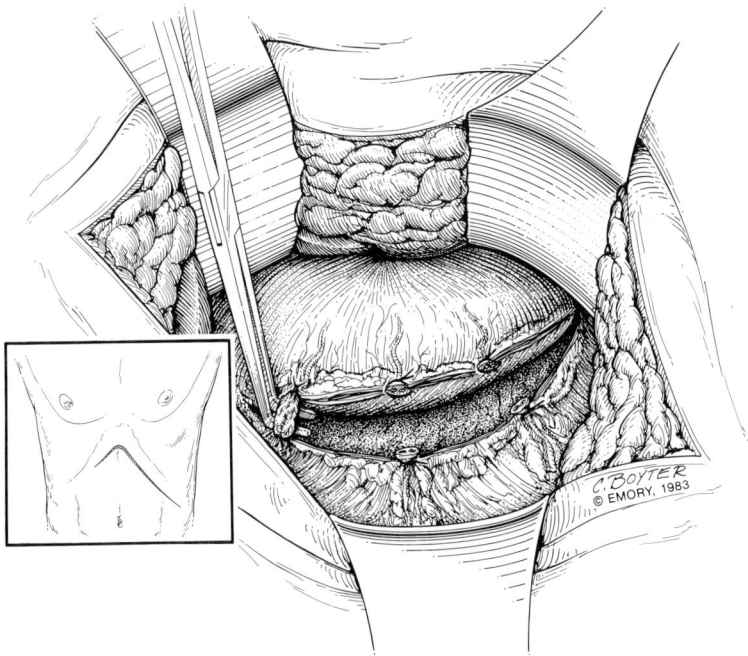

Fig. 9.3 Exposure for open drainage. The left subcostal incision is extended to the right if extensive necrosis is found. A wide approach to the lesser sac through the gastrocolic omentum is favoured over the more restricted transmesocolic route. (Reproduced from Bradley & Fulenwider 1984, by permission of Surgery, Gynecology & Obstetrics)

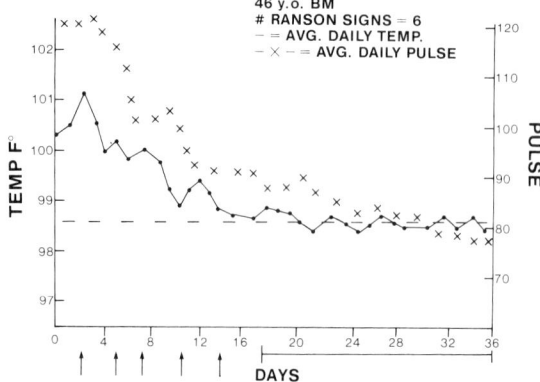

Fig. 9.4 Hospital course of patient no: 28. Single arrows represent open drainage of infected pancreatic necrosis and repeated dressing changes under light anaesthesia. Solid bar represents daily dressing changes on the ward. Despite extensive debridement on each occasion, control of sepsis was not complete until after the fifth dressing change. This observation is consistent with continuing necrosis.

Table 9.3 Experiences with open drainage in management of infected pancreatic necrosis

Author	No. of patients	Clinical severity*	Mortality rate, %
Bradley et al (1981, 1984, 1987)	33	5.3	12
Pemberton et al (1986)	17	5.5	18
Waclawiczek et al (1986)	17	n.s.	17
Wertheimer & Norris (1986)	10	>5	20
Vogel (1987, personal commn.)	11	>5	0
Total	88	>5	13.4

* Average number of Ranson signs (>5 = anticipated mortality in excess of 50%)

Currently, 29 of our 33 patients with infected pancreatic necrosis treated by this method have survived. None of the four deaths were due to sepsis: one death was secondary to autopsy-proved myocardial infarction, one to ventricular arrhythmia, one to massive aspiration, and one to suspected air embolism from a disconnected subclavian catheter. The single most outstanding observation from this series has been the amount and extent of additional infected necrosis removed at the subsequent serial dressing changes. We attribute our good results in these patients with infected necrosis to re-exploration and removal of re-accumulating necrotic tissue.

Some investigators have questioned the necessity for open drainage and have continued to advocate conventional closed drainage (Warshaw & Jin 1985). Others prefer less conventional forms of drainage, such as continuous lavage of the lesser sac (Beger et al 1985). However, comparatively favourable experiences with the technique of open drainage for infected pancreatic necrosis are now being accumulated by a number of other investigators and other institutions (Pemberton et al 1986, Waclawiczek et al 1986, Wertheimer & Norris 1986, Vogel 1987 (personal communication)) (Table 9.3). Perhaps because of the comparatively small number of patients with infected pancreatic necrosis in a single institution, no randomized

studies have been done comparing open drainage versus closed drainage. However, in view of a 60% mortality for closed drainage of infected necrosis in our own institution before beginning open drainage, we plan to continue the procedure in appropriate cases and feel that this technique has much to offer this difficult group of patients.

Acute pseudocyst

By definition, an acute pseudocyst is one that develops in conjunction with an episode of acute pancreatitis and is less than six weeks old (Bradley et al 1976). These pseudocysts presumably arise from necrosis of a portion of the pancreatic duct system as a result of inflammation from acute pancreatitis. Acute pseudocysts behave in an entirely different fashion from chronic counterparts (pseudocysts present longer than six weeks) (Bradley et al 1976, Crass & Way 1981). Spontaneous resolution of acute pseudocysts is common, occurring in 20–40% of cases (Bradley et al 1979, Aranha et al 1983), but it is rare in chronic pseudocysts. Furthermore, complications such as haemorrhage, secondary infection, rupture and obstruction are much less common than in chronic pseudocysts (Bradley et al 1979).

The diagnosis of an acute pseudocyst is often suggested by clinical evidence of persistence of pancreatic inflammation beyond the customary seven days. Suspicions that an individual episode of acute pancreatitis has become complicated are best confirmed by CT scanning (dynamic pancreatography). While ultrasonography will reliably demonstrate peripancreatic fluid collections, it is unreliable in detecting pancreatic necrosis (Bradley & Fulenwider 1984, Silverstein et al 1981, Warshaw & Jin 1985). CT scanning with contrast enhancement is capable of recognizing both conditions. Once an acute pseudocyst is identified by CT, serial ultrasound can be used to follow its progress.

In view of the frequency of spontaneous resolution, and after considering the low complication rate, interventional drainage for acute pseudocysts is seldom required. An expectant approach toward the management of pseudocysts arising in association with acute pancreatitis has much to offer. Indications for surgery in acute pseudocysts are usually restricted to the infrequent development of a complication.

Correlation of the CT findings with the clinical course of these patients is a prerequisite for optimum management. Even using dynamic pancreatography, it is often impossible to determine whether or not an acute pseudocyst has become secondarily infected. Even though fever, tachycardia and elevations in white blood cell count can be seen in uncomplicated acute pancreatitis, it is the *trend* in these parameters along with changes in physical findings which suggest that secondary infection has occurred. Repeated CT scans are often advisable (Fig. 9.5). In borderline cases, clinical judgment can be materially assisted by transcutaneous CT-guided aspiration for smear and culture (Gerzof et al 1984). If the smear is positive *and* no pancreatic necrosis can be demonstrated by intravenous contrast enhancement, external drainage of the infected pseudocyst by a CT-guided transcutaneous catheter can be performed. If this approach is chosen, one must be certain that the 'infected pseudocyst' is not, in fact, infected pancreatic necrosis. As we have noted, external drainage in the latter case is ineffective, and persistence with this form of drainage often leads to death. Currently, we prefer to restrict external drainage of infected pseudocysts to those people who are poor candidates for surgical drainage, and

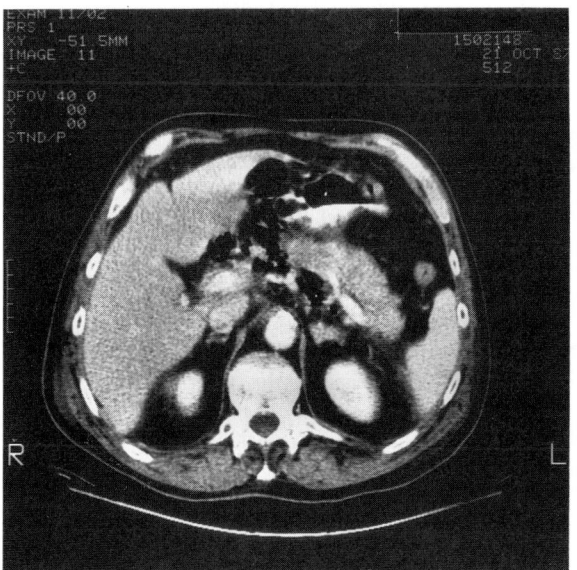 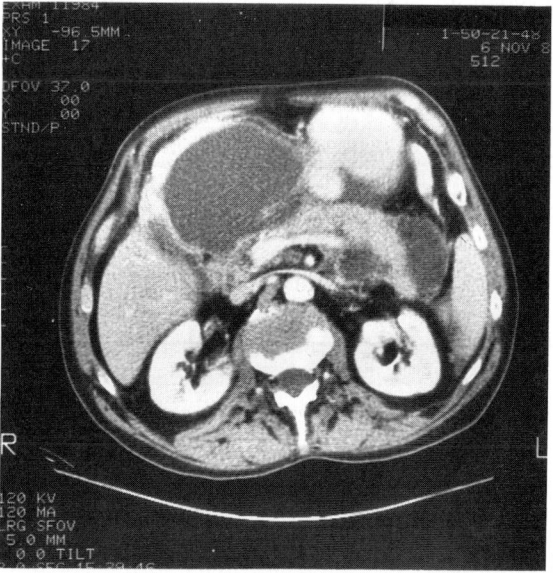

A   B

Fig. 9.5A,B (A) Admission dynamic pancreatogram, remarkable only for pancreatic swelling. C-reactive protein, however, was 35 mg %, suggesting necrosis. Clinical resolution of inflammation was interrupted two weeks later by a fever spike. (B) Repeat dynamic pancreatogram shows normal pancreatic perfusion but fluid-filled structures surrounding the head and tail of the gland. Separate pancreatic abscesses were found in these locations at surgery. Serial CT scanning is mandatory in the absence of clinical improvement.

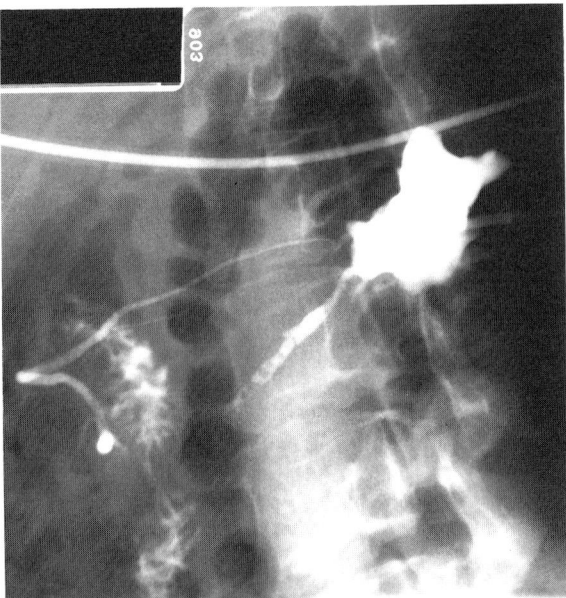

Fig. 9.6 Pancreatic fistula resulting from transcutaneous drainage of an infected pseudocyst. Note residual pseudocyst cavity and communication with pancreatic duct. Premature removal of drain will result in reaccumulation of the pseudocyst.

in whom dynamic pancreatography and C-reactive protein levels do not suggest necrosis.

In the absence of pancreatic or peripancreatic tissue necrosis, surgical drainage of acute infected pseudocysts may safely consist of external drainage by a large-bore catheter. Persistent communication of the pseudocyst with the pancreatic ductal system will result in an external pancreatic fistula (Fig. 9.6). Should a pancreatic fistula develop, premature removal of the drainage catheter may result in reaccumulation of the pseudocyst. Whenever serial fistulograms through the catheter fail to opacify the ductal system, and when the surrounding cavity has shrunk to the diameter of the catheter, it is safe to pull the drain.

Pancreatic abscess

As we have discussed, we prefer to use the term 'pancreatic abscess' in a much more restrictive way than has previously been fashionable. According to our definition, a pancreatic abscess is a collection of classically purulent material in the region of the pancreas enclosed by inflammatory walls. Using this definition, an infected pseudocyst would be a type of pancreatic abscess.

The primary reason we have chosen to restrict the term to those cases of purulence without necrosis is that the clinical courses of infected necrosis and pancreatic abscess are different. Bittner and his colleagues have observed significantly higher mortality rates, as well as greater incidence of renal and pulmonary failure, in patients with infected necrosis as opposed to pancreatic abscess (Bittner et al 1987). Although it is probably true that pancreatic abscess also begins with pancreatic or peripancreatic necrosis (which then becomes secondarily infected), in the case of patients with pancreatic abscess the necrosis is limited and purulence predominates. In contrast, in patients with infected necrosis, the necrosis predominates and purulence is limited. In our view, this distinction is not only important as regards prognosis, but it is also important in choosing the correct form of surgical drainage.

As with secondary infection in acute pseudocysts, we feel that in the absence of appreciable necrosis conventional surgical drainage using large bore catheters is effective for such peripancreatic classically purulent collections.

Intestinal necrosis

Currently, fewer than 50 cases of intestinal necrosis associated with acute pancreatitis have been reported (Bradley 1982b). Since the author has personal knowledge of another 11 unreported cases in this area of the United States, it is likely that limited individual experiences are not reported. As a consequence, the incidence of intestinal necrosis in acute pancreatitis may be underestimated.

While the pathogenesis of intestinal necrosis in patients with acute pancreatitis is uncertain, two separate mechanisms have been implicated. Direct tissue digestion by activated pancreatic enzymes is one such mechanism. Demonstrations of activated pancreatic proteolytic and lipolytic enzymes in the serum, ascitic fluid and pancreatic exudate of patients with acute pancreatitis (Schroder et al 1980, Satake et al 1982, Dubnick et al 1985) suggest that necrosis could result from direct contact of the activated enzymes with adjacent segments of intestine. Another potential mechanism for intestinal necrosis could involve vascular thrombosis of segmental mesenteric blood supply. Both arterial (Katz et al 1974, Ranson et al 1977) and venous mesenteric thrombosis (Gatch & Brickley 1951, Siler & Wulsin 1951) have been reported from histological examination of segments of necrotic intestine resected in patients with acute pancreatitis. In addition, arterial thrombosis has been demonstrated by arteriography to occur in acute pancreatitis (Reuter et al 1969). Vascular thrombosis could result from inflammatory changes in the vascular wall induced by the adjacent broth of proteolytic enzymes.

Regardless of the actual mechanism, it seems clear that the sites of intestinal involvement are controlled by mesenteric reflections (Meyers & Evans 1976). The transverse colon has been the most commonly affected segment of intestine, followed by the duodenum and then the jejunum. A glance at Figures 9.7 and 9.8 offers a satisfactory explanation for these anatomical predilections. Activated pancreatic exudate could easily pass between the mesenteric leaves to reach the sites of intestinal involvement. Fat necrosis of the

transverse mesocolon and root of the mesentery is a common finding in patients with acute pancreatitis requiring surgical exploration. For these reasons a careful search for extension of infected necrosis into the root of the mesentery and transverse mesocolon is an important part of surgical exploration.

Intestinal necrosis should be suspected in any patient with the triad of abdominal mass, sepsis, and gastrointestinal haemorrhage. We found this

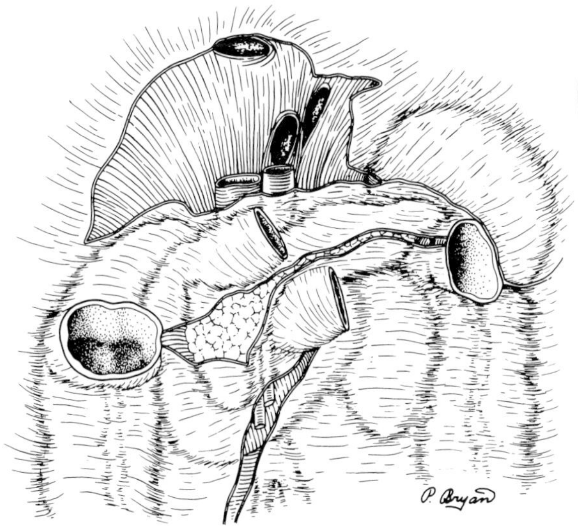

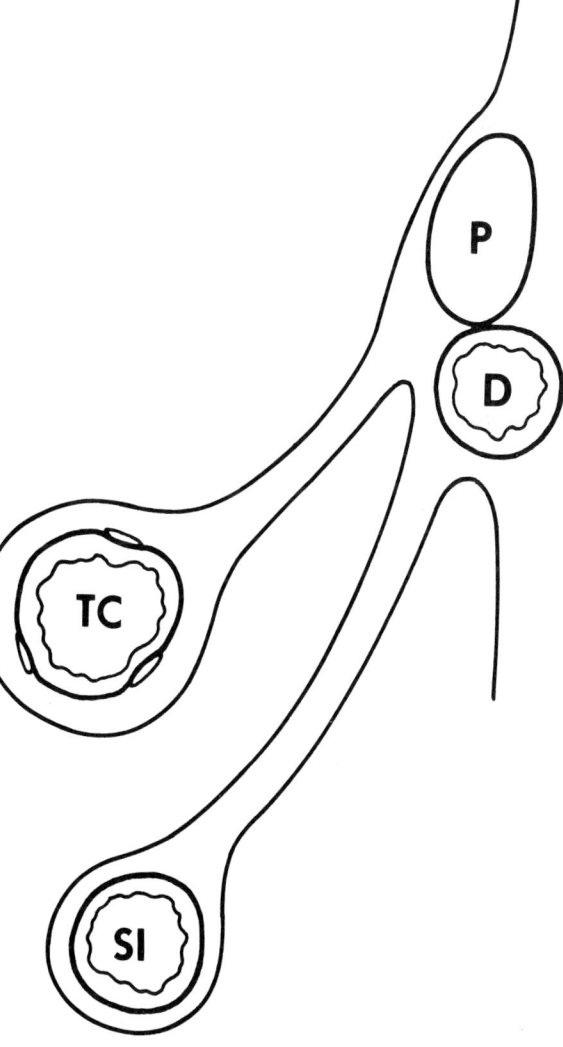

Fig. 9.7 Peritoneal reflections from the retroperitoneum. Note the access of inflammatory pancreatic exudates to the duodenum, transverse mesocolon and small intestinal mesentery.

Fig. 9.8 Schematic lateral view of access routes for inflammatory pancreatic exudate to the intestinal tissue or to intestinal blood supply. P = pancreas, D = duodenum, TC = transverse colon, SI = small intestine.

triad to be present in almost half of the reported cases of intestinal necrosis in acute pancreatitis (Bradley 1982b). Furthermore, patients with infected pancreatic necrosis are particularly susceptible to intestinal involvement. This may reflect extension of the necrotic process between the leaves of the mesentery, with secondary involvement of intestinal blood supply. Diagnosis of intestinal necrosis can be difficult in these patients in the absence of the triad, since many already have signs of sepsis and peritoneal findings. Occasionally, a plain abdominal radiograph (Fig. 9.9) or a CT scan can suggest intestinal involvement. The development of gastrointestinal haemorrhage should be an early warning sign, signifying the possibility of the existence of intestinal necrosis. In doubtful cases, careful water-soluble contrast studies or limited colonoscopy may prove to be of value.

If these studies are positive, or if intestinal necrosis remains a strong possibility, exploration is indicated, because untreated intestinal necrosis is 100% fatal in these patients. At the time of exploration, the best surgical option is removal of the involved segment with proximal enterostomy. Proximal enterostomy alone is associated with haemorrhage from the involved segment in 60% of cases (Bradley 1982b). Although therapeutic embolization for control of massive haemorrhage from intestinal necrosis could be considered in extremely poor risk patients, the author has no experience with this technique in the face of intestinal necrosis. Since embolization could not be expected favourably to affect any associated intestinal necrosis, this manoeuvre cannot be recommended under these circumstances.

Stress ulceration haemorrhage

In addition to bleeding from gastritis and pre-existing peptic ulcers, haemorrhage from stress ulceration is common in patients with severe acute pancreatitis (Siler & Wulsin 1951, Thal et al 1951). In most instances, stress ulceration is associated with the onset of sepsis in these patients (Frey et al 1982). Since the introduction of H_2 blockers to keep gastric pH above 4–5 in all patients with severe acute pancreatitis, this complication is rarely seen. Gastric resection for massive haemorrhage from stress ulceration represents an almost insurmountable hurdle for these patients, and is a situation better prevented than treated.

Vascular necrosis

Loss of vascular wall integrity is an uncommon but dramatic complication of severe acute pancreatitis. This complication is almost always associated with infected pancreatic necrosis. First described by Rich and Duff (1936), the histological changes in the wall of the involved vessel include splitting of the internal elastic lamina, arteritis, and eventual full-thickness necrosis. These pathological changes may be segmental, and can result in either thrombosis or massive haemorrhage. Presumably the arteritis results from a combination of bacterial toxins and activated pancreatic enzymes working directly on the surface of the vessel. In all

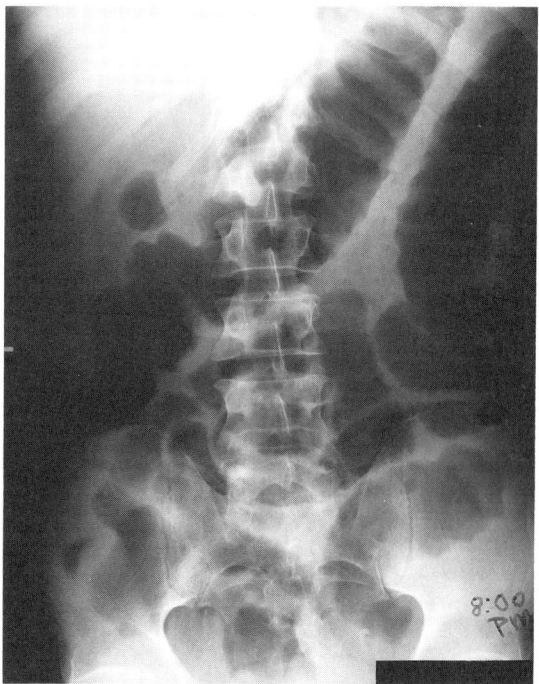

Fig. 9.9 Toxic megacolon in a patient with infected pancreatic necrosis. Necrosis of the transverse and descending portions of the colon was found at exploration.

likelihood, false aneurysms of peripancreatic arteries associated with severe acute pancreatitis are due to weakening of arterial walls by this mechanism.

The most frequently involved vessels are those in close anatomical proximity to the necrotic process in the pancreas. The splenic artery is most commonly involved, followed by the gastro-duodenal, and then the superior and inferior pancreaticoduodenal arteries. Venous necrosis is rare indeed, perhaps reflecting the propensity of veins to thrombose early in the course of involvement.

The resulting haemorrhage may take several directions. It can occur freely into the abdominal cavity, a condition suggested by rapid abdominal distension and shock. Suspicion of such a complication can be rapidly confirmed by paracentesis. Bleeding can also occur directly into a pre-existing

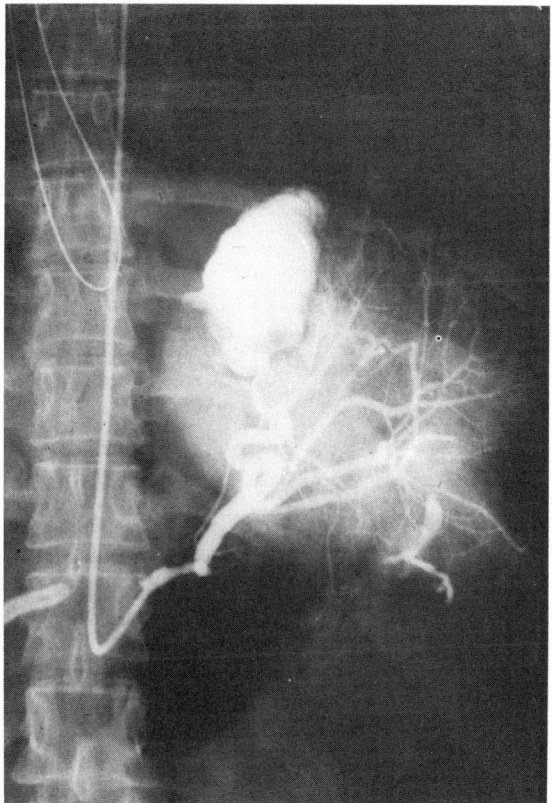

Fig. 9.10 Spontaneous haemorrhage into a pseudocyst resulting in a pseudoaneurysm. The splenic artery is most commonly involved.

acute pseudocyst as a result of erosive arteritis (Léger et al 1976, Stizman & Imbembo 1984) (Fig. 9.10). The sudden appearance of an abdominal mass, or a rapid increase in a pre-existing mass associated with increased abdominal pain, is almost pathognomic of bleeding into a pseudocyst (Bradley 1982b). Under these conditions, the pseudocyst has been converted into a pseudo-aneurysm (Wolstenholme 1974). Urgent control is required before it ruptures freely into the abdominal cavity (Wu et al 1977).

Haemorrhage may also result from incomplete drainage of infected pancreatic necrosis, presumably from prolonged contact of the infected erosive broth of activated enzymes with the regional vessels. Long-term use of inflexible rigid drains may also cause injury to the peripancreatic vessels, as well as producing enteric fistulas. Haemorrhage from drain erosion has been reported from the splenic artery and vein (Caro 1952), the superior mesenteric artery and vein, and the portal vein (Howard & Jordan 1960). Haemorrhage from incomplete drainage and erosion into blood vessels or intestines by rigid drains are two additional reasons to support the use of open drainage in patients with infected necrosis.

Haemorrhage, even from major veins, may often be controlled with packing if the injury cannot be repaired. Major venous bleeding is not infrequently encountered when performing retroperitoneal debridement for infected necrosis. The frequency of this complication can be decreased if sharp dissection is minimized. We use only finger dissection for removal of necrotic tissues, planning to remove any additional necrosis at future dressing changes. Repair of the splenic and superior mesenteric veins can be quite difficult in these patients. Extensive packing, with planned removal in two days, may offer an exit from a sticky situation. We have found this manoeuvre quite useful on occasion.

On the other hand, haemorrhage from erosive arteritis requires direct control. Angiographic localization of the bleeding site is of considerable assistance, if time and conditions permit (Stabile et al 1983). While some have advocated angiographic embolization as primary therapy (Waltman et al 1986, Vugic et al 1980), failure to remove any associated infected necrosis will lead to a high rate of recurrent haemorrhage as the erosive process continues. In those patients in whom infected necrosis is the cause of the erosive arteritis, we use angiographic embolization as part of our preoperative preparation. Widespread and effective drainage is the only assurance against recurrent haemorrhage in these patients. Angiographic embolization for massive haemorrhage could be considered definitive therapy in patients with prohibitive operative risk from other causes, such as recent myocardial infarction or cerebral vascular accident, or in those patients in whom persistent infected necrosis can be ruled out.

In a dire emergency in which operation must be undertaken without delay, there are a number of principles to be followed. If there is blood in the stomach, a prepyloric gastrotomy should be made to search for stress ulceration, followed by an incision in the cardia to look for varices. If these sites are negative, then the ampulla should be visualized. In this setting, bleeding through the ampulla signifies an intrapancreatic lesion. If the haemorrhage is from a pseudocyst or a pseudo-aneurysm which has ruptured into the intestinal tract, the location of the lesion will predict the artery involved. Lesions in the head of the pancreas are usually associated with the gastroduodenal or pancreaticoduodenal arteries. More distal lesions usually involve the splenic artery. Compression of the suspected vessel is the first step in diagnosis and control. Isolation and control of the involved vessel at its origin is the preferred method of treatment, but due to local conditions it may not always be possible. Failure to isolate and control the involved vessel may dictate the need for extensive resection, a situation best avoided if possible in these overstressed patients.

The approach to patients with massive bleeding into the free abdominal cavity differs from gastrointestinal haemorrhage in that aortic compression or occlusion is more frequently necessary before identification and control is attempted. Involved arteries should be ligated proximal to the site of their involvement, in order to place the tie in a section of artery uninvolved with the necrotizing changes in the wall.

The advent of massive haemorrhage in a patient with acute pancreatitis is ominous, with mortality rates ranging up to 75% (Stabile et al 1983); every

effort must be made to prevent it, and, to institute if unavoidable, early and definitive treatment.

Obstruction

Acute cholangiopathy

Common bile duct obstruction in acute pancreatitis is usually associated with biliary calculi, a condition well covered by McMahon in Chapter 7. Less commonly appreciated are two other causes of common duct obstruction in these patients: pericholangitis and compression by acute pseudocysts.

Biochemical and clinical jaundice occurs in approximately 20% of patients with acute pancreatitis (Bradley & Salam 1978). Almost half of these cases have been unassociated with any known cause. Because the resultant hyperbilirubinaemia is mild (usually < 100 μmol/l) and transient (< 10 days), periductular oedema and cholangitis have been implicated as a possible cause (Bradley & Salam 1978). The important point to retain is that transient hyper-

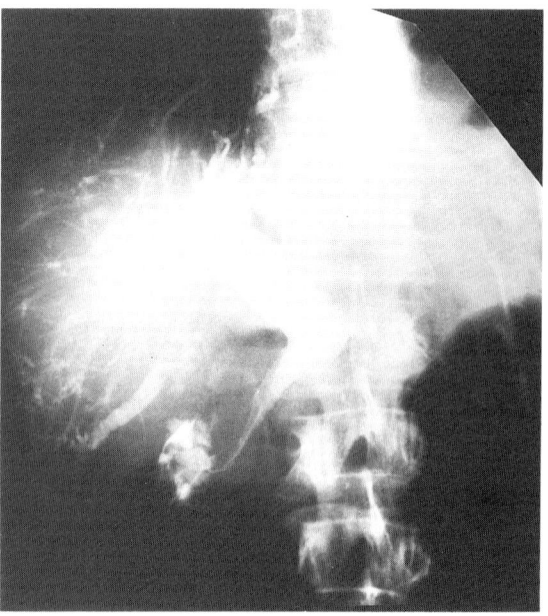

Fig. 9.11 Obstruction of common bile duct by large pseudocyst in head of pancreas.

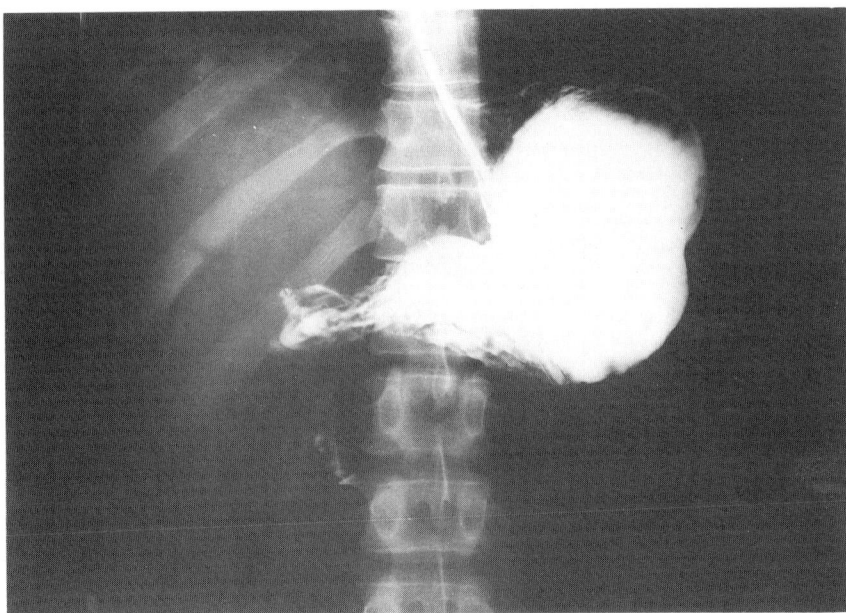

Fig. 9.12   Duodenal obstruction caused by massive pseudocyst. Note antral elevation.

bilirubinaemia is the most common type of jaundice in patients with acute pancreatitis, and in the absence of other demonstrable causes it can be expected to resolve without the necessity for surgery.

Rarely, an acute pseudocyst may result in occlusion of the common duct (Fig. 9.11). In the absence of associated sepsis, this condition may be safely observed for a few weeks in anticipation of spontaneous resolution of the pseudocyst and bile duct obstruction. Persistent obstruction beyond this time or the development of clinical sepsis dictate a more aggressive approach. Transcutaneous CT-guided drainage is quite effective in these circumstances, if the possibility of associated infected necrosis can be eliminated. In doubtful cases, exploration with external drainage of the acute pseudocyst by a large-bore catheter is indicated, along with management of any co-existing necrosis.

Intestinal obstruction

Intestinal obstruction due to acute pancreatitis is a rare event. When it does occur, it is usually the result of small bowel adhesions secondary to peritoneal inflammation. The diagnosis is secured by the characteristic high-pitched rushing bowel sounds of mechanical obstruction rather than the distended quiet abdomen of inflammatory ileus.

Even less common is intestinal obstruction resulting from a massive acute pseudocyst (Fig. 9.12). Gastric outlet obstruction is the most common presentation. Differentiation from other forms of duodenal involvement seen in pancreatitis is easily made by sonography or computed tomography. In the absence of infected necrosis, transcutaneous guided catheter drainage is effective treatment.

In summary, the indications for surgery in patients with acute pancreatitis are becoming clearer. Evidence of necrosis, infection or haemorrhage is required before urgent surgical intervention is considered. With a single exception (cholecystectomy for biliary pancreatitis), the therapy of uncomplicated acute pancreatitis remains supportive, and the principal role of surgery is to manage the complications of the underlying disease process.

REFERENCES

Agarwal N, Pitchumoni C S 1986 Simplified prognostic criteria in acute pancreatitis. Pancreas 1: 69–73

Altemeier W A, Alexander J W 1963 Pancreatic abscess. Archives of Surgery 87: 80–85

Aranha G V, Prinz R A, Greenlee H B 1982 Pancreatic abscess: an unresolved surgical problem. American Journal of Surgery 144: 534–538

Aranha G V, Prinz R A, Esguerra A C, Greenlee H B 1983 The nature and course of cystic pancreatic lesions diagnosed by ultrasound. Archives of Surgery 118: 486–488

Banks S, Wise L, Gersten M 1983 Risk factors in acute pancreatitis. American Journal of Gastroenterology 78: 637–640

Becker J M, Pemberton J H, Dimagno E P, Ilstrup D M, McIlrath D C, Dozois R R 1984 Prognostic factors in pancreatic abscess. Surgery 96: 455–461

Beger H G, Krauzberger W, Bittner R, Block S, Buchler M 1985 Results of surgical treatment of necrotizing pancreatitis. World Journal of Surgery 9: 972–979

Beger H G, Bittner R, Block S, Buchler M 1986 Bacterial contamination of pancreatic necrosis: a prospective clinical study. Gastroenterology 91: 433–438

Bittner R, Block S, Buchler M, Beger H G 1987 Pancreatic abscess and infected pancreatic necrosis: different local septic complications in acute pancreatitis. Digestive Diseases and Sciences 32: 1082–1087

Block S, Maier W, Buchler M et al 1984 Identification of pancreas necrosis in severe acute pancreatitis — imaging procedures versus clinical staging. Digestive Diseases and Sciences 29: 941

Bolooki H, Jaffe B, Gliedman M L 1968 Pancreatic abscesses and lesser sac collections. Surgery Gynecology and Obstetrics 126: 1301–1309

Bradley E L III 1982a Overview. In: E L Bradley (ed) Complications of pancreatitis. Saunders, Philadelphia, pp 1–15

Bradley E L III 1982b Enteropathies, E L Bradley (ed) In: Complications of pancreatitis. Saunders, Philadelphia pp 287–292

Bradley E L III 1987 Management of infected pancreatic necrosis by open drainage. Annals of Surgery 206: 542–550

Bradley E L III, Fulenwider J T 1984 Open treatment of pancreatic abscess. Surgery Gynecology and Obstetrics 159: 509–513

Bradley E L III, Salam A 1978 Hyperbilirubinemia in inflammatory pancreatic disease: natural history and management. Annals of surgery 188: 626–632

Bradley E L III, Gonzalez A C, Clements J L 1976 Acute pancreatic pseudocysts: incidence and implications. Annals of Surgery 184: 734–737

Bradley E L III, Clements J L Jr., Gonzalez A C 1979 The natural history of pancreatic pseudocysts: a unified concept of management. American Journal of Surgery 137: 135–141

Buchler M, Malfertheiner P, Schoetensack C, Uhl W, Beger H G 1986 Sensitivity of antiproteases, complement factors and C-reactive protein in detecting pancreatic necrosis. International Journal of Pancreatology 1: 227–235

Buggy B P, Nostrant T T 1983 Lethal pancreatitis. American Journal of Gastroenterology 78: 810–814

Camer S J, Tan E G C, Warren K W, Braasch J W 1975 Pancreatic abscess. A critical analysis of 113 cases.

American Journal of Surgery 129: 426–431

Caro D B 1952 An unusual case of acute pancreatitis. British Medical Journal i: 1070–1072

Crass R A, Way L W 1981 Acute and chronic pseudocysts are different. American Journal of Surgery 142: 660–664

Crass R A, Meyer A A, Jeffrey R B et al 1985 Pancreatic abscess: impact of computerized tomography on early diagnosis and surgery. American Journal of Surgery 150: 127–131

Davidson E D, Bradley E L 1981 Marsupialization in the treatment of pancreatic abscess. Surgery 89: 252–256

Donohue P E, Nyhus L M, Baker R J 1980 Pancreatic abscess after alcoholic pancreatitis. Archives of Surgery 115: 905–909

Dubnick M A, Geokas M C, Mar G, McMahon M J, Mayer A D, Majmudar A P N 1985 Digestive enzymes and protease inhibitors in ascites fluid from patients with acute pancreatitis. Gastroenterology 88: 1370

Frey C F, Lindenauer S M, Miller T A 1979 Pancreatic abscess. Surgery Gynecology and Obstetrics 149: 722–726

Frey C F, Stanley J C, Eckhauser F 1982 Hemorrhage. In: E L Bradley (ed) Complications of pancreatitis. Saunders, Philadelphia, pp 96–119

Gatch W D, Brickley R A 1951 Perforation of colon following acute necrosis of the pancreas. Archives of Surgery 63: 698–703

Gebhardt C, Gall F P 1981 Importance of peritoneal irrigation after surgical treatment of hemorrhagic necrotizing pancreatitis. World Journal of Surgery 5: 379–385

Gerzof S G, Johnson W C, Robbins A H, Spechler S J, Nasbeth D 1984 Percutaneous drainage of pancreatic pseudocysts. Archives of Surgery 119: 888–892

Geokas M C, Rinderknecht H, Walberg C B, Weissman R 1974 Methemalbumin in the diagnosis of acute hemorrhagic pancreatitis. Annals of Internal Medicine 81: 483–486

Gerzof S G, Banks P A, Robbins A H et al 1987 Early diagnosis of pancreatic infection by CT guided aspiration. Gastroenterology 93: 1315–1320

Gregg J A, Maher L, DeGirolami P C, Gregg J A Jr 1985 Secretion of beta lactam antibiotics in pure human pancreatic juice. American Journal of Surgery 150: 333–335

Hiatt J R, Fink A S, King W III, Pitt H A 1987 Percutaneous aspiration of peripancreatic fluid collections: a safe method to detect infection. Surgery 101: 523–530

Hill M C, Dach J L, Barkin J, Isikoff M B, Morse B 1984 The role of percutaneous aspiration in the diagnosis of pancreatic abscess. American Journal of Roentgenology 141: 103–108

Holden J L, Berne T V, Rosoff L Sr 1976 Pancreatic abscess following acute pancreatitis. Archives of Surgery 111: 858–861

Howard J M, Jordan G L Jr 1960 Surgical diseases of the pancreas. Lippincott, Philadelphia

Hunter T B, Haber K, Pond G D 1982 Phlegmon of the pancreas. American Journal of Gastroenterology 77: 949–952

Jacobs M L, Daggett W M, Civetta J M, Vasu M A 1977 Acute pancreatitis: Analysis of factors influencing survival. Annals of Surgery 185: 43–51

Karlson K B, Martin E C, Frankuchen E I, Mattern B F,

Schultz R W, Casarella W J 1982 Percutaneous drainage of pancreatic pseudocysts and abscesses. Radiology 142: 619–624

Katz P, Dorman M J, Aufses A H Jr 1974 Colonic necrosis complicating post operative pancreatitis. Annals of Surgery 179: 403–408

Kivisarri L, Sommer K, Standertskjold-Nordenstam C-G, Schroder T, Kivilaakso E, Lempinen M 1980 Early detection of acute fulminant pancreatitis by contrast-enhanced computed tomography. Scandinavian Journal of Gastroenterology 15: 633–635

Kune G A 1968 Abscesses of the pancreas. Australian and New Zealand Journal of Surgery 38: 125–129

Kune G A, King R 1973 The late complications of acute pancreatitis — pancreatic swelling, cyst and abscess. Medical Journal of Australia 1: 1241–1246

Léger L, Lenriot J P, Hovasse P 1976 Les hémorrhagies intra-kystiques des pseudokystes pancréatiques. Journal de Chirurgie 111: 137–162

Léger L, Chiche B, Louvel A 1981 Pancreatic necrosis and acute pancreatitis. World Journal of Surgery 5: 315–317

McMahon M J, Bower M, Mayer A D, Cooper E H 1984 Relation of alpha-2- macroglobulin and other antiproteases to the clinical features of acute pancreatitis. American Journal of Surgery 147: 164–169

Maier W 1987 Early objective diagnosis and staging of acute pancreatitis by contrast enhanced computed tomography. In: Beger H, Buchler M (eds) Acute pancreatitis. Springer, Berlin, pp 132–140

Mendez G, Isikoff M B, Hill M C 1980 CT of acute pancreatitis: interim assessment. American Journal of Roentgenology 135: 463–465

Meyers M A, Evans J A 1976 Effects of pancreatitis on the small bowel and colon spread along mesenteric planes. Radiology 149: 151–160

Miller T A, Lindenauer S M, Frey C F, Standley J C 1974 Pancreatic abscess. Archives of Surgery 108: 545–551

Nuutinen P, Kivisarri L, Standertskold C G, Lempinen M, Schroder T, Larmi T 1986 Contrast enhancement of the pancreas in CT during acute experimental pancreatitis compared to pancreatic microangiography. Digestive Diseases and Sciences 31: 361

Onderdonk A B, Weinstein W M, Sullivan N M 1974 Experimental intra-abdominal abscesses in rats. Infection and Immunity 10: 1256–1259

Owens B J, Hamit H F 1977 Pancreatic abscesses and pseudocyst. Archives of Surgery 112: 42–45

Pemberton J, Nagorney D M, Becker J M, Ilstrup D, Dozois R, Remine W H 1986 Controlled open lesser sac drainage for pancreatic abscess. Annals of Surgery 203: 596–604

Ranson J H C, Spencer F C 1977 Prevention, diagnosis, and treatment of pancreatic abscess. Surgery 82: 99–106

Ranson J H C, Rifkind K M, Roses D F, Fink S D, Eng K, Spencer F C 1974 Prognostic signs and the role of operative management in acute pancreatitis. Surgery Gynecology and Obstetrics 139: 69–81

Ranson J H C, Lackner H, Berman T R, Schinella R 1977 The relationship of coagulation factors to clinical complications of acute pancreatitis. Surgery 81: 502–506

Ranson J H C, Balthazar E, Caccavale R, Cooper M 1985 Computed tomography and the prediction of pancreatic abscess in acute pancreatitis. Annals of Surgery 201: 656–665

Renner I G, Savage W T III, Pantoja J L, Renner V J 1985 Death due to acute pancreatitis: A retrospective analysis of 405 autopsy cases. Digestive Diseases and Sciences 30: 1005–1018

Reuter S R, Redman H C, Joseph R R 1969 Angiographic findings in pancreatitis. American Journal of Roentgenology 107: 56–67

Rich A R, Duff G L 1936 Experimental and pathologic studies on pathogenesis of acute hemorrhagic pancreatitis. Bulletin of the Johns Hopkins Hospital 58: 212–228

Rotman N, Bonnet F, Larde D, Fagniez P 1986 Computerized tomography in the evaluation of the late complications of acute pancreatitis. American Journal of Surgery 152: 286–289

Sarles H, (ed) 1965 Pancreatitis: symposium of Marseille 1963. Karger, Basel

Sarner M, Cotton P B 1984 Definitions of acute and chronic pancreatitis. Clinical Gastroenterology 13: 865–870

Satake K, Chung Y S, Umeyama K 1982 Serum elastase levels in pancreatic disease. American Journal of Surgery 144: 239–241

Schroder T, Kivilakso E, Kianunen D K J, Lempinen M 1980 Serum phospholipase A_2 in human acute pancreatitis. Scandinavian Journal of Gastroenterology 15: 633–635

Schroder T G, Kivisarri L, Standertskjold-Nordenstam C-C, Somer K, Kivialakso E, and Lempinen M 1984 The clinical significance of contrast enhanced computed tomography (CT) in acute pancreatitis. Annales Chirurgiae et Gynaecologiae 73: 268–272

Siler V E, Wulsin J H 1951 Consideration of the lethal factors in acute pancreatitis. Archives of Surgery 63: 496–502

Silverstein W, Isikoff M B, Hill M C, Barkin J 1981 Diagnostic imaging of acute pancreatitis: prospective study using CT and sonography. American Journal of Roentgenology 137: 497–502

Singer M V, Gyr K, Sarles H 1985 Revised classification of pancreatitis. Report of the second international symposium on the classification of pancreatitis in Marseille, France March 28–30, 1984. Gastroenterology 89: 683–690

Sostre C F, Flournoy J G, Bova J G, Goldstein H, Schenker S 1985 Pancreatic phlegmon, Clinical features and course. Digestive Diseases and Sciences 30: 918–927

Stabile B E, Wilson S E, Haile T D 1983 Reduced mortality from bleeding pseudocysts and pseudoaneurysms caused by pancreatitis. Archives of Surgery 118: 45–51

Stizman J V, Imbembo A L 1984 Splenic complications of a pancreatic pseudocyst. American Journal of Surgery 147: 191–196

Thal A P, Perry J F Jr, Egner W 1951 A clinical and morphologic study of 42 cases of fatal acute pancreatitis. Surgery Gynecology and Obstetrics 105: 191–198

Vugic I, Anderson M C, Meridith H C 1980 Successful embolization of the dorsal pancreatic artery to control massive upper gastrointestinal hemorrhage. American Surgeon 46: 184–187

Waclawiczek H W, Pimpl W, Chelizek F 1986 Perioperative interdisciplinary management in acute necrotizing pancreatitis. Digestive Diseases and Sciences 31: 359

Wallace, J R, Cushing R D, Bawdon R E, Sugawa C, Lucas C E, Ledgerwood A M 1986 Assessment of antimicrobial penetration into the pancreatic juice in humans. Surgery Gynecology and Obstetrics 162: 313–316

Waltman A C, Luers P R, Athanasoulis C A, Warshaw A L

1986 Massive arterial hemorrhage in patients with pancreatitis. Archives of Surgery 121: 439–443

Warshaw A L 1974 Inflammatory masses following acute pancreatitis. Surgical Clinics of North America 54: 621–632

Warshaw A L, Jin G 1985 Improved survival in 45 patients with pancreatic abscess. Annals of Surgery 202: 408–415

Warshaw A L, Lee K-H 1979 Serum ribonuclease elevations and pancreatic necrosis in acute pancreatitis. Surgery 86: 227–234

Wells C L, Rotstein O D, Pruett T L, Simmons R L 1986

Intestinal bacteria translocate into experimental intra-abdominal abcesses. Archives of Surgery 121: 102–107

Wertheimer M D, Norris C S 1986 Surgical management of necrotizing pancreatitis. Archives of Surgery 121: 484–487

Wolstenholme J T 1974 Major gastrointestinal hemorrhage associated with pancreatic pseudocyts. American Journal of Surgery 127: 377–383

Wu T K, Zaman S N, Gullick H D, Powers S R 1977 Spontaneous hemorrhage due to pseudocysts of the pancreas. American Journal of Surgery 134: 408–410

10 Adhesion obstruction of the small bowel

M. LAVELLE-JONES and A. CUSCHIERI

Adhesion obstruction complicates about 5% of all laparotomies and is currently the most frequent cause of small bowel obstruction. Two-thirds of all episodes of adhesive obstruction will settle using conservative measures; the remainder require operative intervention. For most patients needing surgery, adhesion obstruction is a single event cured by the division of adhesive bands; only 5–10% will suffer recurrent attacks. Unfortunately, this group derives least benefit from repeated adhesiolysis, and further episodes of obstruction are almost inevitable. The optimum treatment for these patients with recurrent adhesion obstruction continues to be controversial. Currently, plication of the small bowel mesentery or intraluminal tube stenting appear to be more effective than simple division of adhesions in such cases. Success, however, is at the cost of a higher postoperative morbidity and mortality.

Incidence

The incidence of acute intestinal obstruction in adults in the UK has decreased by 50% over the last 20 years, and it now comprises only 3% of all emergency surgical admissions (Bevan 1982). This decline reflects the increased emphasis in hospital practice on elective surgery (for example hernia repair) together with the trend towards early detection and treatment of colorectal cancer. As a result neglected, strangulated hernia and obstructed colonic cancer — previously common causes of acute intestinal obstruction — have become less frequent (Ellis 1971). In contrast, adhesive obstruction is becoming an increasingly

common cause of acute intestinal obstruction. Whereas adhesions caused 23% of all obstructions reviewed during the period 1960–75 and ranked second to carcinoma (48%), their relative incidence was reversed within a decade. Currently, adhesive obstruction is encountered twice as often as obstructed cancer (Bevan 1984). In an analysis of a large number of cases (Ellis 1982), one-third of all intestinal obstructions were caused by adhesions, and 60% of small bowel obstructions were secondary to adhesive disease.

In addition to this relative increase in adhesion obstruction, it is likely that the increasing number of laparotomies performed annually has also led to an absolute increase in adhesion obstruction in Western countries (Ellis 1971). Conversely, in Nigeria and other third-world countries where elective abdominal surgery continues to be infrequent, adhesions are still an uncommon cause of obstruction (Chiedozi et al 1980).

Although adhesions can affect any viscus within the peritoneal cavity, they almost inevitably involve the small bowel, particularly the ileum. Usually the large bowel is spared (Miller & Winfield 1959). It has been estimated that about 5% of all laparotomies are complicated by adhesive small bowel obstruction (Krook 1947). However, certain operations, e.g. total colectomy plus omentectomy, are complicated by a much higher (10%–20%) incidence of adhesive obstruction (Lockhart-Mummery 1967, Ritchie 1972). In addition, patients who require laparotomy for multiple organ injury after trauma or who have had severe intra-abdominal sepsis are also at an increased risk of adhesion formation (Bevan 1984).

In a recent series of over 1400 laparotomies in

neonates and children the incidence of adhesion obstruction requiring surgical intervention was 3.3% (Festen 1982). Overall, the pattern of disease in this age group is similar to that in adults with adhesive obstruction, being more common after repeated laparotomy or following peritonitis (Festen 1982).

Congenital adhesions

Rarely, congenital adhesions can cause obstruction of the duodenum or duodenojejunal flexure (Ladd 1937). Although more usual in neonates and young children, congenital adhesions can also present in adulthood (Christensen & Jensen 1975). Many aetiological factors have been proposed to explain the development of congenital adhesive bands, but it seems likely that they represent persistent peritoneal folds and are a sequel to an abnormal rotation of the duodenum (Slavensky 1969). Barium studies are not always helpful in establishing this diagnosis, which can remain undetermined until laparoscopy or laparotomy is performed (Christensen & Jensen 1975).

Postoperative adhesions

The vast majority of intra-abdominal adhesions are the sequel to a previous laparotomy (Raf 1969). In a recent postmortem analysis (Weibel & Majno 1973) adhesions were present in 67% of individuals following a single laparotomy, their incidence increasing to 93% after multiple procedures.

Various theories have been proposed to explain adhesion formation. Traditionally, it has been taught that fibrous adhesions develop from the organization of a fibrinous exudate which develops between small bowel loops and the abdominal wall after surgery. This organization, in turn, was considered dependent upon the coexistence of breaches in the parietal or visceral peritoneum (Behan 1920). This theory led to the principle that peritoneal defects should be closed at all costs. More recently, the observations that raw peritoneal surfaces healed rapidly (Williams 1955) and that oversewing serosal defects did not reduce the incidence of adhesion formation (Singleton et

al 1952) suggested that additional factors might be involved. Subsequently, Ellis has demonstrated, in a series of elegant experiments (Ellis 1962; Ellis et al 1965), the importance of avoiding tissue ischaemia and the role of adhesions acting as vascular grafts preserving the viability of injured and ischaemic segments of bowel.

Ischaemia is not, however, the only cause of postoperative adhesions. Excessive adhesions will form in response to infection, walling of areas of sepsis within the peritoneal cavity or sealing an enteric anastomosis.

Other causes of adhesions

While most symptomatic adhesions fall into this 'postoperative' category, there are, in addition, several well-defined syndromes characterized by adhesive disease, namely, starch granuloma syndrome, chronic radiation enteritis, 'burned-out' Crohn's disease, and sclerosing peritonitis.

Since their management differs from that of 'simple' postoperative adhesive disease these conditions are considered separately.

Starch granuloma syndrome

Certain peroperative intraperitoneal contaminants promote an intense foreign-body reaction, the 'starch granuloma syndrome', characterized by: 1. cramp-like abdominal pains; 2. nausea and vomiting; 3. fever; and 4. abdominal distension with local or generalised tenderness typically occurring 10–30 days after abdominal surgery (Taft et al 1970). This intense foreign-body reaction can cause ascites, dense adhesion formation and small bowel obstruction. Granuloma-forming agents include talc or corn starch glove-dusting powder (Fraser 1982) and non-absorbable suture or gauze remnants (Myllarniemi 1967). The diagnosis of starch peritonitis can be confirmed by the detection of starch granules, using iodine staining or polarised light microscopy, in fresh ascitic fluid obtained by paracentesis (Warshaw 1972) (Fig. 10.1). Confirmation of this diagnosis is important, as the majority of cases will settle with conservative management and unnecessary reoperation can

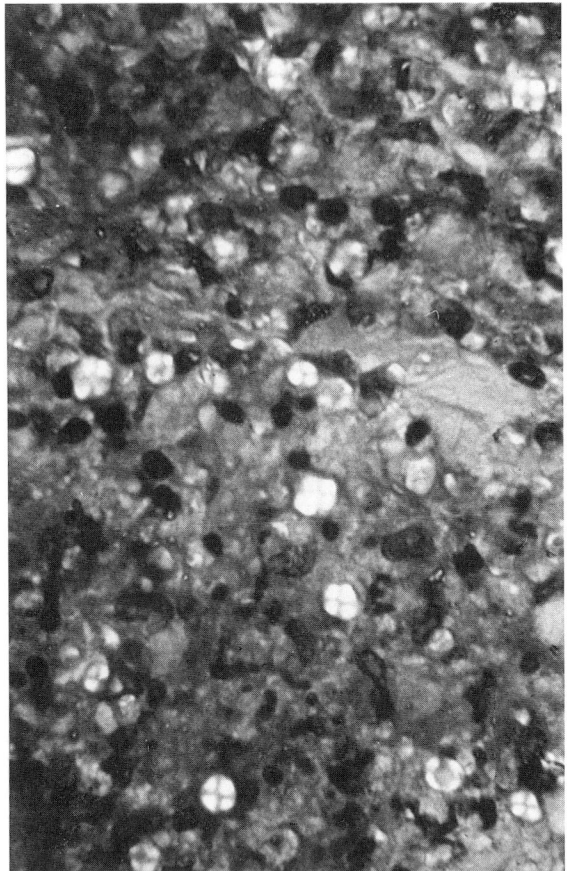

Fig. 10.1 Photomicrograph showing starch granules.

be avoided (Warshaw 1972). The importance of avoiding starch granuloma formation is emphasised by the high incidence (>60%) of significant foreign-body reactions detected in a series of over 300 cases of postoperative adhesions requiring laparotomy (Myllarniemi 1967).

Chronic radiation enteritis

The small bowel is highly radiosensitive and most patients who undergo abdominal or pelvic irradiation will experience a transient, acute radiation enteritis causing nausea, abdominal cramps and diarrhoea (Cox et al 1986). These symptoms, induced by radiation damage to the intestinal mucosa (Smith & DeCosse 1986), occur within weeks of irradiation. In contrast, damage to the vascular and interstitial small bowel connective tissue is slowly progressive (Berthrong 1986). As a result, chronic radiation enteritis producing obstructive symptoms typically presents 2–24 years after treatment (Schofield et al 1983). It is characterized by dense, fibrotic enteroenteric adhesions and tapered stricture formation. Each contributes to the mechanical small bowel obstruction (Berthrong 1986).

Chronic radiation enteritis is a dose-related phenomenon, increasing in frequency when a total dose of 80 Gy is exceeded (Perez et al 1984). It is more frequent in those patients who undergo combined external beam and intracavitary irradiation (Berthrong 1986). Other important risk factors include pre-existing intra-abdominal adhesions causing fixity of small bowel loops in the pelvis, previous pelvic inflammatory disease and a slender build (Smith & DeCosse 1986). Overall, up to 5% of patients may develop late gastrointestinal complications following radiotherapy (Perez et al 1984).

Various measures will lead to a decreased incidence of obstructive radiation enteritis in the future. These include improvements in radiation dosimetry, simple measures to displace the small intestine out of the field of irradiation (e.g. prone or head-down positioning during pelvic irradiation), and small bowel contrast radiography before irradiation to detect areas of small bowel fixity in patients with an antecedent laparotomy. Affected areas can either be freed operatively or excluded from the field of irradiation.

Partial small bowel obstruction caused by radiation damage may respond to dietary manipulation, steroids or salicylazosulphapyridine therapy (Smith & DeCosse 1986). The optimum operative treatment for those who do not settle is debatable. High morbidity and mortality rates following resectional surgery have led some authors to recommend intestinal bypass of the involved small bowel segments in those patients who do not respond to conservative measures (Swann et al 1976). Since the disease process is itself progressive, this approach will leave the patient at the risk of recurrent enteritis or the subsequent development of a blind loop syndrome. Furthermore, a bypass does not obviate the risk of anastomotic dehiscence — a major cause of mortality in these patients. Indeed the observation that microscopic degenerative vascular changes extend into bowel that appears macroscopically normal (Ledda et al 1981) suggests that the poor results previously obtained after resection may have been caused by the surgeon underestimating the extent of resection necessary to provide a safe anastomosis (Smith & DeCosse 1986). Thus a satisfactory compromise may be to resect widely the affected segment of small bowel and protect any anastomosis, at least temporarily, with a defunctioning stoma (Schofield et al 1983).

'Burned-out' Crohn's disease

Acute or subacute small bowel obstruction in Crohn's disease is usually caused by a flare-up of the small bowel or ileocolic patterns of the disease. For most Crohn's patients, an episode of adhesive obstruction is the consequence of a previous laparotomy performed to treat the complications of the disease. However, there is a distinct subgroup in whom the disease follows an indolent course and ultimately becomes 'burned out' (Kandel & Prokipchuk 1987). In these people, the persistence of enteroenteric adhesions and/or fibrostenotic segments of small bowel can lead to recurrent bouts of small bowel obstruction or bacterial overgrowth in the chronically obstructed, stagnant loops. Clearly, it is important to differentiate between those patients with subacute obstruction caused by active Crohn's disease, who warrant conservative management, and those in whom the obstruction is due to adhesive disease, who would benefit from adhesiolysis. Currently, a small bowel enema is the best method of demonstrating adhesions and thus selecting patients for early surgery (Bartram 1980).

Sclerosing peritonitis

Infrequently, adhesive small bowel obstruction has been the sequel to sclerosing encapsulating peritonitis (abdominal cocoon syndrome) induced by practolol, a beta-blocker, which has since been withdrawn (Brown et al 1974). Subsequently this condition has been identified as a complication of peritoneal dialysis (Pusateri et al 1986). Sclerosing

peritonitis is characterized by the deposition of a layer of dense, cellular fibroconnective tissue on the peritoneal surface of small bowel loops. The agents responsible remain unknown although acetate-containing dialysate, intraperitoneal contamination by formaldehyde disinfectant, and antibiotic instillation have all been implicated (Pusateri et al 1986).

The management of sclerosing peritonitis is also debatable. Some (Jackson 1983) recommend peritoneal stripping i.e. peeling off the fibroconnective plaque in confluent sheets, while others (Pusateri et al 1986), citing the high mortality rate (>80%) after operative intervention, recommend conservative management with long-term parenteral nutrition and restricted oral fluid intake.

Preventing postoperative adhesions

There is a variety of measures that the surgeon can adopt to reduce postoperative adhesion formation. Most of these have to do with technique.

At operation all attempts should be made to prevent contamination of the peritoneal cavity. Surgical gloves should be washed free of visible starch or, alternatively, starch-free gloves (Hydragel) may be substituted. Packs should be employed to prevent enteric contents causing peritoneal soiling during intestinal anastomoses and, perhaps most important of all, handling of tissues and operative trauma should be kept to a minimum.

Every anastomosis needs to be performed with meticulous surgical technique and must be completed without vascular compromise. In addition, to minimize the risk of ischaemic adhesions forming between an anastomotic line and adjacent loops of small bowel the anastomosis, where possible, should be wrapped with omentum (Ellis 1982). In this way, the risk of adhesive band formation, which can later kink and obstruct the small intestine, will be kept to a minimum.

At the end of each operation efforts should be made to achieve absolute haemostasis, thus avoiding postoperative collections which may act as a nidus for infection and promote adhesion formation. Any necrotic or dubiously viable tissue should be excised prior to closure. An attempt should be made to remove all foreign material, including stray gauze fibres and redundant non-absorbable suture remnants from the peritoneal cavity. Finally, the loops of bowel should be returned to the abdominal cavity in an orderly fashion and the omentum drawn over them before closure in an attempt to reduce adhesion formation between the small intestine and the abdominal wall. The importance of the omentum in preventing adhesions may be gauged from the high incidence of postoperative adhesion formation (up to 20%) after removal of the omentum during total colectomy (Ellis 1982).

Recognition of the rapid regenerative capacity of mesothelium has reduced the emphasis on the importance of closing peritoneal defects (Ellis 1982). Most surgeons would now agree that denuded areas of parietal or visceral serosa are best left to re-epithelialize (Bevan 1982, Ellis 1982, Jones & Munro 1985). No attempt should be made to close the peritoneum under tension. Under these circumstances, we favour mass closure of the abdominal wall using a nonabsorbable suture, leaving the peritoneum unsutured in order to reduce the risk of ischaemia and adhesion formation.

In addition to the technical measures outlined above, numerous agents, usually introduced peroperatively, have been proposed in an attempt to prevent postoperative adhesion formation. These have been extensively reviewed elsewhere (Ellis 1971). Essentially, they fall into three categories designed to:

1. inhibit fibrin and fibroblast activity; these include heparin (Lehman & Boyes 1940); dicoumarol (White 1949) and, more recently, low molecular weight dextrans (Kapur et al 1968), aprotinin (Trasylol) (Ellis, 1982) and steroids (Luttwak et al 1957);
2. promote fibrinolysis; e.g. streptokinase (Wright et al 1950), actase (James et al 1965), pepsin and trypsin (Kubota 1922);
3. sustain small bowel separation. Numerous methods have been proposed to prevent prolonged contact between small bowel loops after surgery. They include air insufflation (Bainbridge 1909),

neostigmine-stimulated intestinal motility (Cone 1951) and a variety of 'lubricating' agents ranging from amniotic fluid (Johnson 1927) to olive oil (Claypool et al 1910). More recently, hydrophobic polymer coatings have been proposed as a means of reducing peritoneal adhesions (Goldberg et al 1980).

Although these measures may appear theoretically attractive, so far none have been effective in reducing postoperative adhesion formation (Ellis 1971, Jones & Munro 1985).

The effects of adhesions

Adhesions themselves probably do not cause obstruction. However, by anchoring the small bowel at a second point, in addition to the root of the mesentery, they provide an axis around which the intestines may kink, twist or form a volvulus loop leading to an obstructive episode.

Postoperative adhesions promote acute intestinal obstruction, recurrent intestinal obstruction, and bacterial overgrowth

Acute adhesion obstruction of the small bowel

Since the overall incidence of symptomatic adhesions after laparotomy is only 5%, it follows that the vast majority of postoperative adhesions are silent. Although adhesions can become symptomatic at any time after operation, it has been estimated that one-third of obstructive episodes occur within 12 months of the antecedent laparotomy (Raf 1969) and that up to 80% are evident within 5 years (Weigelt et al 1980).

Clinical features

Abdominal colic is the most constant feature of adhesive small bowel disease; other symptoms depend on the site of obstruction (Le Quesne 1976). In general, distal small bowel obstruction is associated with progressive abdominal distension and dehydration. Mid small bowel obstruction is often associated with severe colic, whereas high small bowel obstruction may be deceptively pain-free though at the cost of profuse vomiting and rapid dehydration. Absolute constipation may or may not be present, irrespective of the level of obstruction. In addition to these cardinal features of intestinal obstruction, adhesions are characterized by the frequent (10%, Bizer et al 1981) and rapid (Bevan 1984) development of strangulation. Detection of this life-threatening complication is imperative with regard to the timing of operative intervention. Unfortunately, existing clinical and biochemical indices differentiate poorly between simple and strangulating obstruction (Sarr et al 1982). The following criteria (Lefall & Syphax 1970) are a helpful, although not a foolproof (Sarr et al 1982), guide to the detection of strangulation:

Localized abdominal tenderness
Tachycardia
Leucocytosis
The onset of constant abdominal pain
Fever

Although the presence of these risk factors does not invariably indicate strangulation, their continued absence generally supports the lack of strangulation. Most would agree that the presence of one or more of these features in an obstructed patient is an indication for urgent laparotomy (Wolfson et al 1985).

Investigation of patients with adhesion obstruction

The initial management of the patient presenting with adhesive obstruction follows the principles established for intestinal obstruction of any cause.

Admission haematocrit, white cell count and urea and electrolyte values may all be normal. Without adequate rehydration, a progressive haemoconcentration and electrolyte imbalance will supervene if the obstruction is unrelieved. Serial haematocrit and electrolyte determinations should be obtained, compared against the baseline values, and used to monitor fluid balance and rehydration. The development of a leucocytosis that cannot be accounted for by simple haemoconcentration may herald the onset of strangulation.

An erect and supine plain abdominal radiograph is useful, in conjunction with the physical findings, in determining the level of obstruction. Appearances on the erect film may vary little from normal in early high small bowel obstruction, or may reveal the classical 'ladder' pattern of dilated small bowel loops with multiple air-fluid levels in a long-standing distal obstruction. Additional information regarding the level of obstruction may be provided by the supine abdominal film, showing either the ringed pattern (valvulae conniventes) of the jejunum or the plain pattern of the terminal ileum. Scattered fluid levels throughout the abdomen may warn the surgeon of multiple diffuse adhesions, whereas a localized group of fluid levels and gas shadows is more in keeping with obstruction due to a single adhesive band (Bevan 1984). Finally, a closed loop obstruction may be implicated by a coexistence on plain abdominal X-ray of a single distended loop and a solitary pair of fluid levels on the erect film.

Management

The timing of operative intervention in adhesion obstruction remains controversial. Several recent American reports have advocated early laparotomy in all cases of adhesive obstruction, citing the hazards of overlooking strangulating obstruction and the difficulties in clinically differentiating strangulating from simple obstruction (Shatila et al 1976, Laws 1978). However, a policy of mandatory exploration in all cases of adhesion obstruction, apart from producing even more adhesive disease, will lead to unnecessary surgery being performed in the 50–65% of patients who could be expected to settle using conservative measures (Bizer et al 1981). Furthermore, recent evidence suggests that a delay in operation does not inevitably lead to an increase in mortality nor is it always associated with an increased incidence of strangulated intestine (Tanphiphat et al 1987).

It is not unreasonable, therefore, for patients with adhesion obstruction to undergo a period of conservative management unless there is overwhelming evidence of strangulation, closed loop obstruction, high level small bowel obstruction, or clinical deterioration despite resuscitation.

Conservative management

Alimentary tract decompression, intravenous fluid replacement and serial clinical reassessment are the essentials of conservative treatment in acute adhesion obstruction.

Restrictions on oral intake must be supplemented with nasogastric suction even if the patient is not vomiting. An accurate fluid balance should be maintained, taking into account that up to 8 l of fluid/day (comprising saliva, gastric, pancreatic, biliary and intestinal secretion) can be sequestered in the proximal small bowel during an episode of acute intestinal obstruction (Bevan 1984). It is our practice to replace 50% of this estimated deficit with isotonic saline and the balance with 5% dextrose solution. Regular determinations of haematocrit, blood urea and electrolytes, and the urine output are used to regulate the fluid balance. Potassium replacement is administered as appropriate.

Many bouts of adhesion obstruction will settle using this or similar régimes. In a recent series of 127 obstructive episodes, two-thirds responded to nonoperative treatment (Wolfson et al 1985). Notably, patients with incomplete or recurrent bouts of obstruction are more likely to respond to conservative measures (Wolfson et al 1985).

Nasogastric or long tube gastrointestinal decompression?

Long intestinal tubes introduced via the nose or mouth were originally designed as a means of intubating the upper intestine for physiological or radiological studies (Miller & Abbott 1934). Later, this same technique was championed as a means of decompressing the intestine in nonstrangulating small bowel obstruction, obviating the need for laparotomy. Particular emphasis was placed on the ability to provide intestinal decompression by direct intubation beyond the pylorus. However, early experience taught that its application often led to a delay in surgical intervention, particularly in the presence of strangulation, and consequently to unacceptably high mortality rates. Despite these observations, its use continues to be recommended (Wolfson et al 1985). In a recent study (Bizer et al, 1981) there was no difference overall in the ability of conventional nasogastric tubes or long tubes to avert operative intervention (45% and 47% avoiding surgery, respectively) in a group of 262 patients all with small bowel obstruction treated primarily by tube decompression. In the same study, resolution of obstruction was more frequently achieved in patients treated with long tubes if the duodenum was successfully negotiated than in those in whom intubation beyond the pylorus failed. Taken together, these observations suggest that patients whose adhesions resolved following successful passage of a long tube could have been treated with equal success if a conventional nasogastric tube had been used. Thus, long-tube decompression possesses few advantages over simple nasogastric decompression, which relies on reflux of intestinal contents into the stomach. Indeed, the major advantage of continuous nasogastric aspiration in the obstructed patient may be to provide gaseous decompression of the gastrointestinal tract by preventing the build-up of swallowed air.

Operative management

Up to two-thirds of patients with adhesion obstruction can be expected to settle using conservative measures. The optimum duration for a trial of non-operative treatment remains debatable, but most recent series (Bizer et al 1981, Wolfson et al 1985) recommend that patients who do not improve within 72 h warrant operative intervention. Obviously, should the patient's clinical status deteriorate, or if strangulation is suspected, immediate surgery becomes mandatory. The high incidence (>50%) of vascular compromise in adhesive small bowel obstruction in children (Festen 1982) suggests that for them, early surgical intervention is essential and should be undertaken as soon as preoperative resuscitation is completed.

Operative intervention for adhesive obstruction can be a hazardous and technically difficult procedure. For this reason it is best dealt with by the experienced surgeon who is familiar with the hazards of operating on the obstructed abdomen. Although it is recognized that, in many instances, division of a single adhesive band may be all that is required, the presence of multiple dense adhesions cannot always be predicted.

Generally, it is best to reopen any existing vertical abdominal scar. Only when obstruction presents following a subcostal or Pfannenstiel incision is there merit in creating a new upper or lower midline abdominal incision. As adhesions are frequently adherent to the internal surface of a previous incision, extreme care is necessary to avoid damaging the adherent small bowel on entering the peritoneal cavity. For this reason, it is often safer to open the abdomen above or below the existing limits of an old scar by extending the incision in the appropriate direction. In this manner, offending bowel loops may be detached under direct vision from the abdominal wall. Only when the small bowel has been completely freed from the anterior abdominal wall and the existing scar extended to expose the entire peritoneal cavity can any attempt be made to examine the small bowel methodically and relieve the obstruction.

The basic aim in adhesive small bowel obstruction is to completely free each loop of small bowel from the ligament of Treitz to the ileocaecal valve. Any segment found to be gangrenous or of doubtful viability is resected. Fibrotic, strictured segments of small bowel at the site of longstanding fibrous adhesions should be dealt with either by resection or stricturoplasty, depending on the extent of the stricture. Simple bypass of these areas is avoided.

It is frequently helpful at an early stage to empty congested distended small bowel loops by milking their contents in a retrograde fashion into the stomach where they can be aspirated, in turn, via a wide bore nasogastric tube fed into the stomach by the anaesthetist. This method obviates the need for an enterotomy or needle puncture associated with Savage (1960) or open decompression of the obstructed loops.

At operation, four main patterns of adhesions can be found (Bevan 1984): single band; multiple bands; incisional; and omental bowstring — the latter implying herniation of small bowel loops between the anterior abdominal wall and an omental band stretching into the pelvis or iliac fossae (Bevan 1984).

Obviously, a single band adhesion can be dealt with either by division or excision. Multiple adhesions, in contrast, often require a long and tedious dissection. When they are encountered, a start should be made at the point within the abdomen that appears most promising. Frequently, the dissection has to be approached from several sites before the anatomy can be clearly defined and adherent small bowel loops safely unravelled. As a general guide the dissection, using a combination of blunt and sharp techniques, should adhere to an avascular areolar plane. Adhesions are least vascular at their point of insertion. If bleeding is encountered, it indicates that a false plane has been created, with the imminent risk of mesenteric damage or enteric perforation. Should the small bowel be inadvertently breached — an event that may occur despite meticulous dissection — the defect should be immediately repaired using interrupted seromuscular non-absorbable sutures.

Obviously, areas of non-viable bowel require resection using conventional techniques. Similarly, areas of anastomotic narrowing or segments of bowel damaged by dense fibrosis and adhesion formation may require formal resection. There is no place for a simple bypass of these areas; this would simply predispose the patient to bacterial overgrowth in the bypassed loops, with an ongoing risk of strangulation in the unresected anchored loops. Occasionally, a stricturoplasty may be used to relieve a single isolated ring stricture, particularly if there have been numerous previous resections, for example in a Crohn's patient where conservation of the small bowel is essential.

Recurrent small bowel obstruction

For the majority of patients with adhesive small bowel obstruction, operative intervention is a single event and a cure is frequently achieved by adhesiolysis alone. The other 5–10% will suffer recurrent attacks (Jones & Munro 1985).

Clinical features

Most recurrent obstructive episodes will settle using conservative measures. A few patients will require further operative intervention to relieve their symptoms. Others will develop symptoms due to bacterial overgrowth caused by stasis in chronically obstructed loops. These individuals may present with malabsorption, steatorrhoea, hypoproteinaemia and a megaloblastic anaemia (Banwell et al 1981). In these cases the detection of bacterial overgrowth can be difficult, relying on a combination of standard malabsorption tests (e.g. Schilling; 5-day faecal fat collection), radiological features (small bowel enema), and non-invasive breath tests (^{14}C-glycocholate; hydrogen; ^{14}C-xylose;) to differentiate bacterial overgrowth and terminal ileal disease (SeHCAT test). When the nutritional status is poor, patients will require a period of intravenous hyperalimentation before the operation.

Occasionally, adhesions may be held to account for chronic, nonspecific abdominal pains, invariably in patients who have undergone previous laparotomy and who have been extensively investigated, often without cause being found to account for their symptoms. At our own institution, we have employed laparoscopy as the final arbiter in those individuals in whom extensive noninvasive investigation has failed to reveal a cause for their abdominal pain. In of a group of 16 such cases in whom postoperative adhesions were discovered and divided at laparoscopy, no symptomatic relief was obtained unless the patient described a clear history of colicky abdominal pain. Inevitably, poorly localized intermittent abdominal aches continued despite complete laparoscopic division of adhesions. Based on these observations, we are of the opinion that long-standing postoperative adhesions do not cause chronic, poorly defined abdominal pain.

For the unfortunate minority (~5%) who will require repeated laparotomy for adhesive obstruction, there is evidence that division of adhesions alone is of little value. The recurrence rate after multiple operations for adhesive obstruction is high. By the third laparotomy, although in an admittedly small group of patients, the incidence of recurrent symptomatic adhesions approaches 30% (Krook 1947). It is within this group that dense multiple adhesions are most common, and simple lysis of adhesions of least value.

In these patients, two approaches are currently used in an attempt to promote orderly formation of adhesions, namely mesenteric plication and intraluminal tube stenting.

Mesenteric plication

In 1937, Noble proposed small bowel enteric plication to obviate the development of adhesive obstruction. As originally described, this operation approximated adjacent segments of small bowel by suture apposition. Noble recommended using absorbable catgut sutures, running the stitch from the root of the mesentery along the free edge of the adjacent mesenteric folds to be continued, in turn, along the mesenteric border of the adjoining loops of small bowel. Various subsequent reports emphasized variations in technique, including the use of nonabsorbable sutures (Lord et al 1949) and placement of the plicating sutures on the antimesenteric border of the bowel wall (Seabrook & Wilson 1954). From the outset, this time-consuming operation appeared successful in relieving adhesive obstruction. However, enteric plication was not without complication itself. Most serious was the development of postoperative interloop fistulae and peritonitis as a result of damage to the bowel wall by the plicating suture and the almost universal postoperative complaint of intermittent cramp-like abdominal pains without radiological evidence of obstruction. These observations led Childs and Phillips (1960) to propose transmesenteric plication of the small bowel, principally to avoid fistula formation. These authors advocated the use of a non-absorbable plicating suture threaded in turn through each leaf of mesentery, close to the bowel wall, and then threaded back to the starting point to be tied to form a loop. A total of three sutures was recommended, one being placed at either end of the mesentery and one in the middle (Fig. 10.2A). When these sutures are tightened, the loops of bowel take on the organized appearance of a closed fan (Fig. 10.2B). Subsequently, this technique has been further simplified (McCarthy & Sharf 1965), employing a single suture at each site of plication, passed through the mesentery several centimetres from the bowel wall and tied in turn to its neighbour. Thirty-one patients with recurrent small bowel obstruction who had been operated on using this method were followed up for an average of 5.9 years: with one exception, they had had no further episodes of intestinal obstruction (McCarthy 1975). A major contraindication to the

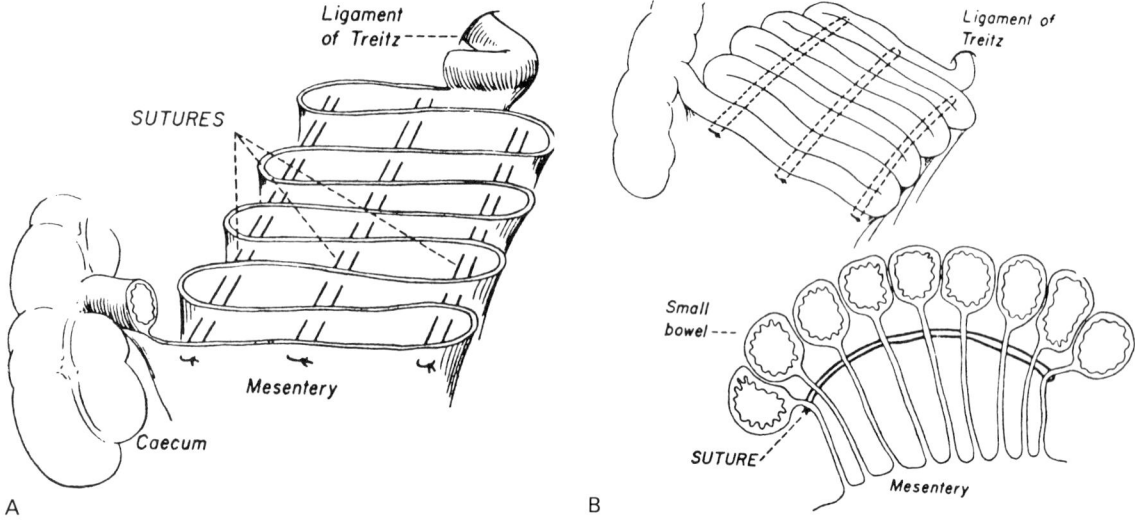

Fig. 10.2 (A) Transmesenteric sutures of the Childs-Phillips plication. (B) When there sutures are tied, the loops of bowel simulate a closed fan.

performance of this operation appears to be intra-abdominal sepsis. In this series, 7/8 patients with generalized peritonitis at the time of plication succumbed during the postoperative period.

At our own institution, we have employed a further modification of this technique in 13 patients with recurrent generalized small bowel adhesive disease (Fig. 10.3). Rather than plicate the mesentery throughout its entire length, adjacent loops of bowel are simply plicated using non-absorbable sutures at the free margins of their mesentery. This minimizes puncture of the mesentery with its attendant risk to the mesenteric vascular supply. As a further safety measure, the

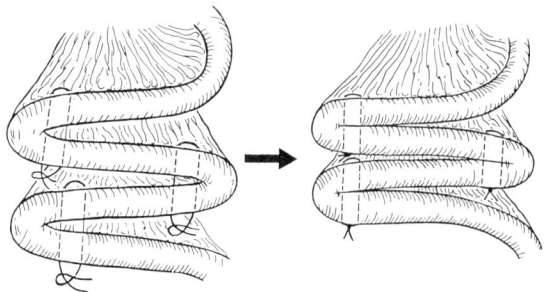

Fig. 10.3 Ninewells' modification of mesenteric plication: interrupted sutures are used to approximate the pleated adjacent (50 cm) loops of small intestines on alternate sides. With this technique, the risk of damage to the mesenteric vessels is virtually abolished.

site of puncture is chosen following careful trans-illumination of the mesentery. In each case, the sutures are tightened sufficiently to hold the bowel loops in the closed fan position but without compromise to the vasculature.

Intraluminal tube stenting

Intraluminal small bowel tube stenting was originally described by White (1956) as a means of reducing symptomatic adhesion formation. Later this procedure was popularized by Baker (1959) primarily as a peroperative means to relieve advanced mechanical small bowel obstruction. This alternative method of creating 'orderly' adhesions employs a long balloon-tipped catheter, introduced into the bowel lumen usually via a jejunostomy sited some 200–300 mm distal to the ligament of Treitz. Thereafter, the catheter is threaded distally, with the balloon partially inflated to aid its manipulation until a point is reached beyond the ileocaecal valve. The proximal end of the catheter is exteriorized via the jejunostomy site, where it is secured either by a Witzel tunnel (Baker 1959) or a double purse string suture (Close & Christensen 1979). In either case it is recommended that the adjacent jejunum be secured to the anterior abdominal wall at the point

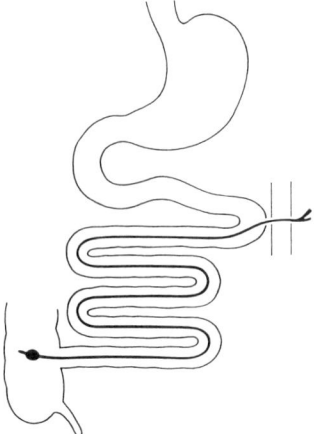

Fig. 10.4 Intestinal tube plication. (Reproduced from Essential Surgical Practice, 2nd edn, 1988, Cuschieri A, Giles G R, Mossa A R, (eds), by permission of Butterworths)

of exit of the tube from the abdomen (Fig. 10.4). Once in position, the tube is usually allowed to drain by gravity (Weigelt et al 1980, Jones & Munro 1985). Most authors recommend leaving the tube in situ, with the tip in the caecum, for a period of 2–3 weeks. Generally, the balloon is simply used to guide the catheter through the intestinal lumen, although some authors choose to leave it inflated within the caecum for a variable length of time (Close & Christensen 1979, Jones & Munro 1985). After 2–3 weeks have elapsed, the catheter is withdrawn in retrograde fashion. It is recommended that the tube be spigotted once intestinal function recovers (Jones & Munro 1985).

Numerous variations on this basic technique have been proposed (Fig. 10.5). Since introduction of the intestinal tube via a jejunostomy does not allow adequate decompression of the stomach, some (Thow 1972) have recommended insertion of the tube via a gastrostomy or via the nasogastric route (Nelson & Nyhus 1979). However, persistent gastric fistula formation (Robbins et al 1980) or airway complications (McMillin et al 1981) have left these approaches with little to recommend them. Occasionally, retrograde insertion via an ileostomy in the patient who has undergone total colectomy, or via the anal canal following ileorectal anastomosis, will obviate the need for an enterotomy (Jones & Munro 1985). Others (Sanderson 1971) prefer to introduce the tube via the caecum.

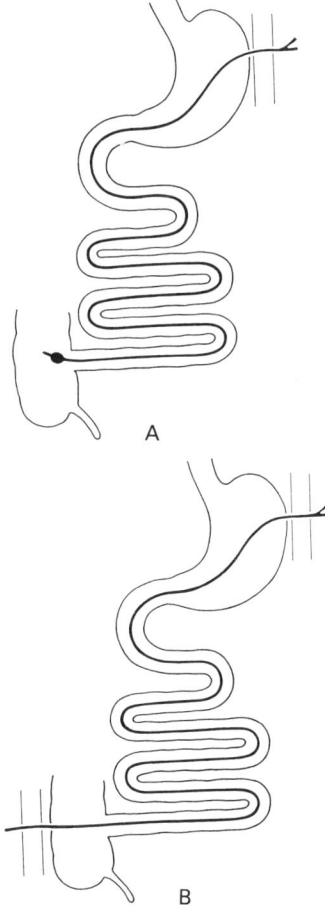

Fig. 10.5 Alternatives of operative intestinal tube plication. (Reproduced from Essential Surgical Practice, 2nd edn, 1988, Cuschieri A, Giles G R, Mossa A R (eds), by permission of Butterworths)

The complications inherent in performing a jejunostomy are a major drawback to the performance of tube plication. Most contemporary series (Close & Christensen 1979, Weigelt et al 1980) have reported intra-abdominal abscess formation during tube stenting or the development of a jejunal fistula after removal of the tube. To combat these difficulties, all proponents of this technique emphasize the importance of careful suture apposition of the jejunostomy against the anterior abdominal wall in order to avoid kinking and distal obstruction, factors that may predispose to fistula formation after extubation. It is also essential that the jejunostomy itself is carefully constructed, ensuring a watertight seal around the catheter exit site to avoid leakage of enteric contents.

In addition several complications may arise related to the tube itself, namely occasional difficulties encountered in removing the tube and, less often, the intussusception of small bowel along the tube axis (Weigelt et al 1980). Finally, it has been suggested that tube stenting may not provide adequate plication in the long term. Small-bowel barium studies taken after mesenteric plication with absorbable sutures demonstrated disruption of the small bowel plication and recurrence of obstruction within six months (Ferguson et al 1967). By inference, the limited duration (2–3 weeks) of tube stenting may be insufficient to promote permanent orderly adhesion formation (Close & Christensen 1979).

The advantages of the .Baker tube 'sutureless' plication are its obvious simplicity and the relative ease with which distended small bowel loops can be decompressed. It can also be used in the presence of peritonitis.

Transmesenteric or tube plication?

Comparison of these techniques based on the available literature is difficult. Clearly, each operation has its proponents and few authors have attempted critical comparison of the relative merits of either procedure. A report by Close & Christensen (1979) has compared 28 plications with 37 intubations and 107 patients who underwent division of adhesions alone. Their results suggested that plication (no recurrence) was more effective than intubation (8% recurrence) or simple enterolysis (9% recurrence), although at a cost of a greater mortality (10.7%, 2.7% and 3.7%, respectively). Tables 10.1, 10.2 and 10.3 summarize the results of several recent major series of recurrent small bowel obstruction treated by plication, stenting, or enterolysis alone. Clearly, direct comparison of the data is not possible, but several trends are apparent. Although neither procedure emerges clearly superior, both mesenteric plication (3.3%) and tube stenting (5.5%) appear to reduce the need for reoperation as compared to

Table 10.1 Mesenteric plication, major series

Series	Patients	Reoperations	Deaths	Follow-up, years
Calvet et al 1966	45	0	7	
Ferguson et al 1967	12	1	0	2–5
Moreaux et al 1968	26	0	0	
Thomeret 1970	31	0	2	
Hollander et al 1971	48	2	2	
Papadimitriou et al 1972	17	0	0	
McCarthy 1975	42	1	8	1–13
Close & Christensen 1979	28	0	3	1–12
Somell 1978	29	5	3	1–11
Total	278	9 (3.3%)	25 (8.9%)	

Table 10.2 Intraluminal tube stenting, major series

Series	Patients	Reoperations	Deaths	Follow-up, yrs
White 1956	16	1	1	1–6
Baker 1968	52	1	0	2–15
Markee & Uhlig 1971	49	2	—	—
Grosfeld et al 1975	20	0	0	2–3
Brightwell et al 1977	28	9	0	1–7
Close & Christensen 1979	37	1	0	1–12
Weigelt et al 1980	154	13	20	1–5+
Jones & Munro (1985)	140	0	0	1–13
Total	496	27 (5.5%)	21 (4.2%)	

Table 10.3 Enterolysis alone, major series

Series	Patients	Reoperations	Deaths	Follow-up, years
Brightwell et al 1977	30	4	0	1–7
Close & Christenson 1979	107	10	4	1–12
Total	137	14 (10.2%)	4 (3%)	

enterolysis (10.2%) alone. But the mortality rate following mesenteric plication (8.4%) is twice that observed after intubation (4.2%) or simple enterolysis (3%).

A management plan for recurrent adhesive obstruction

Single or localized multiple adhesions

These should be simply divided. This approach will ensure minimal trauma to the bowel. Mesenteric plication is not recommended under these circumstances, or prophylactically, because of the higher morbidity with this procedure than with simple enterolysis.

Multiple generalized adhesions with or without gross small bowel obstruction

It is our practice to treat all such cases by mesenteric plication, after enterolysis and decompression of the small bowel by retrograde emptying of enteric contents into the stomach. A specific advantage of this method is that it obviates the enterotomy required for intestinal intubation. Others recommend mesenteric plication only in cases of generalized small bowel adhesions without marked obstruction and hold-up, in which cases they favour tube decompression (Close & Christensen 1979).

Adhesive obstruction and generalized peritonitis

Transmesenteric plication in the presence of infection is associated with a high (>80%) mortality and should not be performed in the presence of gross intraperitoneal contamination. Although some recommend tube stenting if generalized peritonitis coexists with severe adhesions (Close & Christensen 1979), it is our policy, under these conditions, to simply treat the underlying cause of sepsis and to deal only with those adhesions that have precipitated the obstructive episode. The remainder, if sufficiently symptomatic, can be dealt with electively at a later date.

REFERENCES

Bainbridge W S 1909 The intra-abdominal administration of oxygen. Annals of Surgery 49: 305–308

Baker J W 1959 A long jejunostomy tube for decompressing intestinal obstruction. Surgery Gynecology and Obstetrics 109: 519–520

Baker J W 1968 Stitchless plication for recurring obstruction of the small bowel. American Journal of Surgery 116: 316–324

Banwell J G, Kistler L A, Giannella R A, Weber F L, Lieber A, Powell D E 1981 Small intestinal bacterial overgrowth syndrome. Gastroenterology 80: 834–841

Bartram C I 1980 The radiological demonstration of adhesions following surgery for inflammatory bowel disease. British Journal of Radiology 53: 650–653

Behan R J 1920 Intraperitoneal adhesions; their origin and prevention. American Journal of Medical Science 160: 375–380

Berthrong M 1986 Pathological changes secondary to radiation. World Journal of Surgery 10: 155–170

Bevan P G 1982 Acute intestinal obstruction in the adult. British Journal of Hospital Medicine 28: 258–265

Bevan P G 1984 Adhesive obstruction. Annals of the Royal College of Surgeons of England 66: 164–169

Bizer L S, Liebling R W, Delany H M, Gliedman M L 1981 Small bowel obstruction: The role of nonoperative treatment in simple intestinal obstruction and predictive criteria for strangulation obstruction. Surgery 89: 407–413

Brightwell N L, McFee A S, Aust J B 1977 Bowel obstruction and the long tube stent. Archives of Surgery 112: 505–511

Brown P, Baddeley H, Read A E, Davies J D, McGarry J 1974 Sclerosing peritonitis: an unusual reaction to a beta-adrenergic blocking drug (practolol). Lancet 2: 1477–1481

Calvet J P, Fellus P H, Setbon L, Answorth J W, Hirtz H R 1966 Emploi de la plicature mésentèrique (procédé de Childs-Phillips simplifié à titre prophylactique). Memoires de L'Académie de Chirurgie (Paris) 92: 200–206

Chiedozi L C, Aboh I O, Piserchia N E 1980 Mechanical bowel obstruction. Review of 316 cases in Benin City. American Journal of Surgery 139: 389–393

Childs W A, Phillips R B 1960 Experience with intestinal plication and a proposed modification. Annals of Surgery 152: 258–265

Christensen V, Jensen H E 1975 Congenital duodenal adhesions. Acta Chirurgica Scandinavica 141: 759–762

Claypool J R, Vance B M, Robertson F S, Field C W 1910 A study in the prevention of post-operative adhesions. Journal of the American Medical Association 55: 312–314

Close M B, Christensen N M 1979 Transmesenteric small bowel plication or intraluminal tube stenting. American Journal of Surgery 138: 89–96

Cone D F 1951 The effect of intestinal motility on the formation of adhesions. Bulletin of the John Hopkins Hospital 105: 9–11

Cox J D, Byhardt R W, Wilson F, Haas J S, Komaki R, Olson L E 1986 Complications of radiation therapy and factors in their prevention. World Journal of Surgery 10: 171–188

Ellis H 1962. The aetiology of post operative adhesions. British Journal of Surgery 50: 10–16

Ellis H 1971 The cause and prevention of postoperative intraperitoneal adhesions. Surgery, Gynecology and Obstetrics 133: 497–511

Ellis H 1982 The causes and prevention of intestinal adhesions. British Journal of Surgery 69: 241–243

Ellis H, Harrison W, Hugh T B 1965. The healing of peritoneum under normal and abnormal conditions. British Journal of Surgery 52: 471–476

Ferguson A T, Reihmer V A, Gaspar M R 1967 Transmesenteric plication for small bowel obstruction. American Journal of Surgery 114: 203–208

Festen C 1982 Post-operative small bowel obstruction in infants and children. Annals of Surgery 196: 580–583

Fraser I 1982 Simple and effective method of removing starch powder from surgical gloves. British Medical Journal 284: 1835

Goldberg E P, Sheets J W, Habal M B 1980 Peritoneal adhesions: Prevention with the use of hydrophobic polymer coatings. Archives of Surgery 115: 776–780

Grosfeld J L, Cooney D R, Csicsko J F 1975 Gastrointestinal tube stent plication in infants and children. Archives of Surgery 110: 594–599

Hollander L F, Otteni F, Klein A 1971 La plicature mésentèrique selon Childs et Phillips. Lyon Chirurgical 67: 24–29

Jackson B T 1983 Sclerosing peritonitis. In: Adhesions — the problems: Royal College of Obstetricians and Gynaecologists Symposium 16th June 1983

James D C O, Ellis H, Hugh T B 1965 The effect of streptokinase on experimental intraperitoneal adhesion formation. Journal of Pathology and Bacteriology 90: 279–281

Johnson H L 1927 Observations on the prevention of post operative peritonitis and abdominal adhesions. Surgery, Gynecology and Obstetrics 45: 612–616

Jones P F, Munro A 1985 Recurrent adhesive small bowel obstruction. World Journal of Surgery 9: 868–875

Kandel G, Prokipchuk E J 1987 Bowel obstruction in "burned out" Crohn's disease. Hospital practice 22: 142–145

Kapur B M L, Gulati S L, Talwar J R 1968 Prevention of peritoneal adhesions by low molecular weight dextran in the monkey. Indian Journal of Medical Research 56: 1406–1409

Krook S S 1947 Obstruction of the small intestine due to adhesions and bands. Acta Chirurgica Scandinavica 95 (suppl 125) 1–200

Kubota T 1922 Peritoneal adhesions. Japan Medical World 11: 226–228

Ladd W E 1937 Congenital duodenal obstruction. Surgery 1: 878–881

Laws H L 1978 Management of small bowel obstruction. American Surgeon 44: 313–317

Ledda P, Shaw J F L, Everett W G 1981 Journal of the Royal College of Surgeons of Edinburgh 26: 348–356

Lefall L D, Syphax B 1970 Clinical aids in strangulation intestinal obstruction. American Journal of Surgery 120: 756–759

Lehman E P, Boyes F 1940 Heparin in the prevention of postoperative adhesions; report of progress. Annals of Surgery 112: 969–973

Le Quesne L P 1976 Acute intestinal obstruction In: Hadfield J G Hobsley M (eds) Current surgical practice. Edward Arnold, London Vol 1, pp 168–176

Lockhart-Mummery H E 1967 Intestinal polyposis: The present position. Proceedings of the Royal Society of Medicine 60: 381–388

Lord J W, Hoews E L, Joliffe N 1949 The surgical management of chronic recurrent small bowel obstruction. Annals of Surgery 129: 315–322

Luttwak E M, Behar A J, Saltz N J 1957 Effect of fibrinolytic agents and corticosteroid hormones on peritoneal adhesions. Archives of Surgery 68: 69–75

McCarthy J D 1975 Further experience with the Child-Phillips plication operation. American Journal of Surgery 130: 15–19

McCarthy J D, Scharf T J 1965 A simple intestinal plication. Surgery Gynecology and Obstetrics 121: 1340–1342

McMillin R D, Bivins B A, Griffen W O 1981 Intra-luminal stenting in the management of recurrent intestinal obstruction. American Surgeon 47: 74–77

Markee R K, Uhlig B E 1971 Baker tube jejunostomy: management of small bowel obstruction. Minnesota Medicine 54: 981–984

Miller E M, Winfield J M 1959 Acute intestinal obstruction secondary to post-operative adhesions. Archives of Surgery 78: 952–957

Miller T G, Abbott W D 1934 Intestinal intubation: Practical technique. American Journal of Medical Science 187: 595–599

Moreaux J, Testart J, Bismuth H, Hepp J 1968 La plicature-fixation du mésentère selon Childs et Phillips. Annales de Chirurgie (Paris) 22: 1939–1943

Myllarniemi H 1967 Foreign material in adhesion formation after abdominal surgery. Acta Chirurgica Scandinavica Suppl 377: 1–48

Nelson R L, Nyhus L M 1979 A new long intestinal tube. Surgery Gynecology and Obstetrics 149: 581–582

Noble T B 1937 Plication of small intestine as prophylaxis against adhesions. American Journal of Surgery 35: 41–44

Papadimitriou J, Marselol A, Kyriaou K, Tountas C 1972

Childs versus Nobel plication. Chirurgica Gastroenterologica 6: 29–34

Perez P A, Breaux S, Bedwinek J M et al 1984 Radiation therapy alone in the treatment of carcinoma of the uterine cervix. Cancer 54: 235–246

Pusateri R, Ross R, Marshall R, Meredith J H, Hamilton R W 1986 Sclerosing encapsulating peritonitis: Report of a case with small bowel obstruction managed by long-term home parental hyperalimentation, and a review of the literature. American Journal of Kidney Diseases 8: 56–60

Raf L E 1969 Causes of abdominal adhesions in cases of intestinal obstruction. Acta Chirurgica Scandinavica 135: 67–72

Ritchie J K 1972 Ulcerative colitis treated by ileostomy and excisional surgery. British Journal of Surgery 59: 345–351

Robbins R D, Hayes S R, Thow G B 1980 Long-tube gastrostomy with internal splinting. Diseases of the Colon and Rectum 23: 10–16

Sanderson 1971 Decompression of small intestine by retrograde intubation. Surgery Gynecology and Obstetrics 132: 1073–1075

Sarr M G, Bulkley G B, Zuidema G D 1982 Preoperative recognition of intestinal strangulation obstruction. American Journal of Surgery 145: 176–182

Savage P T 1960 The management of acute intestinal obstruction; a critical review of 179 personal cases. British Journal of Surgery 47: 643–654

Schofield P F, Holden D, Carr N D 1983 Bowel disease after radiotherapy. Journal of the Royal Society of Medicine 76: 463–466

Seabrook D, Wilson N 1954 Prevention and treatment of intestinal obstruction by use of the Noble procedure. American Journal of Surgery 88: 186–193

Shatila A H, Chamberlain B E, Webb W R 1976 Current status of diagnosis and management of strangulation small bowel obstruction. American Journal of Surgery 132: 299–303

Singleton A O, Rowe E B, Moore W 1952 Failure of reperitonealization to prevent abdominal adhesions in the dog. American Surgeon 18: 7–10

Slavensky E 1969 Developmental anomalies of the duodenal loop. Munksgaard, Copenhagen

Smith D H, DeCosse J J 1986 Radiation damage to the small intestine. World Journal of Surgery 10: 189–194

Somell A 1978 Mesenteric plication in the treatment of adhesive intestinal obstruction. Acta Chirurgica Scandinavica 144: 255–259

Swann R W, Fowler W C, Boronow R C 1976 Surgical management of radiation injury to the small intestine. Surgery Gynecology and Obstetrics 142: 325–327

Taft D A, Lasershom J T, Hill L D 1970 Glove starch granulomatous peritonitis. American Journal of Surgery 120: 231–236

Tanphiphat C, Chittmittrapap S, Prasopsunti K 1987 Adhesive small bowel obstruction. American Journal of Surgery 154: 283–287

Thomeret G 1970 La plicature de l'intestin grêle. Annales de Gastroentérologie et Hépatologie (Paris) 6: 407–411

Thow G B 1972 Long tube gastrostomy with internal intestinal splinting in inflammatory disease of the small intestine. Diseases of the Colon and Rectum 15: 7–10

Warshaw A L 1972 Diagnosis of starch peritonitis by paracentesis. Lancet i: 1054–1056

Weibel M A, Majno G 1973 Peritoneal adhesions and their relation to abdominal surgery. American Journal of Surgery 126: 345–353

Weigelt J A, Snyder W H, Norman J L 1980 Complications and results of 160 Baker tube plications. American Journal of Surgery 140: 810–815

White R R 1956 Prevention of recurrent small bowel obstruction due to adhesions. Annals of Surgery 143: 714–719

Williams D C 1955 The peritoneum: a plea for a change in attitude towards this membrane. British Journal of Surgery 42: 401–404

Wolfson P J, Bauer J J, Gelerent I M, Kreel I, Aufses A H Jr, 1985 Use of the long tube in the management of patients with small-intestinal obstruction due to adhesions. Archives of Surgery 120: 1001–1006

Wright L T, Smith D H, Rothman M, Quosh E T, Metzger W I 1950 Prevention of post operative adhesions in rabbits with streptococcal metabolites. Proceedings of the Society for Experimental Biology and Medicine 75: 602–604

11 Malignant obstruction of the large bowel

A. R. BERRY and N. J. McC. MORTENSEN

Epidemiology

Colorectal cancer is the second most common malignancy in the UK (Waldron et al 1986). Some 22 000 men and women in England and Wales are found to have the condition each year (Office of Population Censuses and Surveys 1981). Around 15% of these will present with intestinal obstruction; reports range from 8 to 29% (Ohman 1982, Umpleby & Williamson 1984, Phillips et al 1985, Stower & Hardcastle 1985). In Aberdeen 48% of colorectal surgical emergency admissions were patients with cancer (Valerio & Jones 1978), and obstruction accounted for 85% of emergencies and 90% of deaths. In the St Mary's Large Bowel Cancer Project (Aldridge et al 1986) the peak age was in the eighth decade. Patients over the age of 70 years are also more likely to be admitted with complications, and intestinal obstruction is the most common reason for emergency admission (Waldron et al 1986).

So not only is intestinal obstruction a common complication of colorectal cancer, but it also carries a high morbidity and mortality compounded by the increasing age of the patients. Emergency colonic surgery in such patients remains one of the greatest challenges to clinical judgement in surgical gastroenterology.

Site of disease

Although the highest incidence of malignant obstructing lesions is in the right colon (Valerio & Jones 1978), the risk of a tumour causing obstruction is greater on the left side (Goligher 1984), 40% compared to 27% on the right. The risk is greatest at the splenic flexure (Aldridge et al 1986, Phillips et al 1985) followed by the left colon and transverse colon (Ohman 1982), where stenosing lesions are most frequently found. All authors agree that tumours of the rectosigmoid area are the least likely to obstruct (Ohman 1982, Goligher 1984, Phillips et al 1985, Aldridge et al 1986). In the Large Bowel Cancer Study (Phillips et al 1985, Aldridge et al 1986) the risk of obstruction at various sites is shown in Table 11.1.

Table 11. 1 The risk of obstruction of colonic tumours (Reproduced, with permission, from Phillips et al 1985)

Site	No. at risk	No. obstructed	Risk of obstruction
Right colon	1099	242	22%
Splenic flexure	164	80	49%
Left colon	1020	236	23%
Rectosigmoid	2009	128	6%

Waldron et al (1986) demonstrated that the number of so-called Dukes' 'D' cases presenting electively was significantly less than those presenting as emergencies (Table 11.2). The majority of patients have Dukes' B or C lesions (Phillips et al 1985, White & Macfie 1985, Waldron et al 1986), but the most favourable Dukes' A tumours rarely present with obstruction. An appreciable proportion of patients presenting with malignant large bowel obstruction will have disseminated disease. In a recent study from Leeds 23% (8/35) had disseminated disease, seven with hepatic metastases and one with an omental metastasis (White and Macfie 1985), and in the Large Bowel Cancer

Table 11.2 The distribution of Dukes' staging: emergency compared with elective presentation (from Waldron et al 1986)

Group	Dukes' stage A	B/C	D	Unknown	Total
Emergency	2(0.2%)	347(33.6%)	154(14.9%)	20(1.9%)	523(50.6%)
Elective	12(1.2%)	377(36.5%)	92(8.9%)	29(2.8%)	510(49.4%)
			$p < 0.05$		1033(100%)

Project 27% (193/713) were due to Dukes' D lesions (Phillips et al 1985).

Perhaps surprisingly, unfavourable histological grading or the presence of vascular invasion do not seem to be associated with an increased risk of obstruction (Phillips et al 1985, Umpleby & Williamson 1984).

Presentation

The earliest symptoms of large bowel obstruction are a change in bowel habit, usually with increasing constipation, and abdominal distension. Initially these symptoms may not cause concern. Even suprapubic large bowel colic may be tolerated in the early stages before the patient contacts the general practitioner. Eventually however, as the constipation becomes absolute even for gas, the pain becomes more severe and the abdomen tensely distended. The patient may then experience vomiting and seek medical help. It is often two or three days before the patient is admitted to hospital.

Patients with obstructing tumours of the right colon, however, will present more acutely, with a short history of severe central crampy abdominal pain and profuse vomiting — the typical features of small bowel obstruction. Apart from external hernias, carcinoma of the right side of the colon is the commonest cause of small bowel obstruction in patients who have not undergone previous surgery.

By the time patients with colonic obstruction reach hospital, they are likely to be dehydrated because of diminished intake and fluid sequestration in the dilated loops of bowel. There will be some degree of abdominal distension: in the extreme the abdomen will be tensely tympanitic. Tenderness over the right side of the abdomen indicates that the caecum is taking the brunt of the obstruction in the presence of a competent ileocaecal valve. It is at this site that the colon will most commonly tear and rupture when obstructed and distended.

In 18% (22/124) of patients in one reported series (Umpleby & Williamson, 1984), the obstruction was complicated by perforation. In five patients, this was localized, and in 17, it caused generalized peritonitis. Perforation was twice as likely to complicate an obstructing tumour of the left colon. Such patients are gravely ill with systemic signs of sepsis and peritonitis, and not surprisingly, they had twice the hospital mortality rate of non-perforated cases (52% compared to 26%). Five-year survival rates were similar, however, indicating that those who survive the acute event may do better in the long run.

Investigations and diagnosis

The most useful investigation is a plain abdominal radiograph. This may show colonic distension and caecal dilatation if the ileo-caecal valve remains competent (Fig. 11.1), or small bowel dilatation with fluid levels in a right-sided colonic lesion if the ileocaecal valve is incompetent (Fig. 11.2). If perforation has occurred, free intraperitoneal gas may be visible either on an erect chest radiograph or on the abdominal film (Figs. 11.3, 11.4).

The clinical presentation and plain abdominal X-ray alone are usually sufficient to make an accurate diagnosis. The definitive investigation, however, is a barium enema examination, which will accurately demonstrate the site of the lesion (Fig. 11.5). The use of barium or a water-soluble contrast material such as gastrografin is particularly helpful in identifying those patients suffering from pseudo-obstruction of the colon, a condition with which we are becoming increasingly familiar

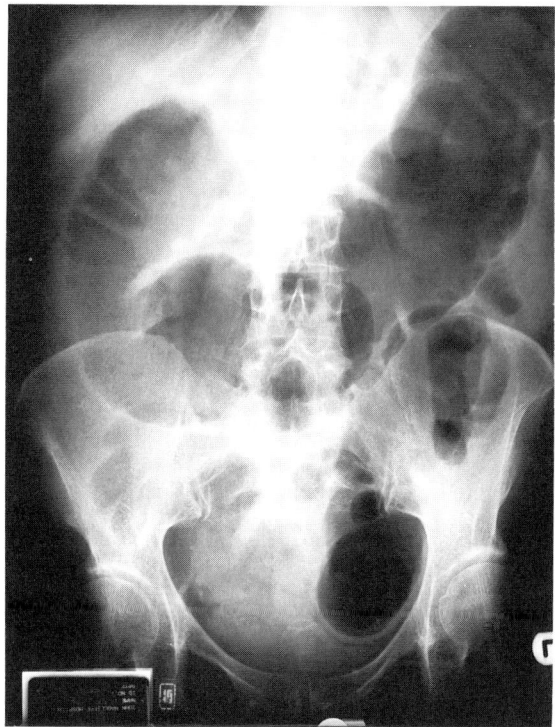

Fig. 11.1 Plain abdominal X-ray. Colonic obstruction due to a carcinoma of the descending colon with dilatation and caecal distension.

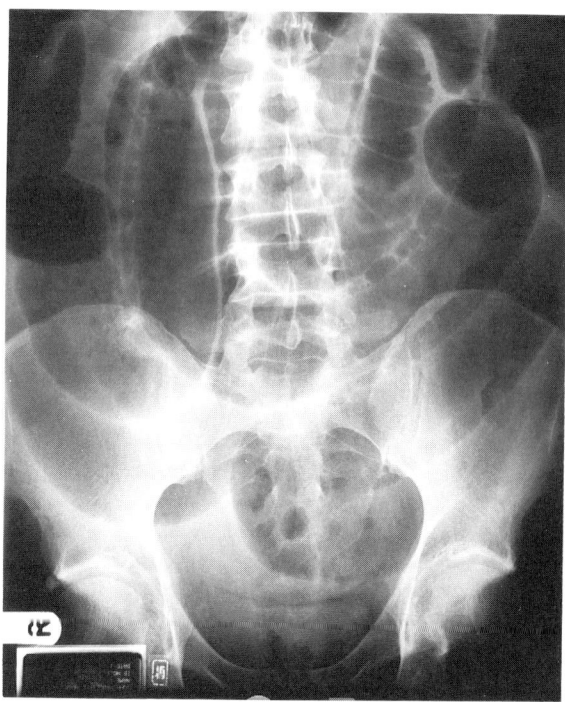

Fig. 11.2 An abdominal film showing small bowel dilatation due to a caecal carcinoma.

(Dudley & Paterson-Brown 1986). This may also be an instance where emergency colonoscopy is helpful in diagnosis and in deflating the dilated colon (Munro & Youngston 1983).

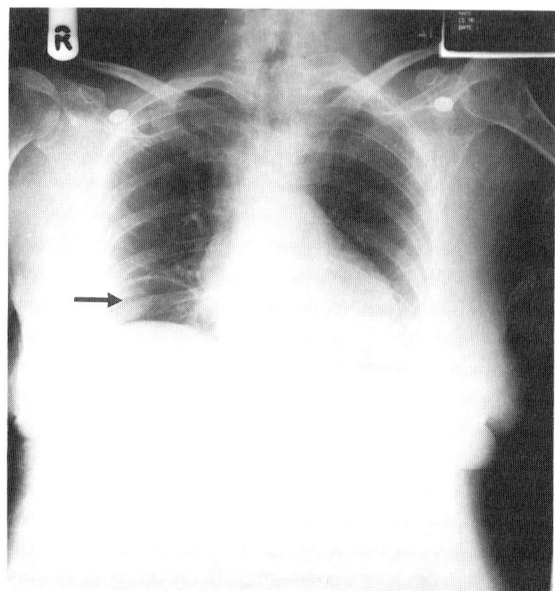

Fig. 11.3 Erect chest X-ray. Free gas in a patient with colonic perforation secondary to an obstructing splenic flexure carcinoma.

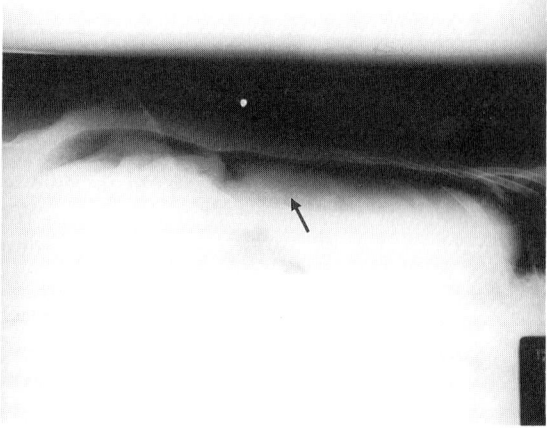

Fig. 11.4 Abdominal film (decubitus) showing free gas in a patient with colonic perforation.

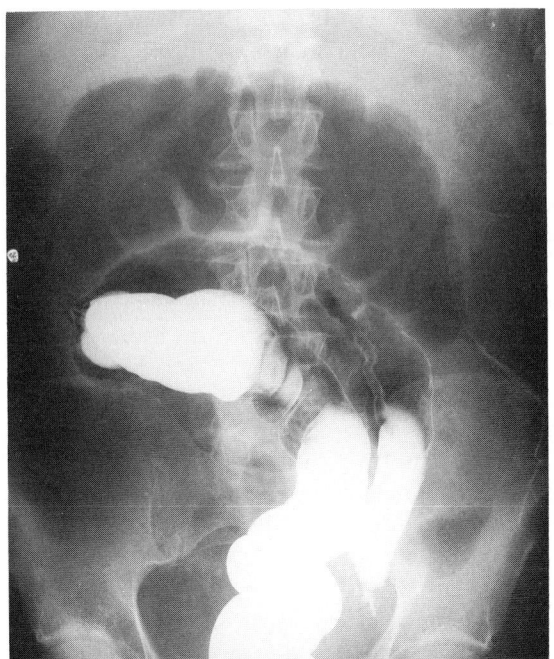

Fig. 11.5 Radiograph after barium enema showing an obstructing carcinoma of the descending colon.

Treatment

Preoperative preparation

Standard principles apply to the emergency management of patients admitted with malignant large bowel obstruction. Prior to surgery, dehydration and electrolyte imbalance should be corrected by intravenous fluids. Nasogastric aspiration will help vomiting, may partially decompress distended bowel and will certainly empty the stomach before general anaesthesia is induced. Preoperative bowel preparation is usually not feasible.

It was established more than a decade ago that prophylactic antibiotics will reduce postoperative septic complications such as wound infection (Evans & Pollock 1973), and these are known to be more frequent following emergency than elective colorectal surgery (Krukowski et al 1984). We give 750 mg cefuroxime and 500 mg metronidazole on induction of anaesthesia and continue this for two days postoperatively. In our

experience a long midline incision will give adequate access in all cases.

Right-sided colonic obstruction

It is generally accepted that lesions in the right side of the colon should be managed by a single operation with resection of the caecum and right colon. An end-to-end anastomosis between terminal ileum and transverse colon is performed in two layers, using continuous absorbable sutures such as surgical catgut, or one of the newer synthetic absorbable materials. Such an anastomosis (Fig. 11.6) involving the well-vascularized small bowel will heal readily (Koruth et al 1985a, Phillips et al 1985).

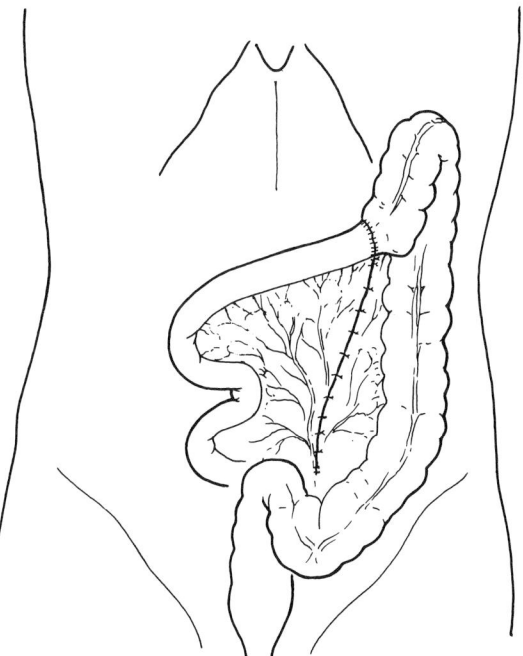

Fig. 11.6 Ileotransverse anastomosis following emergency extended right hemicolectomy for an obstructing carcinoma of the transverse colon.

Left-sided colonic obstruction

There is considerably more debate about the correct surgical treatment of obstructing tumours of the left side of the colon. The results of anastomosing unprepared, probably dilated, obstructed proximal colon to distal colon are poor, with a high incidence of anastomotic dehiscence. Surgeons have wisely preached against the single procedure (Smith et al 1983, Irvin & Goligher 1973), and traditionally a staged resection has been recommended. In a three-stage procedure, the first stage involved raising a proximal defunctioning loop colostomy to relieve obstruction. When the patient recovered, the second stage — consisting of resection of the tumour and anastomosis — was performed. About six weeks later the loop colostomy was closed in the third and final stage. This staged approach was intended to reduce mortality and morbidity, though it is poorly tolerated by some and leads to a prolonged hospital stay (Irvin & Greaney 1977). Most surgeons would now perform an immediate resection by combining the first two operations in a two-stage procedure (Fielding et al 1979). Obstructing carcinomas of the descending and sigmoid colons can be treated by Hartmann's procedure, in which the sigmoid and/or descending colon is resected in the standard radical manner with good tumour and node clearance. After mobilizing the splenic flexure, the proximal bowel is used to form a left iliac fossa colostomy, and the rectal stump is oversewn. An alternative is to bring the upper end of the rectum to the surface, at the lower end of the wound or alongside the colostomy, as a mucous fistula (Fig. 11.7). This manoeuvre may facilitate the second stage of reanastomosis, some six weeks later. This anastomosis should be made with a single layer of interrupted sutures. We prefer to use a synthetic absorbable material or the end-to-end anastomotic stapling gun. The two-stage procedure allows the bowel to be prepared before the anastomosis is fashioned, but even then recent studies have suggested that a disappointingly low proportion of patients successfully have their colostomy closed and reanastomosed: only 61% according to Koruth et al (1985b). This low rate reflects the poor health of many of the elderly patients who present with malignant large bowel obstruction, and the often advanced nature of the disease. For this reason, recent treatment has been aimed at achieving a safe single-stage resection, which can be done in one of two ways.

It is reasonable to perform an extended right hemicolectomy for obstructing lesions around to the splenic flexure or descending colon. The terminal ileum can be anastomosed safely to the proximal sigmoid colon. This technique results in increased frequency of bowel movement and occasionally diarrhoea, but it may be acceptable in preference to a staged procedure in an elderly patient who is a poor operative risk and may have a limited prognosis (Deutsch et al 1983). The procedure can also be lifesaving in those patients with the rare but lethal complication of necrotizing colitis proximal to the obstructing neoplasm (Teasdale & Mortensen 1983).

The second method involves meticulous intraoperative colonic 'cleaning' before anastomosis (White & Macfie 1985). The technique of on-table antegrade colonic lavage to clean unprepared bowel and allow primary anastomosis was described by Radcliffe & Dudley (1983). We have found this method useful in a number of cases (Fig. 11.8), and irrigate with normal saline through a large Foley catheter inserted into the caecum, usually through the base of the appendix

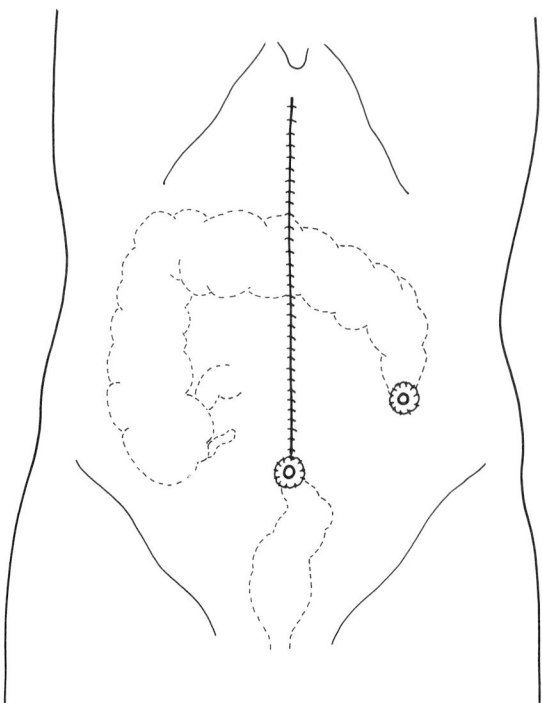

Fig. 11.7 Primary resection with colostomy and mucous fistula.

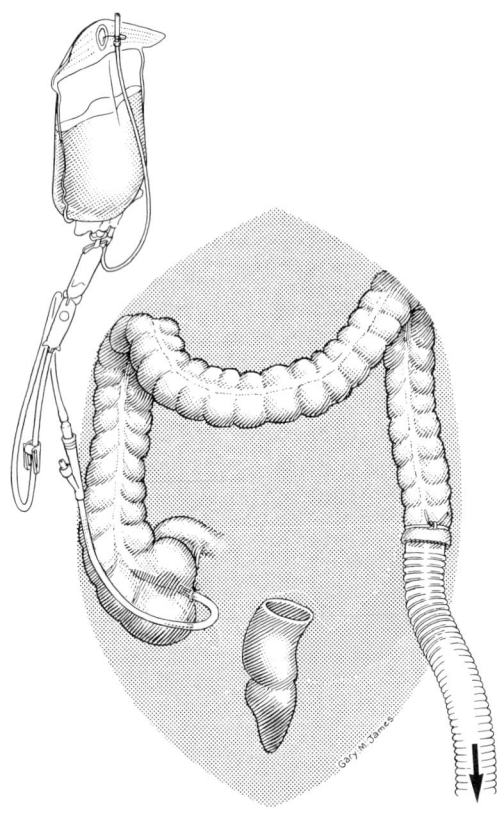

Fig. 11.8 On-table antegrade colonic lavage.

(Klatt et al 1981), though Hughes et al (1985) emphasized the technically demanding nature of the operation.

Results

The results of treatment for malignant obstruction of the colon are generally disappointing in both operative mortality rate and long-term survival. Compared with surgery for non-obstructing tumours, patients have a higher mortality rate (37.7% compared to 11.9%), a higher incidence of lymph node metastases and a lower 5-year survival (22.9% compared to 41.5%, Irvin & Greaney 1977). In an extensive 30-year study from the Karolinska Hospital Stockholm, Ohman (1982) reported only a 16% 5-year survival in patients undergoing surgery for malignant colonic obstruction. In common with other authors (Bulow 1980, Dutton et al 1976, Irvin & Greaney 1977), he found that the prognosis is consistently worse than for patients with non-obstructing colonic tumours. In patients in the Karolinska study undergoing curative resections the overall 5-year survival was 31%, and it was better after staged procedures (35%) than after primary resection (19%).

Various factors have been shown to influence ultimate survival, namely: primary as opposed to delayed resection, the experience of the surgeon, the site of obstruction (Fielding et al 1979) and the presence of coincidental perforation, which is detrimental (Irvin & Greaney 1977).

Umpleby & Williamson (1984) reported an overall mortality rate of 31%, with similar mortality rates for colostomy with delayed resection, resection with colostomy and resection with anastomosis. Koruth et al (1985a), however, reported a reduced mortality of 8.3% (4/48) in patients who underwent primary resection, with or without anastomosis, compared to their 17.2% overall mortality. They also pointed out that primary resection markedly reduced the time spent in hospital. The opposite was reported by Ohman (1982), who described a mortality of 14% for primary resection compared to 5% for staged resection, with a creditable overall mortality of 8%.

Hartmann's procedure is often performed for obstructing left-sided tumours, particularly those

after its removal. The effluent is collected via sterilized corrugated anaesthetic tubing tied into the proximal end of the colon following transection and draining into a closed polythene bag or bucket; the irrigation is continued until the bowel is clean. Following this procedure it is possible to perform a primary anastomosis. Koruth et al (1985b) reported an acceptable 8.5% mortality rate and 8.5% clinical anastomotic leak rate in 47 patients, most of whom had malignant colonic obstruction treated in this way.

The technique is not always practicable however; it adds almost an hour to the length of the procedure (Koruth et al 1985b) and may still not allow anastomosis if the proximal bowel is grossly dilated with dubious viability or in the presence of severe sepsis. An expedient extended right hemicolectomy or subtotal colectomy may be a more suitable procedure in poor risk patients in the distal sigmoid, with a view to reanastomos-ing the bowel at a later date. In fact in one study only 59% of those patients who survived the operation successfully completed the second stage (Koruth et al 1985a), the others retaining their colostomy indefinitely.

Welch & Donaldson (1974), in a ten-year review of experience at the Massachusetts General Hospi-tal, strongly criticized the practice of primary resection, particularly for left-sided lesions which carried a 60% mortality rate, whereas they had a very low (2%) mortality when initial colostomy was followed by later resection. Their overall mor-tality rate was 15%. Fielding also emphasized the high mortality associated with left-sided lesions, but these results were before the days of on-table lavage and prophylactic antibiotics.

It is clear from these conflicting reports from a variety of authors that the safety of primary resec-tion with or without immediate anastomosis in the left colon has not been completely established. Much still depends upon the experience of the sur-geon, the condition of the patient and the severity of obstruction. The problem will only be resolved by prospective studies involving larger numbers of patients. In particular the place of on-table an-tegrade colonic lavage deserves careful scrutiny. Looking further into the future, there are un-published reports from Germany on the use of colonoscopic laser therapy for obstructing car-cinomas. A channel through the lesion is vaporized with the laser, relieving the obstruc-tion. The patient is then prepared for elective surgery in the usual way. Twenty-three such pro-cedures have been carried out with only two perforations. In due course endoscopic manage-ment may have a role, particularly in elderly patients.

It also remains to be seen whether, as a result of earlier symptomatic diagnosis and population screening with occult blood tests, the incidence of malignant large bowel obstruction can be reduced and the morbidity and mortality from this serious complication improved.

REFERENCES

Aldridge M C, Phillips R K S, Hittinger R, Fry J S, Fielding L P 1986 Influence of tumour site on presentation, management and subsequent outcome in large bowel cancer. British Journal of Surgery 73: 663–670

Bulow S 1980 Colorectal cancer in patients less than 40 years of age in Denmark, 1943–1967. Diseases of the Colon and Rectum 23: 327–336

Deutsch A A, Zelikovski A, Sternberg A, Reiss R 1983 One stage subtotal colectomy with anastomosis for obstructing carcinoma of the left colon. Diseases of the Colon and Rectum 26: 227–230

Dudley H A F, Paterson-Brown S 1986 Pseudo obstruction. British Medical Journal 292: 1157–1158

Dutton J W, Hreno A, Hampson L G 1976 Mortality and prognosis of obstructing carcinoma of the large bowel. American Journal of Surgery 131: 36–41

Evans C, Pollock A V 1973 The reduction of surgical wound infection by prophylactic parenteral cephaloridine. British Journal of Surgery 60: 434–437

Fielding L P, Stewart-Brown S, Blesovsky L 1979 Large bowel obstruction caused by cancer: a prospective study. British Medical Journal ii: 515–517

Goligher J C 1984 Surgery of anus, rectum and colon, 5th ed. Ballière Tindall, London, pp 436, 479

Hughes E S R, McDermott F T, Polglase A L, Nottle P 1985 Total and Subtotal colectomy for colonic obstruction. Disease of the Colon and Rectum 28: 162–163

Irvin T T, Goligher J C 1973 Aetiology of disruption of intestinal anastomosis. British Journal of Surgery 60: 461–464

Irvin T T, Greaney M G 1977 The treatment of colonic cancer presenting with intestinal obstruction. British Journal of Surgery 64: 741–744

Klatt G R, Martin W H M, Gillespie J T 1981 Subtotal colectomy with primary anastomosis without diversion in the treatment of obstructing carcinoma of the left colon. American Journal of Surgery 141: 577–578

Koruth N M, Hunter D C, Krukowski Z H, Matheson N A 1985a Immediate resection in emergency large bowel surgery: a 7 year audit. British Journal of Surgery 72: 703–707

Koruth N M, Krukowski Z H, Youngson G G et al 1985b Intra-operative colonic irrigation in the management of left-sided large bowel emergencies. British Journal of Surgery 72: 708–711

Krukowski Z H, Stewart P M P, Alsayer H M, Matheson N A 1984 Infection after abdominal surgery: 5 year prospective study. British Medical Journal 288: 1, 278–280

Munro A, Youngston G G 1983 Colonoscopy in the diagnosis and treatment of colonic pseudo-obstruction. Journal of the Royal College of Surgeons of Edinburgh 28: 391–393

Office of Population Censuses and Surveys 1981 Cancer research campaign: Cancer statistics. Incidence, survival and mortality in England and Wales. Studies on medical and population subjects no 43. HMSO, London pp vii, xii, 22–29

Ohman U 1982 Prognosis in patients with obstructing colorectal carcinoma. American Journal of Surgery 143: 742–747

Phillips R K S, Hittinger R, Fry J S, Fielding L P 1985 Malignant large bowel obstruction. British Journal of Surgery 72: 296–302

Radcliffe A G, Dudley H A F 1983 Intra-operative antegrade irrigation of the large intestine. Surgery Gynecology and Obstetrics 156: 721–723

Smith S R G, Connolly J C, Gilmore O J A 1983 The effect of loading on colonic anastomotic healing. British Journal of Surgery 70: 49–50

Stower M J, Hardcastle J D 1985 The results of 1115 patients with colrectal cancer treated over a 8 year period in a single hospital. European Journal of Surgical Oncology (London) 11: 119–123

Teasdale C, Mortensen N J McC 1983 Acute necrotizing colitis and obstruction. British Journal of Surgery 70: 44–47

Umpleby H C, Williamson R C N 1984 Survival in acute obstructing colorectal carcinoma. Diseases of the Colon and Rectum 27: 299–304

Valerio D, Jones P F 1978 Immediate resection in the treatment of large bowel emergencies. British Journal of Surgery 65: 712–716

Waldron R P, Donovan I A, Drumm J, Mottram S N, Tedman S 1986 Emergency presentation and mortality from colorectal cancer in the elderly. British Journal of Surgery 73: 214–216

Welch J P, Donaldson G A 1974 Management of severe obstruction of the large bowel due to malignant disease. American Journal of Surgery 127: 492–499

White C M, Macfie J 1985 Immediate colectomy and primary anastomosis for acute obstruction due to carcinoma of the left colon and rectum. Diseases of the Colon and Rectum 28: 155–157

12 *Colonic pseudo-obstruction*

S. PATERSON-BROWN and H. A. F. DUDLEY

Most surgeons will have encountered patients who present with features suggestive of acute large bowel obstruction but who, at operation, have no demonstrable mechanical cause. Until fairly recently (say the '40s or '50s) this occurrence, recognized since the end of the 19th century, was accepted as an inevitable diagnostic error. Such complacency is now unjustified. These patients, in whom obstruction is undoubtably present but whose problem is not amenable to surgery, do badly after an exploratory laparotomy for at least two reasons: first because they are often ill from an underlying cause such as hypoxia (the result for example of pneumonia), blood loss or immobilization, consequent upon an orthopaedic procedure such as pinning a fractured neck of femur or replacing a hip; second, because with the abdomen open, and no evident cause, the surgeon may make the wrong decision and so precipitate disaster.

History

In 1896 J B Murphy of Chicago operated upon a patient with clinical intestinal obstruction and chronic lead poisoning in whom he did not discover a mechanical cause. He noted a 'spastic' segment of colon for which he then coined the term 'spastic ileus' (Murphy 1896). Similar observations were reported by others in the early decades of the twentieth century (Zimmerman 1930, Wangensteen 1937), but it was not until 1948 that Ogilvie identified one definite cause for this 'functional' obstruction, when he described it

in two patients with retroperitoneal infiltration by malignant disease (Ogilvie 1948).

The more general term 'pseudo-obstruction' was not introduced until 10 years later when one of us, with his Edinburgh surgical colleagues, described a group of patients who presented in medical, surgical or orthopaedic wards with appearances resembling acute mechanical obstruction, usually but not always of the large bowel, and in whom a mechanical cause was not found (Dudley et al 1958). The patients in this series were diagnosed only at operation, and because spastic segments of intestine could not be demonstrated the term 'spastic ileus' was considered inappropriate and was replaced by 'pseudo-obstruction'. Before this time other causes of this clinical entity, which included Ogilvie's syndrome, had been reported (McFarlane & Kay 1949, Dunlop 1949, Handley 1949).

Since then interest in pseudo-obstruction has been widespread, with many case reports and reviews published in both the surgical and medical literature. Other causes have been identified and the mechanisms of their effect discussed.

Definition

We must make it clear that though we introduced the term 'pseudo-obstruction' we should have been more precise and said 'pseudo-mechanical obstruction'. These patients are functionally obstructed — as are those with neuropathy and chronic obstruction — but they do not have a surgically remediable cause.

Etymologically, the word 'syndrome' means a

'running together' and in modern parlance this implies 'many causes'. That the term 'pseudo-obstruction' is applied to a syndrome therefore implies that what is observed clinically may have diverse antecedents. We consider here only that subgroup of patients who present acutely with features suggestive of established or imminent large bowel obstruction. There is a further group of patients (usually with neuropathy elsewhere in the body) who have either chronic symptoms of gastrointestinal malpropulsion or, rarely, episodic acute features (Hohl & Nixon 1965, *British Medical Journal* 1973, Bogomoletz et al 1979, *Lancet* 1979). Though the term 'pseudo-obstruction' is increasingly applied to this subgroup we think it would be more appropriate to use 'enteroneuropathic obstruction' for them.

Pathophysiology

Debate on cause has centred around on the one hand inferences from the clinical circumstances and on the other hand what is known of the intrinsic and nervous control of intestinal propulsion. As to the first, systemic factors that could affect neural and smooth muscle function — lead levels (Wanebo et al 1971), hypoxia (Dudley et al 1958), hypovolaemia (Bardsley 1974) and renal impairment (Stephens 1962) — are well-known to be associated with the syndrome. As to the second, Catchpole's work on the relative importance of parasympathetic versus sympathetic supply to the colon is relevant. He showed that in the cat, colonic motility was inhibited by activity of the sympathetic nervous system, and in comparison with the small bowel the intrinsic parasympathetic drive only played a minor role in instigating contraction (Neely & Catchpole 1967). In addition, the circular muscle and taenia coli of the colon were highly sensitive to catecholamines and the sympathetic inhibition was mediated mainly through β-adrenergic receptors. Further investigation showed that guanethidine — a catecholamine antagonist — largely abolishes postoperative ileus in an experimental model (Smith et al 1965). Though no controlled trials have been carried out, guanethidine appears useful in idiopathic (i.e. without such identifiable causes as intraperitoneal sepsis) postoperative ileus in man (Catchpole 1969). It is debatable if there is a relationship between such ileus and pseudo-obstruction, though Wilson's radiological observations on the colon in ileus support the view that it is this part of the intestine that is chiefly involved (Wilson 1975). We may tentatively conclude that the main disorder in the functionally obstructed large bowel seen in pseudo-obstruction is an imbalance between perhaps excessive sympathetic inhibitory influence on the one hand and perhaps decreased stimulatory effect of the parasympathetic nervous system on the other hand.

The fact that in pseudo-obstruction the transition from dilated to collapsed bowel most commonly occurs in the region of the splenic flexure or sigmoid colon has led some authors to postulate that the primary lesion is one of 'kinking' between mobile and fixed bowel (Byrne 1960). We discount this on the basis that it is extraordinarily difficult to cause large bowel obstruction by extrinsic compression without infiltration. An alternative explanation for the appearance of the transition zone, which integrates with the concept of parasympathetic–sympathetic imbalance, is decreased parasympathetic activity (as opposed to sympathetic overactivity) to that region of colon (Bachulis & Smith 1978). This area of bowel is where the transition from vagal to sacral parasympathetic innervation occurs. In spite of the fact that parasympathetic influence on motility in the distal colon is said to be minimal, it is known to be responsible for the mass contraction which occurs in the descending colon and rectum during defaecation. With the exception of a stimulatory action on the internal sphincter, the sympathetic nervous system takes no part in these reflexes (Koizumi & Brooks 1980).

All this would suggest that disruption of parasympathetic activity, particularly from the sacral outflow, could be the primary disorder, rather than sympathetic overactivity, so explaining the relatively high proportion of patients who develop pseudo-obstruction following pelvic trauma (Bachulis & Smith 1978). In addition, the similarity of the syndrome in the adult to Hirschsprung's disease may also imply sacral parasympathetic involvement.

The malignant infiltration of the retro-peritoneum which results in 'spastic ileus', as described by Ogilvie, was considered by him to result from disruption to the sympathetic outflow from the coeliac plexus. Although this would explain a contracted gut, it would not automatically produce the dilated colon commonly seen in pseudo-obstruction. An alternative explanation is excessive stimulation of the sympathetic outflow resulting from the the close proximity of the tumour or disruption to the parasympathetic nerves, either in the same region or from a more widespread disease involving the pelvis. Unfortunately Ogilvie does not mention whether pelvic disease was present in either of his cases.

It is of interest to observe that elevated prosta-glandin-E levels have been recorded in a patient with idiopathic pseudo-obstruction primarily of the small bowel, with resolution following a return to normal levels (Luderer et al 1977). The effect of prostaglandins on colonic contractions in the dog is contradictory, but, in man, administration of prostaglandin-E leads to vomiting, watery diarrhoea and abdominal cramps (Lee 1981), suggesting increased rather than decreased motility. Markedly elevated levels of prostaglandin E_2, A_1, $F_{1,2\alpha}$ and B_1 have however been reported in a patient with alcoholic liver disease who developed pseudo-obstruction, which again resolved when the levels returned to normal (Chousterman et al 1977). This relationship between alcoholism and pseudo-obstruction has been noted by others (Wanebo et al 1971, Norton et al 1974, Karani et al 1979).

Causes

Because the principal pathophysiological mechanism leading to the clinical syndrome of pseudo-obstruction involves an abnormality in neurological influences on either extrinsic or intrinsic intestinal activity, the main causes can be divided into three groups:

1. Idiopathic pseudo-obstruction — where there appears to be no precipitating factor

and all other measurements are normal;
2. Pseudo-obstruction secondary to systemic disorders;
3. Pseudo-obstruction secondary to local disorders affecting either the extrinsic or intrinsic nerve supply of the intestine.

We have listed these causes in Table 12.1.

Table 12.1 Causes of colonic pseudo-obstruction

Idiopathic		
Systemic disease	Cardiac disease	
	Renal disease and uraemia	
	Hypovolaemia	
	Hypoxia	
	Alcoholic liver disease	
	Burns	
	Lead poisoning	
	Electrolyte abnormalities	
	Puerperium	
	Myxoedema	
	Acute stress (burns)	
	Drugs (psychotrophic agents and bronchodilators)	
Local disease		
Affecting the extrinsic plexuses	Retroperitoneal injuries	Vertebral fractures
		Spinal surgery
		Endoscopic sphincterotomy
	Retroperitoneal disease	Haematoma
		Malignant infiltration
		Acute pancreatitis
	Pelvic injuries and surgery	
	Intra-abdominal inflammation and sepsis	
Affecting the intrinsic plexuses	Strongyloidiasis	
	Amyloidosis	
	Scleroderma	
	Radiation	

Idiopathic

As understanding of the syndrome increases, the first 'cause' is more and more rare.

Systemic causes

Why the visceral nerves should be affected by systemic disorders while other autonomic fibres are spared remains obscure. However in any major illness there is increased sympathetic activity and this may be a factor in the development of pseudo-obstruction (Addison 1983); observations of pseudo-obstruction in thermally injured patients would support this concept (Lescher et al 1978). It is not surprising, therefore, that pseudo-obstruction has been observed in patients taking sympathomimetic agents such as salbutamol (Catchpole 1986).

Elderly patients are especially susceptible to pseudo-obstruction following episodes of hypoxia, electrolyte abnormalities (particularly hypokalaemia) and uraemia that follow pre-existing cardiorespiratory and renal disease. This group is also at risk because of the high rate of hospital admissions for hip surgery and spinal injuries (Bullock & Thomas 1984). The mechanism behind the functional obstruction seen in these patients is not fully understood, but because hypoxia and electrolyte abnormalities affect neuromuscular activity in cardiac smooth muscle, so producing arrhythmias, perhaps the gut is affected in a similar fashion. In addition, intracellular loss of potassium leads to generalized muscle weakness and depression of intestinal propulsive activity (Streeten & Vaughan Williams 1952), and hypokalaemia has been found in patients with pseudo-obstruction (Stephens 1962, Rothwell-Jackson 1963, Wanebo et al 1971, Bullock & Thomas 1984). One of our patients survived two episodes of pseudo-obstruction resulting from diuretic-induced hypokalaemia for which caecal decompression was required for patchy gangrene.

Pseudo-obstruction has been reported in connection with myxoedema (Hohl & Nixon 1965) because these patients often suffer from intestinal atony and hypomotility, probably from a disturbance of neuromuscular function. Haley reported a patient with intestinal obstruction and myxoedema who survived three exploratory laparotomies in the space of one week (Haley et al 1962) and whose hypothyroidism was not recognized for a further 9 weeks.

The syndrome may also occur as the consequence of the local effects of a systemic disease. Infiltration of the bowel wall from amyloidosis (Legge et al 1970) and systemic sclerosis (Peachey et al 1969) or damage to it from radiation (Perino et al 1986) have also resulted in the clinical features of pseudo-obstruction, presumably from a direct effect on the intrinsic myenteric plexuses of Meissner and Auerbach. Pseudo-obstruction has also been observed in patients with strongyloidosis (Spencer 1986, personal communication). In a review of the syndrome from 1948 to 1980 Nanni et al (1982) identified seven patients who had developed pseudo-obstruction in association with a normal pregnancy or delivery.

Local effects

It is much easier to understand the mechanism of pseudo-obstruction following retroperitoneal injuries and disease in which there is a local disorder affecting the parasympathetic and sympathetic outflow.

Pseudo-obstruction can complicate pelvic surgery and injury, in particular hysterectomy and Caesarian section, pelvic fractures and hip surgery (Bachulis & Smith 1978). In addition it may occur after spinal surgery, fractured vertebrae (Bullock & Thomas 1984) and other causes of retroperitoneal effusion (including Ogilvie's syndrome) and occasionally acute pancreatitis in the presence of severe retroperitoneal inflammation and necrosis (Adams 1974). In regard to the latter, in the last few years we have treated two patients with acute intestinal pseudo-obstruction associated with severe acute pancreatitis. In the first the pseudo-obstruction was the presenting problem, and in the second it followed endoscopic retrograde choledochopancreatography (ERCP) and sphincterotomy which had been complicated by acute pancreatitis and possibly a small retroduodenal perforation. However, caution must be observed in ascribing colonic distension in severe acute pancreatitis to pseudo-obstruction only, because our experience suggests that colonic blood supply is not infrequently imperilled (Aldridge et al 1987). Intra-abdominal sepsis is known to decrease intestinal motility (Aird 1957), and pseudo-obstruction has been observed in patients with acute inflammatory conditions such as acute cholecystitis (Caves & Crockard 1970, Addison 1983). Systemic disturbances can often compound these local factors, but many are associated with pseudo-obstruction in their own right.

Incidence

As a result of misdiagnosis and under-recognition, the incidence of pseudo-obstruction can only be a guess. However it would appear from two recent studies which examined the role of contrast enemas in the diagnosis and management of large bowel obstruction (Stewart et al 1984, Koruth et al 1985) that the condition is more common than generally thought: 25–31% of all patients admitted to a major hospital with the diagnosis of suspected acute large bowel obstruction were ultimately found to have the condition. The peak incidence occurs in the over-60 age group without predisposition for either sex (Addison 1983).

Our own clinical experience is that the condition is still under-appreciated (Dudley & Paterson-Brown 1986). Too many patients undergo a laparotomy because large bowel obstruction is suspected and the surgeon fears an error of omission. We enter here a plea for more careful evaluation and more precise decision-making in patients with suspected large bowel obstruction.

Clinical picture

The syndrome has many characteristic features which help to raise suspicion of its presence in patients with intestinal obstruction. The context is most helpful. The patients, often elderly, may present on a medical or orthopaedic service where they have been admitted with other disease or an injury such as a fractured hip or pelvis, and the emergency surgeon is usually called once the syndrome has become established. A high index of suspicion and an accurate diagnosis allow appropriate measures to be instituted, and operation is seldom required. Frequently those presenting on

the orthopaedic service have nitrogen retention, often as a result of concomitant renal and cardiac disease. The same may be true for direct admissions to the surgical service when an elderly patient has become ill at home, say with pneumonia, and has been unable to sustain an adequate water intake. Alternatively the patient may be a woman who has undergone recent pelvic surgery such as hysterectomy or is in the puerperium after Caesarian section. Abdominal pain is not necessarily a feature (Adams 1974, Bardsley 1974) until perforation becomes imminent and even then may not be elicited. The abdomen distends gradually, becomes tympanitic and the passage of both faeces and flatus diminishes. Bowel sounds — which originate in the small bowel (Baker & Dudley 1961) — can usually be heard, often becoming high-pitched as the small bowel works normally to expel its contents into an increasingly distended caecum. Some generalized but mild tenderness is common. Tenderness and guarding localized to the RIF should be regarded with great suspicion, particularly if the caecum is found to be grossly dilated on subsequent X-ray. Radiographs of the abdomen reveal diffuse gaseous distension, predominantly of the large intestine, compatible with obstruction, and a left-sided cut-off point may be seen in the region of the splenic flexure or sigmoid colon (Adams 1974). Occasionally however the presence of small amounts of gas in the rectum (Adams 1974, Addison 1983) provides a clue that the obstruction is incomplete (Figs. 12.1, 12.2).

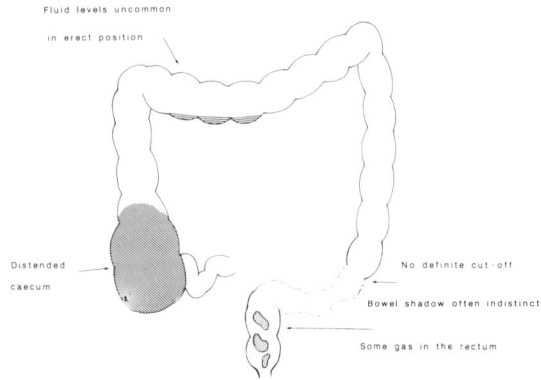

Fig. 12.1 Diagram illustrating the radiological features of pseudo-obstruction.

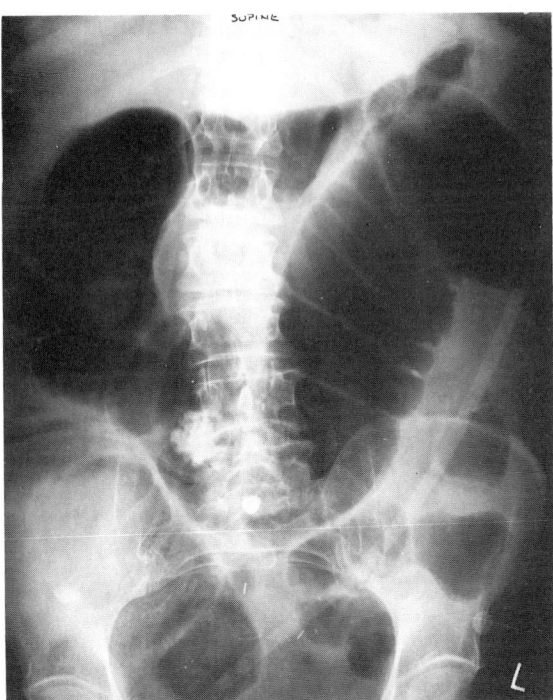

Fig. 12.2 Plain abdominal radiograph of a patient with acute colonic pseudo-obstruction. Note distension of the caecum and transverse colon, with gas present most of the way round to the rectum.

Diagnosis

Following detailed clinical examination and the use of plain radiology in a patient with suspected large bowel obstruction, the diagnosis of either mechanical or pseudo-obstruction can only be tentative. Rigid or flexible sigmoidoscopy will resolve the issue in a small number of patients with low left-sided lesions but it is, as every clinician knows, often difficult to carry out a satisfactory examination in such circumstances. Insufflation of large quantities of air may also confuse subsequent radiological investigation. Confirmation must therefore be sought by further investigation of the colon by a contrast enema. Two studies (Stewart et al 1984, Koruth et al 1985) have demonstrated the value of performing such a study in *all* patients with suspected large bowel obstruction. In addition to revealing pseudo-obstruction in 16% of patients in whom the obstruction was thought to have a mechanical cause, contrast studies also demonstrated a mechanical cause in 13% of patients considered initially to have pseudo-obstruction. An equivocal barium enema (Corder 1986) would indicate the need for colonoscopy.

Therefore we strongly recommend — insist, in our own service — that a patient with suspected large bowel obstruction is not submitted to laparotomy without this investigation having been done. The matter is rarely so urgent that delay is harmful. Middle-of-the-night procedures, often entrusted to relatively junior staff, have little or no place in the emergency surgery of the large bowel.

Management

Once the diagnosis of intestinal pseudo-obstruction has been made, the management is essentially nonoperative. Rehydration, correction of electrolyte abnormalities and restoration of adequate oxygenation may all be required. Since the syndrome was originally described three additional measures have become invaluable.

First, parenteral nutrition removes the need for haste in re-establishing gastrointestinal function. In a malnourished patient we do not hesitate to begin at once; in those who enter hospital in a better state, our cut-off point is no more than five days.

Second, the regimen of guanethidine-physostigmine introduced by Catchpole (1969) for postoperative ileus may have a small part to play. We tend to reserve it for patients with retroperitoneal haemorrhage where progress is slow, but we have no strong logical grounds for so doing.

Third, therapeutic endoscopy. Sigmoidoscopy has long been used in the diagnosis and treatment of sigmoid volvulus (Shepherd 1968, Taha & Suleiman 1980, Anderson & Lee 1981, Goligher 1984), and the advent of colonoscopy allows similar principles to be used, not only in the treatment of this condition (Ghazi et al 1976) but also in decompressing the colonic distension seen in pseudo-obstruction. Recent reports suggest that this technique is gaining in popularity (Kukora & Dent 1977, Bachulis & Smith 1978, Munro & Youngston 1983, Bullock & Thomas 1984). In addition, some haul up a long tube on a thread passed down the operating lumen of the colono-scope before it is inserted in order to provide longer-term decompression (Groff 1983), or alter-natively place an overtube over the colonoscope before insertion (Burke & Shellito 1987). Colonos-copy with or without such therapeutic tricks is not commonly needed, but it may have a useful role in shortening the patient's illness.

Caecal rupture

This is a rare but well-recognized complication (Gierson et al 1975). The caecum and right colon are much more distensible than the left side (Gill et al 1986) and, as with mechanical obstruction, may become stretched to the point of devas-cularization. In a patient who does not respond or whose girth is increasing, caecal tenderness should be tested for at regular intervals and plain X-rays taken daily. Progressive distension of the colon up to and beyond 8–9 cm in the ascending and trans-verse sections despite treatment, is an indication for considering operation (Gierson et al 1975) before the caecum reaches 12 cm when perforation is impending (Lowman & Davis 1956). A large pneumoperitoneum from a pinhole perforation of the caecum may be the first and relatively benign sign that something must be done (Addison 1983). As caecal perforation carries a mortality rate of 43% (Gierson et al 1975) compared to an overall figure for pseudo-obstruction of 25% (Norton et al 1974), pre-emptive decompression is essential if this complication is to be avoided. Early recog-nition may be especially difficult in psychotic patients where pseudo-obstruction is not uncom-mon (McCormack 1974).

If an established or impending ruptured caecum is found, it should be exteriorized (Gierson et al 1975, Bachulis & Smith 1978); tube caecostomy is both unsatisfactory and dangerous.

Surgical management

Apart from caecal perforation, the surgeon may occasionally find himself faced with a distended colon at laparotomy for which a mechanical cause is not apparent. If the advice we have given is fol-lowed, then this circumstance is very uncommon.

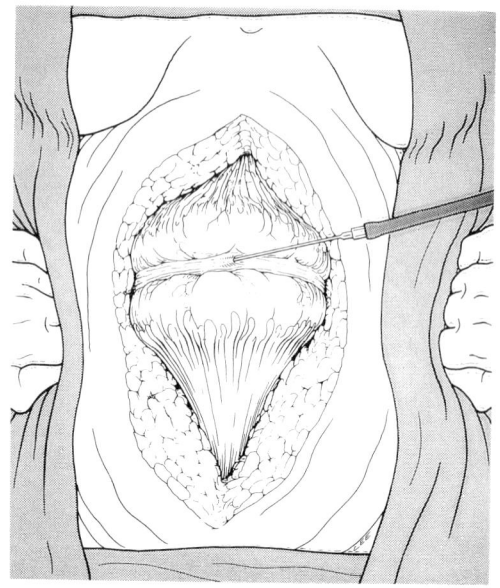

Fig. 12.3 Needle decompression of the transverse colon. A 19 gauge needle is inserted obliquely into the transverse colon through the taenia coli, while maintaining colonic distension by pressure in the flanks.

Nevertheless Jove can nod. There are two choices: first, to perform needle decompression only of the colonic gas by passing a 19-gauge needle attached to a suction source into the transverse colon while maintaining pressure in the flanks (Fig. 12.3); we favour this approach; second, to establish operative colonic decompression. The experience of Caves and Crockard (1970), with which we concur, is that caecostomy is the best manoeuvre. A second operation to close the stoma is not often needed (Addison 1983). Alternatively, and in our opinion less satisfactorily, a transverse colostomy with either operative or endoscopic decompression of the proximal limb can be used (King & Finan 1987). Raising a transverse colostomy in patients who are elderly, distended and often obese creates more problems than it solves and we condemn it.

In conclusion, colonic pseudo-obstruction is an entity more common than is often appreciated. In-judicious laparotomy attracts a high mortality. We now — if clinicians would take it into their dif-ferential diagnosis — have ample means of discrimination between mechanical and functional colonic obstruction. The objective should be to have a zero incidence of 'negative' laparotomy, and we believe that this can be achieved.

REFERENCES

Adams J T 1974 Adynamic ileus of the colon. Archives of Surgery 109: 503–507

Addison N V 1983 Pseudo-obstruction of the large bowel. Journal of the Royal Society of Medicine 76: 252–255

Aird I 1957 A companion in surgical studies. 2nd edn. Livingstone, London, p 825

Aldridge M C, Radcliffe A G, Glazer G, Dudley H A F 1987 Colonic complications of severe acute pancreatitis (abstract). Gut 28: 371

Anderson J R, Lee D 1981 The management of acute sigmoid volvulus. British Journal of Surgery 68: 117–120

Bachulis B L, Smith P E 1978 Pseudo-obstruction of the colon. American Journal of Surgery 136: 66–72

Baker L W, Dudley H A F 1961 Auscultation of the abdomen in surgical patients. Lancet ii: 517–519

Bardsley D 1974 Pseudo-obstruction of the large bowel. British Journal of Surgery 61: 963–969

Bogomoletz W V, Birembaut P, Gaillard D, Dupouy D, Camilleri J P, Phat V N 1979 Chronic idiopathic intestinal pseudo-obstruction with myenteric plexus damage. Lancet ii: 679–680

British Medical Journal 1973 Intestinal pseudo-obstruction. British Medical Journal i: 64–65

Bullock P R, Thomas W E G 1984 Acute pseudo-obstruction of the colon. Annals of the Royal College of Surgeons of England 66: 327–330

Burke G, Shellito P C 1987 Treatment of recurrent colonic pseudo-obstruction by endoscopic placement of a fenestrated overtube. Report of a case. Diseases of the Colon and Rectum 30: 615–619

Byrne J J 1960 Unusual aspects of large bowel obstruction. American Journal of Surgery 103: 62–65

Catchpole B N 1969 Ileus: use of sympathetic blocking agents in its treatment. Surgery 66: 811–820

Catchpole B N 1986 Letter to the Editor. British Medical Journal 292: 1738

Caves P K, Crockard H A 1970 Pseudo-obstruction of the large bowel. British Medical Journal ii: 583–586

Chousterman M, Petite J P, Housett E, Hornych A 1977 Prostaglandins and acute intestinal pseudo-obstruction. Lancet ii: 138–139

Corder A P 1986 Letter to the Editor. British Medical Journal 292: 1463

Dudley H A F, Paterson-Brown S 1986 Pseudo-obstruction. British Medical Journal 292: 1157–1158

Dudley H A F, Sinclair I S R, McLaren I F, McNair T J, Newsam J E 1958 Intestinal pseudo-obstruction. Journal of the Royal College of Surgeons of Edinburgh 3: 206–217

Dunlop J A 1949 Ogilvie's syndrome of false colonic obstruction: case with post-mortem findings. British Medical Journal i: 890–891

Ghazi A, Shinya H, Wolff W I 1976 Treatment of volvulus of the colon by colonoscopy. Annals of Surgery 183: 263–265

Gierson E D, Storm F K, Shaw W, Coyne S K 1975 Caecal rupture due to colonic ileus. British Journal of Surgery 62: 383–386

Gill R C, Cote K R, Bowes K L, Kingma Y J 1986 Human colonic smooth muscle: spontaneous contractile activity and response to stretch. Gut 27: 1006–1013

Goligher J C 1984 Surgery of the anus, rectum and colon. 5th edn. Ballière Tindall, London

Groff W 1983 Colonoscopic decompression and intubation of the cecum for Ogilvie's syndrome. Diseases of the Colon and Rectum 26: 503–506

Haley H B, Leigh C, Bronsky D, Waldstein S S 1962 Ascites and intestinal obstruction in myxedema. Archives of surgery 85: 328–333

Handley R S 1949 Chronic ileus caused by malignant invasion of the posterior abdominal wall. British Medical Journal i: 891–892

Hohl R D, Nixon R K 1965 Myxoedema ileus. Archives of Internal Medicine 115: 145–150

Karani J, Veale D, Rake M O 1979 Intestinal pseudo-obstruction in alcohol abuse: report of two cases. British Medical Journal ii: 1400

King H A, Finan P J 1987 Operative endoscopic decompression of colonic pseudo-obstruction. Journal of the Royal College of Surgeons of Edinburgh 32: 56–57

Koizumi K McC, Brooks C 1980 The autonomic nervous system and its role in controlling body functions. In: Mountcastle V (ed) Medical physiology. 14th edn. C V Mosby, St Louis Vol. 1; pp 914–915

Koruth N M, Koruth A, Matheson N A 1985 The place of contrast enema in the management of large bowel obstruction. Journal of the Royal College of Surgeons of Edinburgh 30: 258–260

Kukora J S, Dent L 1977 Colonoscopic decompression of massive nonobstructive cecal dilation. Archives of Surgery 112: 512–517

Lancet 1979 Intestinal pseudo-obstruction. Lancet i: 535–536

Lee J B 1981 The prostaglandins. In: Williams R H (ed) Textbook of endocrinology. 6th edn. W B Saunders, Philadelphia, p 1057

Legge D A, Wollaeger E E, Carlson H C 1970 Intestinal pseudo-obstruction in systemic amyloidosis. Gut 11: 764–767

Lescher T J, Teegardenz D K, Pruitt B A 1978 Acute pseudo-obstruction of the colon in thermally injured patients. Diseases of the Colon and Rectum 21: 618–622

Lowman R M, Davis L 1956 An evaluation of cecal size in impending perforation of the cecum. Surgery Gynecology and Obstetrics 103: 711–718

Luderer J R, Demers L M, Bonnem E M, Saleem A, Jeffries G H 1977 Elevated prostaglandin E in idiopathic intestinal pseudo-obstruction. New England Journal of Medicine 295: 1179

McCormack M 1974 Caecal rupture in psychotic patients. British Medical Journal iv: 83–84

McFarlane J A, Kay S K 1949 Ogilvie's syndrome of false colonic obstruction: is it a new clinical entity? British Medical Journal ii: 1267–1269

Munro A, Youngston G G 1983 Colonoscopy in the diagnosis and treatment of colonic pseudo-obstruction. Journal of the Royal College of Surgeons of Edinburgh 28: 391–393

Murphy J B 1896 Ileus. Journal of the American Medical Association 26: 15–22

Nanni G, Garbini A, Luchetti P, Nanni G, Ronconi P, Castagneto M 1982 Ogilvie's syndrome (acute colonic pseudo-obstruction): Review of the literature (October 1948 to March 1980) and report of four additional cases. Diseases of the Colon and Rectum 25: 157–166

Neely J, Catchpole B N 1967 An analysis of the autonomic control of gastrointestinal motility in the cat. Gut 8: 230–241

Norton L, Young D, Scribner R 1974 Management of pseudo-obstruction of the colon. Surgery Gynecology and Obstetrics 138: 595–598

Ogilvie W H 1948 Large-intestine colic due to sympathetic deprivation: a new clinical syndrome. British Medical Journal ii: 671–673

Peachey R D G, Creamer B, Pierce J W 1969 Sclerodermatous involvement of the stomach and the small and large bowel. Gut 10: 285–292

Perino L E, Schuffler M D, Mehta S J, Everson G T 1986 Radiation-induced intestinal pseudo-obstruction. Gastroenterology 91: 994–998

Rothwell-Jackson R L 1963 Idiopathic large-bowel obstruction. British Journal of Surgery 50: 797–800

Shepherd J J 1968 Treatment of volvulus of sigmoid colon: a review of 425 cases. British Medical Journal ii: 280–283

Smith M K, Jepson R P, Catchpole B N 1965 Ileus: an experimental study. British Journal of Surgery 52: 381–386

Stephens F O 1962 The syndrome of intestinal pseudo-obstruction. British Medical Journal 1: 1248–1250

Stewart J, Finan P J, Courtney D F, Brennan T G 1984 Does a water soluble contrast enema assist in the management of acute large bowel obstruction: a prospective study of 117 cases. British Journal of Surgery 71: 799–801

Streeten D H P, Vaughan Williams E M 1952 Loss of cellular potassium as a cause of intestinal paralysis in dogs. Journal of Physiology 118: 149–170

Taha S E, Suleiman S I 1980 Volvulus of the sigmoid colon in the Gezira. British Journal of Surgery 67: 433–435

Wanebo H, Mathewson C, Conolly B 1971 Pseudo-obstruction of the colon. Surgery Gynecology and Obstetrics 133: 44–48

Wangensteen O H 1937 Therapeutic problem in bowel obstructions. Ballière, Tindall & Cox, London

Wilson J P 1975 Postoperative motility of the large intestine in man. Gut 16: 689–692

Zimmerman L M 1930 'Spastic ileus'. Surgery Gynecology and Obstetrics 50: 721–732

13 *Complications of small bowel diverticula*

W. E. G. THOMAS

A diverticulum is an abnormal outpouching or cul-de-sac of an organ. Literally, the term 'diverticulum' referred to a 'wayside inn of ill repute', and in the small bowel such diverticula live up to their nefarious reputation. Small bowel diverticula can be congenital or acquired.

Congenital or 'true' diverticula contain all three layers of the bowel wall and develop from an embryological structure, the prime example being Meckel's diverticulum which develops from the vitellointestinal or omphalomesenteric duct. Rarely, a duplication of the alimentary tract may present as a diverticulum. Duplications may or may not communicate with the gut lumen, but when they do, they take on a tubular form like a diverticulum lying within the layers of the mesentery. The commonest site is in the ileum, where nearly 50% of duplications are found. Such lesions are rare, but when they do occur they share the blood supply of the associated gut, which must be taken into consideration if surgical excision is contemplated.

Acquired or 'false' diverticula are outpouches consisting merely of intestinal mucosa and submucosa, but with no muscle in the wall. The majority are thought to be pulsion diverticula, resulting from some mechanical or hydrodynamic force that pushes part of the wall of the gut out through sites of weakness, although rarely is an increase in intraluminal pressure demonstrable. This herniation tends to occur through congenital weak points of the muscle wall where blood vessels (vasa brevia) pierce the muscularis. Such diverticula are seen on the mesenteric border of the bowel and are often associated with muscle hypertrophy of the adjacent bowel wall. Occasionally

traction diverticula can occur, but these are rare in the small bowel although not infrequent in the oesophagus.

Secondary diverticula may develop as a result of long-standing ulceration and fibrosis, such as occurs in the duodenal cap with chronic peptic ulceration. They can also be seen in the distal small bowel secondary to Crohn's disease, idiopathic enteric ulceration or stricture formation from whatever cause. Indeed, a stricture may be the end result of standard acquired jejunal diverticula, which can then in turn lead to secondary diverticulum formation if the fibrosis is severe enough. Secondary diverticula tend to be made up of all three layers of the bowel wall and are simply the result of adjacent cicatrization.

The complications arising in small bowel diverticula depend on their structure, site, size, nature and numerical incidence.

Duodenal diverticula

Duodenal diverticula can be divided into intraluminal and extraluminal varieties.

Intraluminal diverticula

These are extremely rare. They consist of a congenital mucosa-lined sac entirely within the lumen, which is usually sited adjacent to the ampulla of Vater. They were first described by Boyd in 1845, but since then there have only been sporadic case reports. The wall of the sac is lined on both sides by duodenal mucosa, thus distinguishing it from a choledochal cyst which is lined by biliary epithelium. Although it may be regarded as a variant of a duodenal diaphragm, some class it as an entity in its own right, as it is always found attached to the same small segment of duodenal wall in the periampullary region (Mathieu et al 1978). However its embryonic development is not yet established. It appears as a pear-shaped intraluminal barium-filled abnormality on barium meal, and it has been likened to a 'wind-sock' or the 'thumb of a glove' (Silcock 1885).

Extraluminal diverticula

These are the commonest forms of duodenal diverticula. They are usually acquired lesions and may be subdivided into primary and secondary diverticula. Primary extraluminal diverticula tend to occur in elderly patients, and 80% are found on the inner or medial wall of the second part of the duodenum at sites of weakness of the wall. These sites may be where blood vessels pierce the muscle coat of the bowel or in the vicinity of the common bile duct where it runs within the duodenal wall. This factor may explain why the ampulla of Vater

is so commonly found on the rim or in the depths of such a diverticulum, much to the frustration of endoscopists attempting endoscopic retrograde cholangiopancreatography (ERCP). Duodenal diverticula are usually solitary, but can be multiple or multiloculated, and are found coincidentally in approximately 2–5% of barium meals (Fig. 13.1) (Wilk et al 1973, Neill & Thompson 1965) but in up to 22% of all patients at autopsy (Ackerman 1943).

Secondary extraluminal diverticula are usually seen in the duodenal cap and are simply the result of long-standing peptic ulceration with its associated cicatrization and fibrous deformity. The presentation of such a deformity is usually that of the complications relating to the primary peptic ulcer.

Presentation

The majority of duodenal diverticula are asymptomatic, but they can present with vague symptoms of abdominal discomfort or epigastric pain, nausea, vomiting and weight loss. Fortunately major complications are rare, which is just as well, as in one series such complications resulted in a mortality rate of 33% (Munnell & Preston 1966). This high mortality rate may reflect the advanced age of these patients, or the delay in accurate diagnosis by failing to recognize the significance of this condition (Neill & Thompson 1965).

Obstruction to bile and pancreatic ducts

The majority of diverticula lie in the region of the ampulla; indeed the ampulla not infrequently lies within a diverticulum. This situation can lead to obstruction of either the common bile duct or the pancreatic duct or both. The obstruction may be caused by kinking of the ducts or blockage by food debris or enteroliths. It can result in either obstructive jaundice or acute pancreatitis, which has even been reported in association with an intraluminal diverticulum (Fleming et al 1975, Howard et al 1986). Chronic pancreatitis has also been recorded in association with an intraluminal

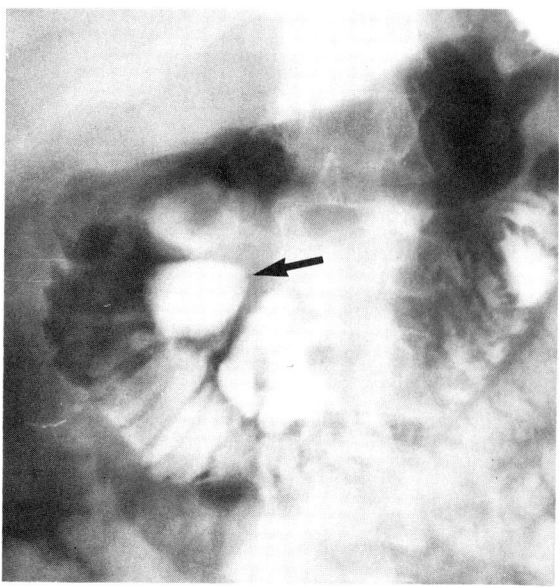

Fig. 13.1 Extraluminal duodenal diverticula outlined by barium.

diverticulum and an annular pancreas (Hirsch et al 1964). It is of interest to note that patients with diverticula in the second part of the duodenum have a higher incidence of gallstones than a comparable normal population (Leinkram et al 1980). Whether this factor is cause or effect is uncertain, but it does suggest that such patients have a degree of chronic obstruction to their common bile duct resulting in biliary stasis.

Perforation

This is one of the commonest complications of duodenal diverticula. It usually occurs as a result of stasis, an enterolith eroding or ulcerating through the very thin mucosal and submucosal wall of the diverticulum, or from peptic ulceration, although it may also occur secondary to acute diverticulitis. Such diverticulitis is uncommon, but when it does occur, it presents as an inflammatory episode in the epigastrium and may be diagnosed either as peptic ulceration, cholecystitis or acute pancreatitis. Unfortunately there are no pathognomonic symptoms or signs.

Perforation tends to occur retroperitoneally. It produces an oedematous bile-stained phlegmon of retroperitoneal tissues, retroperitoneal oedema, emphysema lateral to the duodenum or retroduodenal or retroperitoneal pus (Juler et al 1969). The condition can develop into a retroperitoneal abscess, which may be suggested radiologically by a small fluid level in the vicinity of the duodenum. When the perforation into the peritoneal cavity occurs, it either produces a form of biliary peritonitis or results in fistulation to adjacent organs such as the gallbladder, colon etc. Erythaema has also been reported in the flanks following perforation of a duodenal diverticulum (Stebbings & Thompson 1985) in a similar manner to acute pancreatitis. Failure to recognize such a perforation is the main cause of most deaths from duodenal diverticula (Neill & Thompson 1965).

Perforation is also a hazard of endoscopic sphincterotomy when the ampulla lies within the vicinity of the diverticulum. In the normal anatomy the bile duct runs within the duodenal wall for a limited distance, thus allowing an endoscopic sphincterotomy to be performed, but if the ampulla lies adjacent to or within a diverticulum the muscle wall of the duodenum may be deficient, and therefore there is a greatly increased risk of perforation.

Haemorrhage

When haemorrhage occurs from a duodenal diverticulum, it is usually severe (Sonnenfeld et al 1986) and follows ulceration and erosion into an artery adjacent to the diverticular neck. Slow chronic blood loss is not usually recognized as originating in such lesions, but repeated small bleeds may lead to iron-deficiency anaemia and chronic gastrointestinal blood loss.

Intestinal obstruction

Duodenal obstruction may occur with intraluminal diverticula, as these can fill with food debris and balloon out, thus occluding the lumen. Extraluminal diverticula rarely obstruct locally, although occasionally large enteroliths of inspissated bowel contents can produce distal obstruction when extruded into the bowel lumen, causing a bolus obstruction in a similar manner to gallstone ileus. A rare complication in this category is produced by a phytobezoar formed in a diverticulum (Fanucci et al 1985).

Metabolic disturbances

Metabolic abnormalities resulting from extensive bacterial colonization of a duodenal diverticulum are extremely rare but have been reported (Goldstein et al 1963). Colonization itself is not unusual, but when occurring solely in a duodenal diverticulum it seldom results in malabsorption (Gorbach & Levitan 1970). Such metabolic abnormalities are far commoner in association with jejunoileal diverticula.

Investigation

Duodenal diverticula are very much more accessible to investigation than distal jejunoileal diverticula. Not only are they clearly delineated by barium studies (Fig. 13.1), but they can be viewed directly by endoscopy. Side-viewing endoscopes are valuable for examining the interior of the diverticulum to look for bleeding points or enteroliths that may be responsible for bile or pancreatic duct obstruction. In these latter cases, ERCP is unfortunately all too often technically impossible. However, certain cases of intraluminal diverticula may be outlined by intravenous cholangiography due to the fact that they are so closely associated with the ampulla (Kaftori et al 1966), and extraluminal diverticula can cause initial fear of a leak when outlined by a 'T'-tube cholangiogram (Fig. 13.2).

The diagnosis of perforation of a duodenal diverticulum is usually impossible to make before operation, unless the patient is already known to

have such a diverticulum. In most cases these patients present with symptoms similar to those of a perforated posterior duodenal ulcer or acute pancreatitis. Plain abdominal radiographs may occasionally demonstrate free gas if the perforation ruptures into the peritoneal cavity, or localized retroperitoneal air over an area relating to the duodenum and upper pole of the right kidney (Wolfe & Pearl 1972). Ultrasound may demonstrate a retroperitoneal phlegmon in the region of the head of the pancreas but is unable to differentiate this from acute pancreatitis. A fluid collection may also be seen in the lesser sac or in an abscess cavity or tracking down the right paracolic gutter. An elevated serum amylase is often seen in both a perforated duodenal diverticulum and acute pancreatitis, although in the latter condition it tends to be higher.

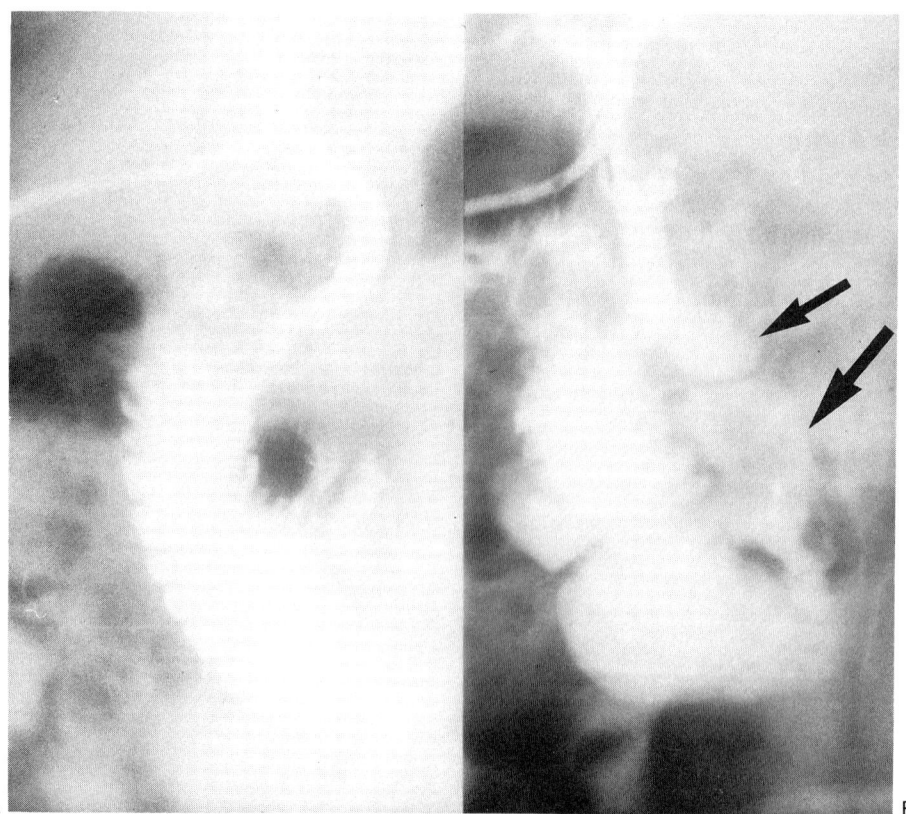

A   B

Fig. 13.2 (B) Duodenal diverticula (arrowed) outlined during a 'T'-tube cholangiogram. Such an appearance may cause concern as it can mimic a leak. (A) An earlier film of the same investigation, showing air in the diverticulum.

Treatment

The vast majority of duodenal diverticula are asymptomatic and should be left entirely alone. It is only a minority in which complications supervene which can require surgery. One of the problems of surgical exploration in many of these cases is recognition of the presence of a duodenal diverticulum. As such lesions are usually found on the medial wall of the duodenum, they may not be easily apparent unless distended by air, fluid or an enterolith, or specifically sought by Kocherization of the duodenum and careful dissection. In those cases in which surgical excision of the diverticulum is indicated, the duodenum should be fully mobilized and the common bile duct exposed and clearly dissected before the diverticulum itself is tackled. If excision is proceeded with, the ampulla should be clearly identified, with cannulation of the bile and pancreatic ducts before closure of the duodenum in two layers. Such a closure may be reinforced by an omental patch, and adequate drainage is essential.

In cases where the common bile duct has been compromised, either by the diverticulum itself or the surgical procedure, then a choledochoduodenostomy or -jejunostomy should be performed. If the patient has coexistent pancreatobiliary disease, it is inadequate simply to perform a cholecystectomy and exploration of the common bile duct (Donald 1979, Manny et al 1981), as the disease will recur in 85% of cases if the diverticulum is left in situ (Lotveit et al 1982). Another approach is to perform a duodenojejunostomy as described by Critchlow et al (1985). In this procedure the duodenum is divided just distal to the pylorus and the distal end closed. The proximal end is then anastomosed to a Roux loop of jejunum. This manoeuvre has the advantage of removing the diverticulum from the food stream, thus solving the problem of recurrent cholangitis or pancreatitis caused by food debris, without having to excise the diverticulum. In the rare cases where haemorrhage occurs in a diverticulum in which both bile and pancreatic ducts open straight into the depths of the diverticulum, then the bleeding point can be tackled intraluminally and oversewn, again taking care not to compromise the two ducts by inserting cannulae into the ampullary orifices.

A perforated duodenal diverticulum usually requires resection, but if this is technically impossible, then it can be treated using a tube duodenostomy (Beech et al 1985). In the unlikely situation of a duodenal defect being created that cannot be closed without compromising the lumen, then a Roux-en-Y loop of jejunum may be used to close the defect.

Intraluminal diverticula can be dealt with either endoscopically or by surgical intervention. Hajiro et al (1979) described an endoscopic technique for such lesions that involves identifying the ampulla and cannulating the ducts and then using the diathermy snare to evert and resect the apex of the diverticulum, thus providing a wide passage for duodenal contents. However many intraluminal diverticula do not lend themselves to such management (Adams 1986) and require operation. This usually involves subtotal resection of the diverticulum via a duodenotomy, after identifying and preserving the ampulla (Howard et al 1986).

Jejunoileal diverticula

Jejunoileal diverticula are in the main acquired thin-walled sacs of mucosa and submucosa found on the mesenteric border of the small bowel (Fig. 13.3). They are thought to be often associated with abnormal intestinal motility (Edwards 1954) with muscle hypertrophy of the adjacent jejunal wall (Phillips 1953). They tend to occur at the point in the jejunal wall at which the vasa recta or vasa brevia pierce the muscle and are usually multiple.

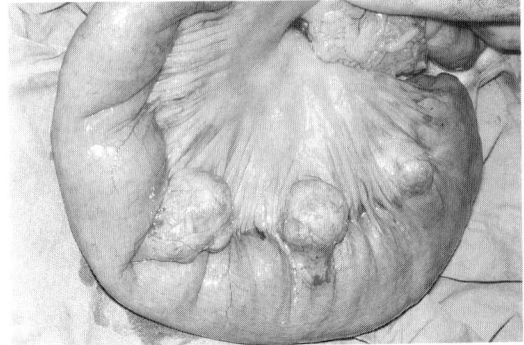

Fig. 13.3 Multiple acquired jejunal diverticula.

They extend into the mesentery and often may not be easy to see unless the jejunum is deliberately distended with air (Welsh 1966). Indeed Rosedale and Lawrence (1936) reported that if the bowel is distended with air at autopsy, considerably more diverticula become apparent than were previously recognized.

Diverticula are most frequent in the jejunum, being commoner in the upper than the lower jejunum, and are only rarely seen in the ileum (Cocks & Zino 1968). They tend to be commoner in men than women and show an increasing incidence with age, occurring almost exclusively in patients over 40 years (Rankin & Martin 1934). Autopsy studies reveal an overall incidence of 0.7% (Geroulakis 1987), while the frequency of detection radiologically ranges from 0.07% to 2.3% (Case 1920, Caplan & Jacobson 1964, Parulekar 1972, Maglinte et al 1986).

The fundamental cause of small bowel diverticula remains unclear. Some are secondary to disease processes such as Crohn's disease, scleroderma, non-specific ulceration (Thomas & Williamson 1985a) or operation (Maglinte et al 1986), but the majority arise from herniation of the mucosa through the muscle layer alongside the penetrating vessels. It has been suggested that most diverticula begin as a pair of small pouches on either side of the mesentery where the vessels pierce the muscular and serosal coats, which enlarge until they coalesce to form a single thin-walled diverticulum. This outpouching may result from raised intraluminal pressure and abnormal intestinal motility (Edwards 1954), possibly due to a visceral myopathy caused by abnormal small bowel smooth muscle function and structure (Krishnamurthy et al 1983). This is supported by finding a 40% incidence of smooth muscle fibrosis, similar to systemic sclerosis in these authors' series.

Presentation

The vast majority of jejunoileal diverticula cause no symptoms and thus require no treatment. Complications of these small bowel diverticula are uncommon, and in one reported series of 87 cases, only 10% experienced complications requiring surgical intervention (Baskin & Mayo 1952). However some cases of jejunal diverticulosis can present with chronic nonspecific symptoms, including abdominal discomfort, flatulence, borborygmi, malabsorption and pseudo-obstruction, giving an overall symptomatic rate of about 40% (Altemeier et al 1963). Major complications include intestinal obstruction, diverticulitis, perforation, peritonitis, intestinal haemorrhage, intestinal stasis or a 'blind loop' syndrome and neoplastic disease. This latter complication is rare, but fibroma, lipoma, carcinoma and sarcoma may be encountered (Maglinte et al 1986).

Intestinal obstruction

Intestinal obstruction associated with jejunal diverticulosis may arise from a number of different mechanisms. The diverticulum may act as a pivot for a volvulus, especially if previous attacks of diverticulitis have produced an adhesion band. Such diverticulitis can also lead to peridiverticular adhesions of the jejunum to other structures, producing obstruction either by direct kinking of the jejunum or by a further loop of bowel being trapped and obstructed under the adhesion (Eckhauser et al 1979, Donald 1979). The diverticulum may also initiate an intussusception (Soofi & Abouchedid 1986).

The small bowel may also be obstructed secondary to enterolith formation (Figs 13.4A, B) (King et al 1985). These enteroliths are usually composed of choleic acid. They cause obstruction either at the site of the diverticulum, or by migrating into the lumen and impacting distally (usually in the terminal ileum) causing a bolus obstruction (Bewes 1967, Ottinger & Carter 1975, Svanes & Halvorsen 1975, Clarke & Kettlewell 1985, Geroulakis 1987). This complication is rare and seldom considered in the preoperative differential diagnosis of obstruction. When encountered at operation, it is advisable to remove the enterolith locally through healthy bowel wall (Fig. 13.5) and search for any further enterolith, but it is usually unnecessary to resect the jejunal diverticulum unless there is evidence of diverticulitis (Clarke & Kettlewell 1985, Geroulakis 1987).

It is also recorded that patients with small bowel

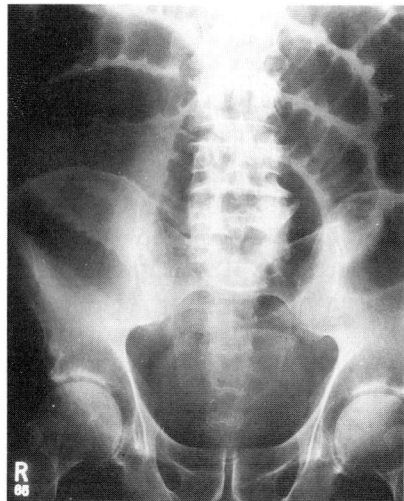

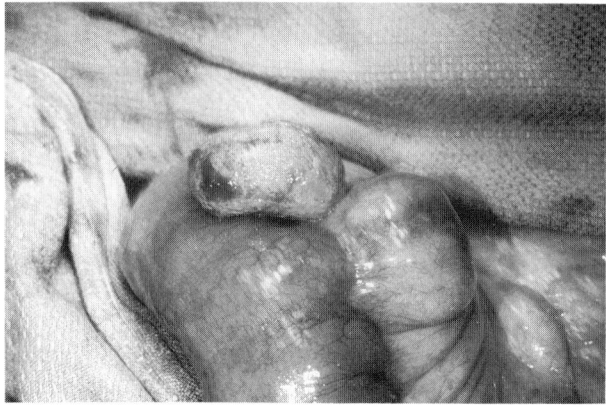

Fig. 13.4 (**A**) Radiological evidence of small bowel obstruction due to enterolith obstruction. (**B**) The enterolith after removal, beside the jejunal diverticulum from which it originated.

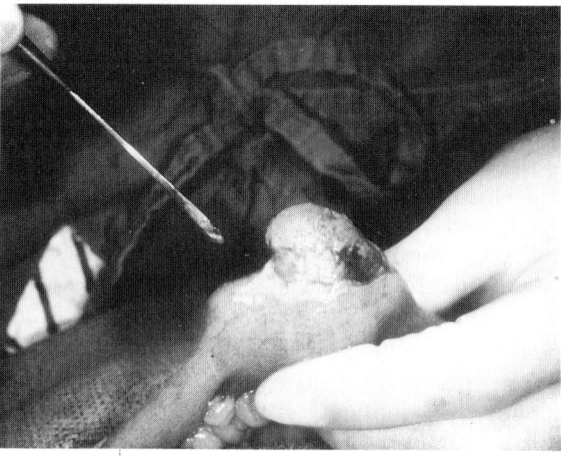

Fig. 13.5 Removal of enterolith by enterotomy through healthy bowel wall.

diverticula may present with a chronic intestinal pseudo-obstruction (Phillips 1953). The patient suffers from recurrent abdominal colic and vomiting and may demonstrate visible peristalsis and a radiological picture of obstruction (Schuffler et al 1981). This is due to abnormal intestinal motility and an intrinsic muscular abnormality, rather than a mechanical blockage (Krishnamurthy et al 1983). However the clinical and radiological picture makes it difficult to distinguish these patients from those with other causes of gradual small bowel obstruction.

Perforation and diverticulitis

These two complications may account for at least 50% of the complications arising in jejunal diverticula (Nobles 1971, Geroulakis 1987). At times it is difficult to separate these two conditions: although perforation itself is well recognized (Herrington 1962, Smith 1976), some patients without an overt diverticular perforation may present with suppurative peritonitis secondary to an acutely inflamed diverticulum and surrounding local abscess (Jones 1974). Indeed some patients present with just such a localized abscess (Brown & Thompson 1985), but usually a perforation presents with peritonitis — either local or general — and most of these will be diagnosed as cases of acute appendicitis, acute colonic diverticulitis or a perforated ulcer. It is therefore especially important to examine the jejunum when laparotomy via a grid-iron incision has been performed for supposed appendicitis and the appendix itself is found to be entirely normal.

Occasionally perforation is precipitated by foreign bodies, parasites, enteroliths or even food particles such as a rolled-up tomato skin (Phillips 1953). The overall mortality of perforation of a jejunal diverticulum may be up to 30% (Babcock et al 1976), so early diagnosis and operative treatment are vital.

In certain cases spontaneous pneumoperitoneum

may be encountered without peritonitis (Dunn & Nelson 1979, Madura & Craig 1981). This complication is caused by transmural passage of air through the semipermeable membrane of a thin-walled diverticulum. It can be exacerbated by air insufflation during gastrointestinal endoscopy, giving a somewhat alarming radiological picture following a straightforward diagnostic procedure (Brown et al 1986).

Haemorrhage

This is an unusual cause of gastrointestinal blood loss and one that is particularly difficult to diagnose. However it should be considered in any case of chronic or recurrent blood loss in a elderly patient in whom endoscopy and barium studies prove normal. The bleeding may be acute and severe (Thomas et al 1967) or chronic and associated with vague abdominal symptoms. In a review of 35 cases (Taylor 1969), the majority passed melaena stool, but a few also produced a haematemesis. There are often no previous medical complaints, although in almost a quarter of the reported cases of acute haemorrhage, bleeding had been chronic prior to surgery (Taylor 1969, Geroulakis 1987). It has been pointed out that in many respects the pattern of bleeding in association with jejunal diverticulosis is similar to that seen with colonic diverticulosis (Jones 1974). The haemorrhage in both cases results from the fact that where the blood vessels penetrate the bowel wall, the lack of muscularis in the diverticular neck exposes the vessel to such an extent that any trauma or diverticulitis may cause bleeding (Shackelford & Marcus 1960).

Malabsorption

Malabsorption may occur in cases of jejunal diverticulosis due to a 'blind-loop' or 'stagnant-loop' syndrome. Why this occurs in some cases and not others is often unclear, but it has been suggested that achlorhydria may permit jejunal colonization in some patients (Murray-Lyon et al 1968). In the normal jejunum the bacterial count is low at 10^1–10^4 organisms/ml, but in the 'blind-loop'

syndrome counts of up to 10^{12} organisms/ml have been reported, with the bacterial population resembling that of the colon (Drasar & Hill 1974). These findings have prompted Gracey (1971) to refer to this condition as the 'contaminated small bowel syndrome'. The organisms found may be many and varied (Drasar & Hill 1974) and the abnormal proliferation may be generalized or localized (Gorbach & Tabaqchali 1969). Such bacterial overgrowth in association with jejunal diverticulosis may result in steatorrhoea, a macrocytic anaemia from malabsorption of vitamin B12, and other absorptive problems such as mineral deficiency and oedema due to hypoproteinaemia (Tabaqchali & Booth 1970). These changes may be the result of bacterial conversion of conjugated bile salts to unconjugated bile salts, although the type and volume of organisms present will determine whether this phenomenon takes place. Indeed, deconjugation has to occur over a significant length of intestine before steatorrhoea occurs.

Cooke et al (1963) found that in a series of 33 patients with small bowel diverticula, 14 had some evidence of malabsorption and vitamin B12 depletion, and 12 of these had a peripheral neuropathy. In some cases this malabsorption state may be accompanied by hypoproteinaemia, weight loss, and a flattened glucose tolerance curve. Therefore this diagnosis should be considered in all elderly patients presenting with unexplained vague abdominal symptoms with steatorrhoea and malabsorption.

The whole concept of a 'blind-loop' syndrome is therefore based upon an increased volume of proximal jejunal contents (the jejunum usually being empty: Latin 'jejunum' means empty), an increased concentration of bacteria in the proximal jejunum and clinical and laboratory test responses to broad-spectrum antibiotic therapy. Diagnosis depends on demonstrating steatorrhoea by means of elevated faecal fat content and finding a low serum vitamin B12 level. A lactulose hydrogen breath test is a valuable non-invasive diagnostic test for confirming bacterial overgrowth (Rhodes et al 1979) but can be attended by false positive and false negative results. However if the results are positive, then attempts should be made to demonstrate a primary causative lesion, such as jejunal diverticulosis, and a trial of broad-spectrum antibiotics should be instituted. It has been clearly demonstrated that administration of such antibiotics to patients with diverticulosis causing 'blind-loop' syndrome relieves chronic gastrointestinal symptoms such as steatorrhoea, bloating and anaemia (Knaver & Svoboda 1968, Christiansen 1969).

Investigation

Jejunoileal diverticula are inaccessible to the standard endoscopes, although instruments have now been designed to traverse the whole length of the small intestine, allowing examination of the lumen during withdrawal (Shinya & McSherry 1982). However the mainstay of diagnosis, other than at laparotomy, is radiology. Occasionally a plain abdominal radiograph may show multiple fluid levels in jejunal diverticula, simulating small bowel obstruction, and indeed the two conditions can coexist. In cases of perforation a plain film may demonstrate a pneumoperitoneum or a fluid level in a localized abscess. However these findings are not specific for jejunal diverticulosis, and the diagnosis is usually only made at laparotomy. In chronic cases the diagnosis depends on barium studies. In 1920 Case was the first to demonstrate small bowel diverticula in vivo by means of barium follow-through studies. He reported an incidence of 0.07% in a series of 6847 studies, but since then the pick-up rate has improved. However it has become apparent that although most cases of diverticulosis are picked up by a standard barium follow-through examination (Fig. 13.6), many other cases are missed (Maglinte et al 1986). Some diverticula are so large that the barium is not retained, and the diverticulum empties too rapidly to be recognized. Others may be so small or narrow-necked that barium does not enter or achieve adequate filling. Therefore intraluminal distension is required by means of enteroclysis, which fills even the smallest diverticulum, and this is now the investigation of choice. It involves the passage of a tube into the duodenum, advancing it as near to the duodenojejunal flexure as possible, and then infusing barium under pressure until all the segments of the small bowel are distended (Maglinte

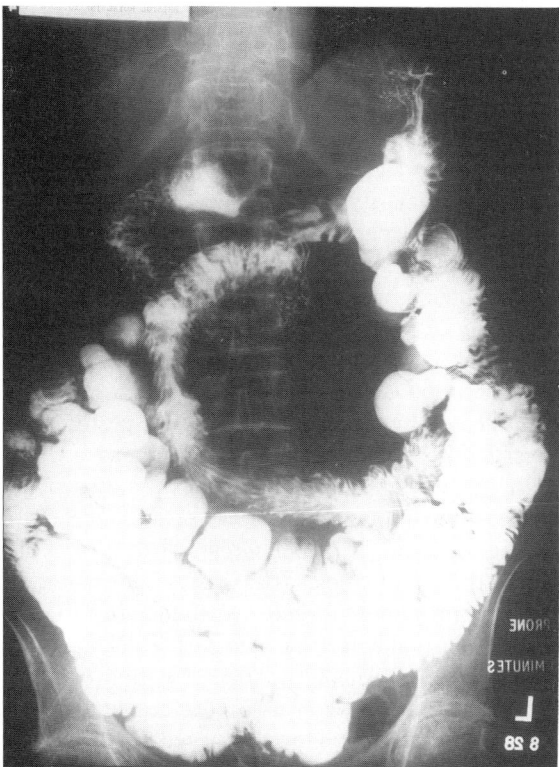

Fig. 13.6 Multiple jejunal diverticula on barium follow-through examination. (Reproduced by kind permission of the publishers of *Hospital Update*)

et al 1984). Use of this technique would seem to show that the prevalence of acquired jejunoileal diverticula is greater than previously reported (Salomonowitz et al 1983, Maglinte et al 1986).

In cases of undiagnosed gastrointestinal blood loss, selective mesenteric angiography when the patient is actively bleeding is of value. However this technique will only pick up bleeding sources if the lesion is bleeding at a rate of 5–6 ml/min for an aortic flush (Jaffe et al 1965) or 0.5–2 ml/min for a selective mesenteric artery catheterization (Balint et al 1977).

Alternatively, a ^{99m}Tc sulphur colloid scan may detect the source of bleeding from jejunal diverticula if the blood loss exceeds 0.1 ml/minute (Alavi 1982). However even at this degree of sensitivity, this technique is still limited by the intermittent nature of the bleeding. With ^{99m}Tc-labelled red cells 100% success rates have been claimed (Winzelberg et al 1982) as opposed to

65% for conventional angiography (Best et al 1979).

Treatment

The vast majority of jejunoileal diverticula encountered at laparotomy are totally asymptomatic and therefore require no treatment. In cases of proven malabsorption and 'blind-loop' syndrome, broad-spectrum antibiotics are all that is required. Operation is seldom indicated or even advisable in this condition except when jejunal diverticulosis is complicated by intestinal obstruction, perforation, diverticulitis, haemorrhage or malignancy.

In many cases simple excision of the diverticula and end-to-end anastomosis has proved most successful (Donald 1979, McGrew et al 1985), but where the diverticulosis is extensive, this is not always appropriate. Where resection of all the diverticula is not feasible due to the considerable length of bowel involved, then resection of those diverticula that have bled or perforated (for example) is indicated. However, even this policy is not easy to follow. The guilty or incriminated diverticulum is not always easy to identify, especially in cases of bleeding. Some surgeons have recommended cross-clamping of the jejunum in cases of acute severe bleeding to localize the actual point of bleeding (Wells 1967). When this procedure is not attended by a satisfactory result, or when the bleeding is chronic, a blind resection of the diverticula may be required, and opening the bowel afterwards will often reveal evidence of diverticulitis plus an ulcer containing a bleeding vessel (Thomas & Williamson 1985b). In patients with diverticulosis so extensive that a blind resection is not a practical option, a bleeding point may be sought by on-table endoscopy of the small bowel by means of an enterotomy.

Intestinal obstruction caused by diverticulitis or intussusception of a diverticulum usually requires resection of the offending lesion. Band adhesion or volvulus obstruction may be correctable without having to resort to resection, and in enterolith obstruction it is usually adequate simply to remove the enterolith (Clarke & Kettlewell 1985), ensuring that there are no more in proximal diverticula that could precipitate further obstructive episodes.

In the cases of troublesome pseudo-obstruction an empirical trial of metoclopramide may prove helpful (Albibi & McCallum 1983).

Meckel's diverticulum

In the third week of pregnancy the yolk sac forms the ventral aspect of the gut, and as the midgut starts to develop from the primitive intestinal loop, it communicates with the exterior by the omphalomesenteric duct. This duct then elongates and narrows and usually becomes completely involuted by the fifth week, but if regression is not complete it results in some of the commonest congenital abnormalities of the gastrointestinal tract. These anomalies of the omphalomesenteric duct (vitellointestinal duct) are remnants of the embryonic yolk sac. When the duct persists in its entirety, it leads to an omphalomesenteric fistula, with the external opening at the umbilicus. When the duct is obliterated at the gastrointestinal end an umbilical sinus remains, but if both ends are obliterated an umbilical cyst or intra-abdominal enterocystoma results. The commonest remnant is Meckel's diverticulum, a partial persistence of the proximal omphalomesenteric duct sited on the antimesenteric border of the terminal ileum. This diverticulum, first described in 1809 by Johann Friedrich Meckel, is a true diverticulum made up of all layers of the intestinal wall. It receives its blood supply from a remnant of the vitelline artery, an end artery of the superior mesenteric artery running in a distinct mesodiverticulum.

Ninety per cent of Meckel's diverticula occur within the terminal 100 cm of the ileum, but they have been found as far as 180 cm from the ileocaecal valve (Dowse 1961, Williams 1981). In about 10% of cases a fibrous cord connects the apex of the diverticulum to the undersurface of the umbilicus (omphalodiverticular band) (Fig. 13.7) or to the ileal mesentery (mesodiverticular band) (Johns et al 1959, Williams 1981).

Meckel's diverticulum is the most prevalent congenital anomaly of the gastrointestinal tract. In autopsy series the incidence ranges from 0.3 to 4% (Christie 1931, Harkins 1933, Kittle et al 1947, Jay et al 1950, Seagram et al 1968, Michas et al 1975), but traditionally it is regarded as occurring

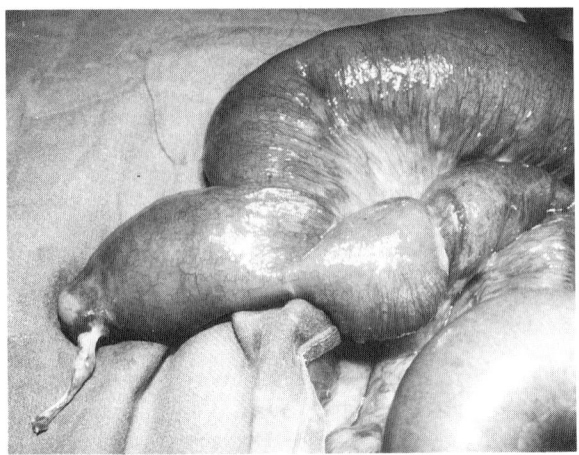

Fig. 13.7 A divided omphalodiverticular band that stretched from the apex of the diverticulum to the undersurface of the umbilicus.

in 2% of the general population. In a prospective study of 1954 appendicectomies a Meckel's diverticulum was found in 3.2% (Soderlund 1959); it is more common in people born with other congenital malformations, especially exomphalos, oesophageal atresia and anorectal atresia (Simms & Corkery 1980). The sex ratio is equal in most autopsy series, but more males do appear to develop complications (Debartolo & Vanheerden 1976, Mackey & Dineen 1983).

Heterotopic tissue is found in 30–50% of Meckel's diverticula (Fig. 13.8), but may be as high as 72% in symptomatic cases (Soderlund 1959, Artigas et al 1986). In a review of 140 diverticula, gastric mucosa was found in 52%, pancreatic tissue in 5%, and a combination in 8%. Ileal mucosa alone was present in 35% (Gross 1953). These areas of ectopic mucosa are often directly or indirectly the main risk factor for the development of the complications that arise in Meckel's diverticulum (Artigas et al 1986).

Presentation

It has been estimated that only about 4% of Meckel's diverticula become symptomatic (Soltero & Bill 1976). Indeed Charles Mayo stated in 1933 that 'Meckel's diverticulum is frequently suspected, often looked for, and seldom found'. This statement remains true, and it has been calculated that to save one patient's life from the complications of Meckel's diverticulum, it would be necessary to remove approximately 800 asymptomatic diverticula (Soltero & Bill 1976), a statistic that is very relevant when considering the management of the Meckel's diverticulum that is a coincidental finding at laparotomy.

The vast majority of Meckel's diverticula are therefore asymptomatic. In a series of 402 cases, 35% were incidental findings at laparotomy, 45% incidental findings at autopsy and 2% incidental findings on barium studies of the small intestine (Mackey & Dineen 1983). In a large series of 202 complicated Meckel's diverticula, the overall complication rate was 4%, a figure that diminished with age (Soltero & Bill 1976). The presenting symptoms of these complications were related to intestinal obstruction, diverticulitis, Littre's hernia, omphalomesenteric fistula, enterocystoma, gastrointestinal haemorrhage, neoplasia and malabsorption. Occasionally Meckel's diverticulum can present with intermittent or incomplete band obstruction or chronic peptic ulceration. This has been termed 'dyspepsia Meckelii' (Williams 1981) and can often produce a puzzling clinical picture.

Intestinal obstruction

Intestinal obstruction associated with a Meckel's

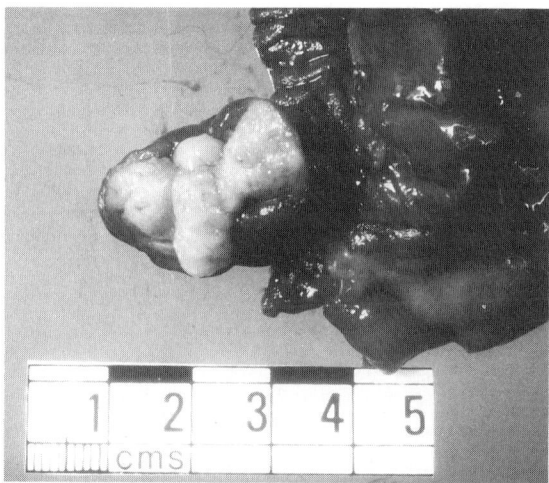

Fig. 13.8 Ectopic gastric and pancreatic tissue in a Meckel's diverticulum.

diverticulum may originate in many ways. It is the commonest presenting feature in most series, occurring in over a third of the symptomatic cases (Soltero & Bill 1976, Williams 1981, Mackey & Dineen 1983). It may occur as a result of volvulus of the bowel around a persistent omphalodiverticular band (Soderlund 1959, Rutherford & Akers 1966, Mackey & Dineen 1983), entrapment of bowel loops under a mesodiverticular band (Rutherford & Akers 1966, Seagram et al 1968), intussusception (Harkins 1933, Williamson et al 1984), inflammatory adhesions (Mackey & Dineen 1983) or incarceration of a Littré's hernia (Soderlund 1959, Mackey & Dineen 1983). Faecaliths or calculi can form in Meckel's diverticulum (Moran et al 1985, Barr 1986) in a similar manner to jejunal diverticula. They can occasionally become dislodged and produce a bolus obstruction.

In most cases the presentation is one of classical small bowel obstruction, without any obvious indication of the underlying cause. However, when intussusception occurs (Fig. 13.9), as in 4–14% of complicated Meckel's diverticula (Moore & Johnston 1976, Yamaguchi et al 1978), it can present without overt small bowel obstruction and thus present a diagnostic conundrum (Williamson et al 1984).

Entrapment of a Meckel's diverticulum in an external hernia is surprisingly common (Weinstein et al 1962, Mackey & Dineen 1983). First described by Littré in 1742, such herniation is found at all ages, and occurs in inguinal (50%), femoral (20%) or umbilical hernias (20%). It is more common in men, on the right side, and is encountered in approximately 1/200 external groin hernias. Intestinal obstruction is relatively uncommon, but it can present in a similar manner to a Richter's hernia or with strangulation and obstruction of the small bowel, especially when the ileum becomes twisted around the hernia neck (Payson et al 1956).

Diverticulitis and perforation

The percentage incidence of acute inflammation in a Meckel's diverticulum is much lower than in the appendix. This is because Meckel's diverticula are usually wide-mouthed (Fig. 13.10), contain little lymphoid tissue and are self-emptying (Rutherford & Akers 1966). When diverticulitis does occur it is usually the result of neck obstruction due to oedema, enteroliths, tumours, foreign bodies or ectopic mucosa (Boothroyd 1967). Most patients present with signs and symptoms indistinguishable from those of acute appendicitis, although the actual tenderness may be more central (Williams 1981), and an occasional clue is cellulitis of the umbilicus. Chronic diverticulitis is uncommon, but tuberculosis and Crohn's disease have been reported (Solomons & Halford 1964, Quint 1986).

Diverticulitis is commonly complicated by perforation (Fig. 13.11), fistulation to adjacent intestine or acute peridiverticulitis (Mackey & Dineen 1983). Perforation however may also be precipitated per se by enteroliths, foreign bodies (especially fish bones) (Rosswick 1965) or peptic ulceration related to ectopic gastric mucosa.

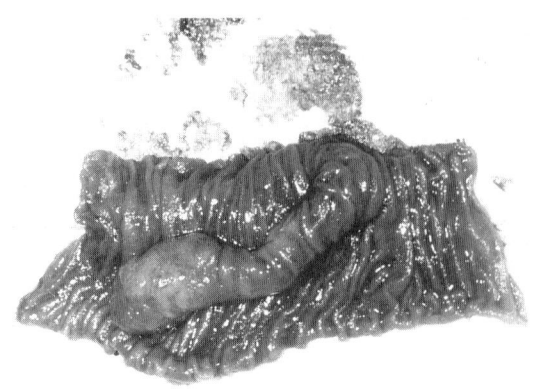

Fig. 13.9   An intussuscepted Meckel's diverticulum.

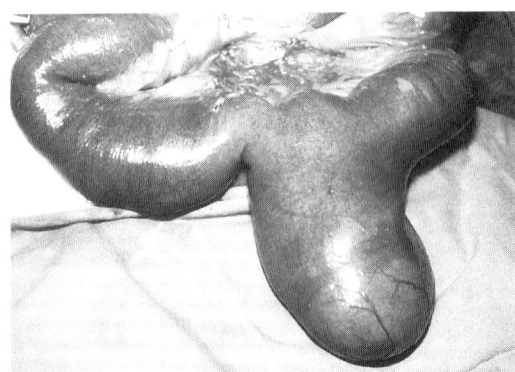

Fig. 13.10   A wide-mouthed Meckel's diverticulum.

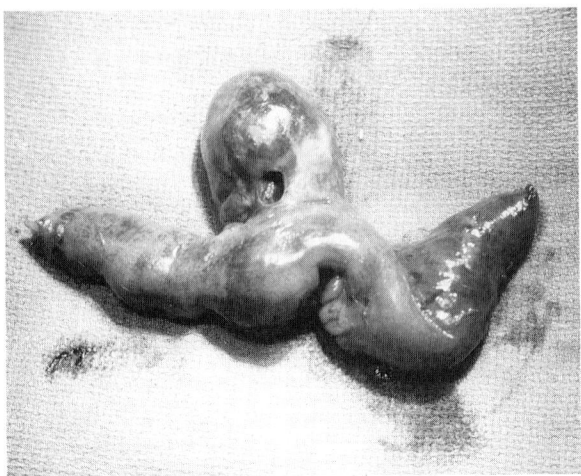

Fig. 13.11 A perforated Meckel's diverticulum. (Reproduced by kind permission of the publishers of the *World Journal of Surgery*)

Haemorrhage

About 25% of patients with symptomatic Meckel's diverticula present with lower gastrointestinal haemorrhage (Mackey & Dineen 1983), usually as a result of peptic ulceration of the ileal mucosa associated with acid secretion from ectopic gastric epithelium. It is the most common cause of severe intestinal bleeding in childhood, and 50% of patients presenting in this way are under 2 years of age. The severity of bleeding can range from chronic occult blood loss (Williamson et al 1984) to passage of large amounts of bright red blood per rectum (Mackey & Dineen 1983). Indeed the bleeding can be so severe that intestinal obstruction secondary to intraluminal thrombus has been reported (Neuss et al 1986). Usually the blood is mixed in with the stool and is dark or bright red; melaena is uncommon. A previous history of a gastrointestinal bleed is elicited in 40% of patients, but in some the initial bleed may be so brisk that they rapidly exsanguinate. Early diagnosis is therefore essential (Long 1986).

Neoplasia

Tumours are uncommon in Meckel's diverticulum, being reported in only 2% of cases (Williams 1981). They may be the same pathologi-cal types as those occurring in the rest of the small bowel or may arise in ectopic mucosal elements in the diverticulum. Malignant tumours are three times as common as benign tumours and are more commonly symptomatic. Such tumours may initiate intussusception (Lie 1966) or volvulus (Niv et al 1986, Sayfan et al 1985) and occasionally can be dual (Traill 1968). The majority are incidental findings at autopsy or laparotomy (Jones et al 1972) and often require careful palpation of the diverticulum to be detected.

Carcinoids of Meckel's diverticulum are usually small (<10 mm) (Weitzner 1969). They are four times more common in men, occurring at a mean age of 55 years (Weitzner 1969, Jones et al 1972, Payne-James et al 1985). They rarely metastasize or produce the carcinoid syndrome, but when they do they can cause intestinal ischaemia due to vascular elastosis produced by the metastatic state (Palvio et al 1985). Other tumours reported include leiomyoma (Hertzog et al 1985, Blamey & Woods 1986), leiomyosarcoma (Niv et al 1986, Saadia & Decker 1986), malignant melanoma (Bloch et al 1986) and neurovascular hamartoma (Stewart 1985).

Miscellaneous

Patients with a Meckel's diverticulum may also present with complications related to a patent omphalomesenteric duct (Fig. 13.12). This may manifest itself in the newborn with a mucoid, purulent or enteric discharge and excoriation around the umbilicus. Although this is usually seen in infants (Mackey & Dineen 1983), it may present late in adults as recurrent cellulitis or a deep-seated abdominal wall abscess representing an infected enterocystoma. A Meckel's diverticulum may also be associated with overt exomphalos (Simms & Corkery 1980). Malabsorption is uncommon in association with a Meckel's diverticulum, but when it does occur, the mechanism is the same as is seen and described for jejunal diverticulosis.

Investigation

Plain abdominal radiographs are rarely of any

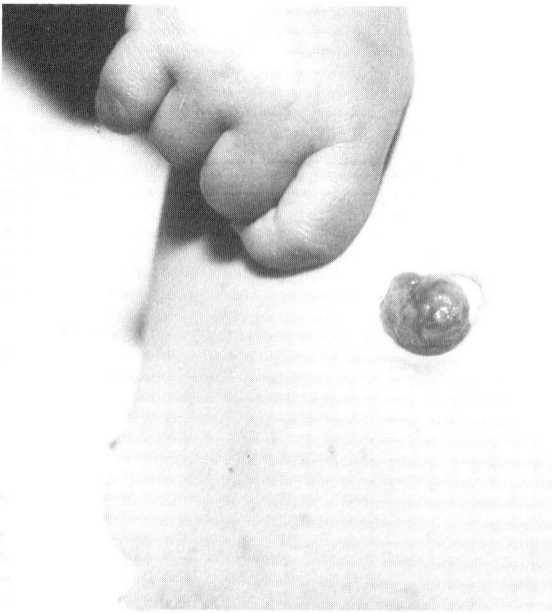

principally from urinary tract obstruction, angiomas, or leiomyomas (Petrokubi et al 1978, Hertzog et al 1985). However, it carries a sensitivity of 85%, a specificity of 95% and a 90% accuracy for detecting ectopic gastric mucosa in a bleeding Meckel's diverticulum (Sfakianakis & Conway 1981).

A Meckel's diverticulum containing gastric

Fig. 13.12   A patent omphalomesenteric duct in an infant manifesting itself as a fistula at the umbilicus. (Reproduced by kind permission of the publishers of *Hospital Update*)

value in the diagnosis of a Meckel's diverticulum, apart from confirming the presence of intestinal obstruction. They are also rarely seen on routine barium studies, only about 1–2% presenting as an incidental finding on follow-through examinations. This is usually because overlying barium-filled loops of bowel prevent an adequate view (Hall 1975). However when intussusception has occurred, a filling defect may be observed (Williamson et al 1984). Superior mesenteric angiography may be successful in diagnosing a bleeding diverticulum (Faris & Whitley 1973, Hall 1975) by demonstrating extravasation or a blush, although the latter finding may be misinterpreted as a leiomyoma (Williamson et al 1984).

In 1970 scintigraphic techniques were introduced to demonstrate a Meckel's diverticulum (Jewett et al 1970). This technique uses ^{99m}Tc pertechnetate to demonstrate the ectopic gastric mucosa that is commonly present in these diverticula. The pertechnetate anion is selectively taken up and excreted into the lumen of the diverticulum by the mucoid cells that line the surface of gastric mucosa (Sfakianakis & Haase 1982). The technique can produce false negative results (Feuerstein et al 1985) or false positive results,

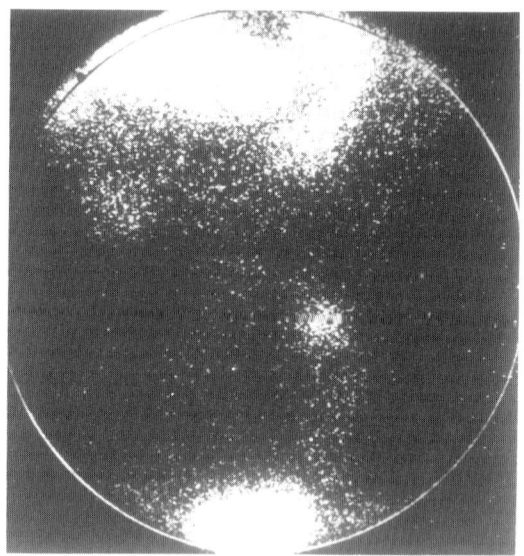

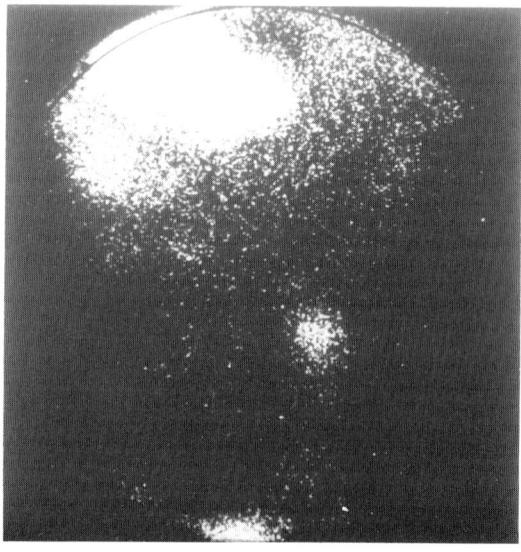

Fig. 13.13   Technetium scan showing activity in the mid-abdomen associated with a Meckel's diverticulum. (Reproduced by kind permission of the publishers of the *World Journal of Surgery*)

mucosa will show up as a 'hot spot' on a technetium scan in the lower abdomen (Fig. 13.13) often to the right of the midline (Jewett et al 1970), and technical improvements have made this the investigation of choice for detecting a Meckel's diverticulum (Petrokubi et al 1978). It is simple, non-invasive and an ideal screening test for patients of all ages, especially for those who are bleeding from an unknown source (Winzelberg 1983).

Treatment

Considerable controversy has existed over what should be done about the asymptomatic Meckel's diverticulum found incidentally at laparotomy. Many surgeons have advocated routine excision (Dowse 1961, Michas et al 1975), but a survey of British surgeons showed that there was no consensus view (Lang-Stevenson 1983). As over 75% of Meckel's diverticula reported are incidental findings, there is a great need for surgical guidelines (*Lancet* 1983).

In a comprehensive study of the risk factors associated with Meckel's diverticulum, Soltero & Bill (1976) predicted that the risk of complications developing in a Meckel's diverticulum was 4.2% in infancy, 3.0% in adulthood, and zero over 75 years of age. They then assumed a possibly excessive mortality rate of 6% from operation for excision of a complicated diverticulum (Benson & Linkner 1956), as opposed to 0% for an incidental diverticulectomy (Soderlund 1959), and calculated that it would be necessary to remove 800 uncomplicated Meckel's diverticula to prevent one death.

Some workers have sought to define diverticula at risk. Such risk factors may include bands, ectopic tissue, tumours, enteroliths and narrow-necked diverticula. Other surgeons base their management on the age of the patient.

Therefore a working policy may suggest that diverticulectomy should be considered for any diverticulum with the above risk factors or found incidentally in a young child. However in an adult, a wide-mouthed diverticulum with no band or palpable ectopic tissue may be left alone.

When complications occur, diverticulectomy is required along with any associated band. Acute bleeding from ectopic gastric mucosa may occasionally be controlled by H2 receptor antagonists, allowing elective resection rather than emergency surgery, but this is uncommon. When excising a Meckel's diverticulum, ligation–excision and invagination of the stump as in an appendicectomy are not advised as the neck is usually too wide (Fig. 13.10) and can initiate an intussusception (Dowse 1961). Simple excision by clamping the diverticulum in the transverse or oblique axis of the ileum and then closing the defect in layers is adequate in most cases, taking care to ligate and divide the diverticular artery coming from the ileal mesentery. However for wide-based diverticula, cases of acute diverticulitis with adjacent ileal inflammation, or tumours, formal ileal resection is required.

Appendicitis remains the commonest preoperative diagnosis for a complicated Meckel's diverticulum (Williams 1981). It is therefore important in cases in which a normal appendix is encountered to seek and remove any small bowel diverticulum that may be responsible for the presenting symptoms. As Meckel's diverticula have been reported up to 180 cm from the ileocaecal valve (Weinstein et al 1962), the common practice of examining the distal 80 cm or so of terminal ileum is inadequate. However when acute appendicitis is found, no such search should be made, as this may disseminate infection, and the co-existence of acute appendicitis and Meckel's diverticulitis is exceedingly rare (Moore & Johnston 1976).

REFERENCES

Ackerman W 1943 Diverticula and variations of the duodenum. Annals of Surgery 117: 403–413

Adams D B 1986 Management of the intraluminal duodenal diverticulum: endoscopy or duodenotomy. American Journal of Surgery 151: 524–526

Alavi A 1982 Detection of gastrointestinal bleeding with 99m Tc sulphur colloid. Seminars in Nuclear Medicine 12: 126–138

Albibi R, McCallum R W 1983 Metoclopramide: pharmacology and clinical applications. Annals of Internal Medicine 98: 86–95

Altemeier W A, Bryant L R, Wulsin J H 1963 The surgical

significance of jejunal diverticulosis. Archives of Surgery
86: 732–741

Artigas V, Calabuig R, Badia F et al 1986 Meckel's
diverticulum: value of ectopic tissue. American Journal of
Surgery 151: 631–634

Babcock T, Hutton J, Salander J 1976 Perforated jejunal
diverticulitis. American Surgeon 42: 568–571

Balint J A, Sarfeh I J, Fried M B 1977 Gastrointestinal
bleeding: Diagnosis and management. J. Wiley, New
York, pp 31–41

Barr H 1986 Meckel's diverticulum. British Journal of
Clinical Practice 40: 301–302

Baskin R H, Mayo C W 1952 Jejunal diverticulosis: a
clinical study of 87 cases. Surgical Clinics of North
America 32: 1185–1196

Beech R R, Friesen D L, Shield C F 1985 Perforated
duodenal diverticulum: treatment by tube duodenostomy.
Current Surgery 42: 462–465

Benson C D, Linkner L M 1956 The surgical complications
of Meckel's diverticulum in infants and children. Archives
of Surgery 73: 393–398

Best E B, Teaford K A, Rader F E 1979 Angiography in
chronic recurrent gstrointestinal bleeding: a nine year
study. Surgical Clinics of North America 59: 811–829

Bewes P C 1967 Surgical complications of jejunal
diverticulosis. Proceedings of the Royal Society of
Medicine 60: 225–226

Blamey S L, Woods S D 1986 Leiomyoma of Meckel's
diverticulum. Medical Journal of Australia 145: 232–234

Bloch T, Tejada E, Brodhecker C 1986 Malignant
melanoma in Meckel's diverticulum. American Journal of
Clinical Pathology 86: 231–234

Boothroyd L S A 1967 The odd Meckel's diverticulum.
Canadian Medical Association Journal 96: 45–49

Boyd R 1845 Description of malformation of the duodenum.
Lancet i: 648

Brown M W, Brown R C, Orr G 1986 Pneumoperitoneum
complicating endoscopy in a patient with duodenal and
jejunal diverticula. Gastrointestinal Endoscopy 32: 120–121

Brown R J, Thompson R L 1985 Perforated jejunal
diverticulum presenting with a psoas abscess. Ulster
Medical Journal 54: 78–79

Caplan H H, Jacobson H G 1964 Small intestine
diverticulosis. American Journal of Roentgenology
92: 1048–1060

Case J T 1920 Diverticula of the small intestine other than
Meckel's diverticulum. Journal of the American Medical
Association 75: 1463–1470

Christiansen M 1969 Jejunal diverticulosis. American
Journal of Surgery 118: 612–618

Christie A 1931 Meckel's diverticulum: a pathological study
of 63 cases. American Journal of Diseases of Children
42: 544–557

Clarke P J, Kettlewell M G W 1985 Small bowel obstruction
due to an enterolith originating in a jejnunal diverticulum.
Postgraduate Journal of Medicine 61: 1019–1020

Cocks J R, Zinco F J 1968 Acute diverticulitis of the
terminal ileum. British Journal of Surgery 55: 45–49

Cooke W T, Cox E V, Fone D J et al 1963 The clinical and
metabolic significance of jejunal diverticula. Gut 4: 115–117

Critchlow J F, Shapiro M E, Silen W 1985
Duodenojejunostomy for the pancreaticobiliary
complications of duodenal diverticula. Annals of Surgery
202: 56–58

Debartolo H M, Vanheerden J A 1976 Meckel's

diverticulum. Annals of Surgery 180: 30–33

Donald J W 1979 Major complications of small bowel
diverticula. Annals of Surgery 190: 183–188

Dowse J L 1961 Meckel's diverticulum. British Journal of
Surgery 48: 392–399

Drasar B S, Hill M J 1974 Human intestinal flora.
Academic Press, London.

Dunn Y, Nelson J A 1979 Jejunal diverticula and chronic
pneumo-peritoneum. Gastrointestinal Radiology
4: 165–168

Eckhauser F E, Zelenok G B, Freider D T 1979 Acute
complications of jejuno-ileal pseudo-diverticulosis: surgical
implications and management. American Journal of
Surgery 138: 320–323

Edwards H C 1954 Intestinal diverticulosis and diverticulitis.
Annals of the Royal College of Surgeons of England
14: 371–388

Fanucci I E, Andreoli A, Davoli M et al 1985 A rare
complication of duodenal diverticulum — phytobezoar.
Radiologia Medica 71: 784–785

Faris J G, Whitley J C 1973 Angiographic demonstration of
Meckel's diverticulum: case report and review of
literature. Radiology 108: 285–286

Feuerstein I M, Mukherji S K, Leftridge C A et al 1985
False negative delayed imaging in Meckel's diverticulum.
Clinical Nuclear Medicine 10: 889–890

Fleming C R, Newcomer A D, Stephens D H et al 1975
Intraluminal duodenal diverticulum. Report of two cases
and review of the literature. Mayo Clinic Proceedings
50: 244–248

Geroulakis G 1987 Surgical problems of jejunal
diverticulosis. Annals of the Royal College of Surgeons of
England 69: 266–268

Goldstein F, Cozzolino H J, Wirts C W 1963 Diarrhoea
and steatorrhoea due to a large solitary duodenal
diverticulum. Report of a case. American Journal of
Digestive Diseases 8: 937–943

Gorbach S L, Levitan R 1970 Intestinal flora in health and
in gastrointestinal disease. In: Glass G B J (ed) Progress in
gastroenterology Vol II Grune & Stratton, New York

Gorbach S L, Tabaqchali S 1969 Bacteria, bile and the
small bowel. Gut 10: 963–972

Gracey M 1971 Intestinal absorption in the 'contaminated
small bowel' syndrome. Gut 12: 403–410

Gross R E 1953 The surgery of infancy and childhood.
Saunders, Philadelphia

Hajiro K, Yamamoto H, Matsui H et al 1979 Endoscopic
diagnosis and excision of intraluminal duodenal
diverticulum. Gastrointestinal Endoscopy 25: 151–154

Hall T J 1975 Meckel's bleeding diverticulum diagnosed by
mesenteric arteriography. British Journal of Surgery
62: 882–884

Harkins H H 1933 Intussusception due to invaginated
Meckel's diverticulum: report of two cases with a study of
160 cases collected from the literature. Annals of Surgery
98: 1070–1095

Herrington J L 1962 Perforation of acquired diverticula of
jejunum and ileum. Surgery 51: 426–433

Hertzog M S, Chacko A K, Pitts C M 1985 Leiomyoma of
terminal ileum producing false positive Meckel's scan.
Journal of Nuclear Medicine 26: 1278–1282

Hirsch F, Halet W, Piront A 1964 Diverticule interne du
duodénum: forme de duplication. Archives des Maladies
de l'Appareil Digestif 53: 839–844

Howard J M, Wynn O B, Lenhart F M et al 1986

Intraluminal duodenal diverticulum: an unusual cause of acute pancreatitis. American Journal of Surgery 151: 505–508

Jaffe B F, Youker J E, Margoulis A R 1965 Aortographic localisation of controlled gastrointestinal haemorrhage in dogs. Surgery 58: 984–988

Jay G D, Margulis R R, McGraw A R et al 1950 Meckel's diverticulum; a survey of 109 cases. Archives of Surgery 61: 158–169

Jewett T C, Duszynski D O, Allen J E 1970 The visualisation of Meckel's diverticulum with 99m Tc pertechnetate. Surgery 68: 467–470

Johns T N P, Wheeler J R, Johns F S 1959 Meckel's diverticulum and Meckel's diverticular disease. Annals of Surgery 150: 241–256

Jones E L, Thompson H, Alexander Williams J 1972 Argentaffin tumour of Meckel's diverticulum. A report of 2 cases and review of the literature. British Journal of Surgery 59: 213–219

Jones P F 1974 Jejunal and ileal diverticula In: Emergency abdominal surgery. Blackwell, Oxford, pp 550–552

Juler G L, List J W, Stemmer E A et al 1969 Perforating duodenal diverticulitis. Archives of Surgery 99: 572–578

Kaftori J K, Munk J, Schramek A 1966 Intraluminal diverticulum of the duodenum demonstrated by intravenous cholangiography. British Journal of Radiology 39: 388–390

King P M, Bird D R, Eremin O 1985 Enterolith obstruction of the small bowel. Journal of the Royal College of Surgeons of Edinburgh 30: 269–270

Kittle C F, Jenkins H P, Dragstedt L R 1947 Patent omphalomesenteric duct and its relation to the diverticulum of Meckel. Archives of Surgery 54: 10–31

Knaver M, Svoboda A 1968 Malabsorption and jejunal diverticulosis. American Journal of Medicine 44: 606–610

Krishnamurthy S, Kelly M M, Rohrman C A et al 1983 Jejunal diverticulosis. Gastroenterology 85: 538–547

Lancet 1983 Meckel's diverticulum. Surgical guidelines at last? (editorial) Lancet ii: 438–439

Lang-Stevenson A 1983 Meckel's diverticulum: To look or not to look: To resect or not to resect. Annals of the Royal College of Surgeons of England 65: 218–220

Leinkram C, Roberts-Thompson I C, Kune G A 1980 Juxtapapillary duodenal diverticula: association with gallstones and pancreatitis. Medical Journal of Australia 1: 209–210

Lie J T 1966 Leiomyosarcoma of Meckel's diverticulum. British Journal of Surgery 53: 336–339

Long B W 1986 Early diagnosis and management of bleeding Meckel's diverticulum. Journal of the Mississipi State Medical Association 27: 149–154

Lotveit T, Osnes M, Larsen S 1982 Recurrent biliary calculi — duodenal diverticulum as a predisposing factor. Annals of Surgery 196: 30–32

McGrew V, Patel J, Miller P 1985 Jejunal diverticulosis: medical and surgical management. South African Medical Journal 78: 533–535

Mackey W C, Dineen P 1983 A fifty year experience with Meckel's diverticulum. Surgery Gynecology and Obstetrics 156: 56–64

Madura M J, Craig R M 1981 Duodenal and jejunal diverticula causing a pneumo-peritoneum. Journal of Clinical Gastroenterology 3: 61–63

Maglinte D D T, Hall R, Miller R E et al 1984 Detection of surgical lesions of the small bowel by enteroclysis.

American Journal of Surgery 147: 225–229

Maglinte D D T, Chernish S M, Deweese R et al 1986 Acquired jejuno-ileal diverticular disease; subject review. Radiology 158: 577–580

Manny J, Muga M, Eyal Z 1981 The continuing clinical enigma of duodenal diverticula. American Journal of Surgery 142: 596–600

Mathieu B, Salducci J, Remacle J P et al 1978 Intraluminal duodenal diverticulum; report of a case investigated by fiberoptic endoscopy. American Journal of Digestive Diseases 23: 1

Mayo C W 1933 Meckel's diverticulum. Proceedings of the Mayo Clinic 8: 230

Meckel J F 1809 Über das Divertikel am Darmkanal. Archives of Physiology 9: 421–453

Michas C A, Cohen S E, Wolfman E F 1975 Meckel's diverticulum. American Journal of Surgery 129: 682–685

Moore T, Johnston A O B 1976 Complications of Meckel's diverticulum. British Journal of Surgery 63: 453–454

Moran K T, Flynn J R, McCormack M 1985 Unusual presentation of a stone in a Meckel's diverticulum in association with acute appendicitis. Irish Medical Journal 78: 320–321

Munnell E R, Preston W J 1966 Complications of duodenal diverticula. Archives of Surgery 92: 152–156

Murray-Lyon I M, Finlayson N D C, Shearman D J C 1968 Studies on two patients with concomitant intrinsic factor secretory defect and jejunal diverticulosis. Scandinavian Journal of Haematology 5: 383–389

Neill S A, Thompson N W 1965 The complications of duodenal diverticula and their management. Surgery Gynecology and Obstetrics 120: 1251–1258

Neuss M N, Garbutt J T, Leight G S et al 1986 Intraluminal thrombus and bowel obstruction in acute leukemia due to bleeding Meckel's diverticulum. American Journal of Medicine 80: 1194–1196

Niv Y, Abu-Avid S, Kopelman C et al 1986 Torsion of leiomyosarcoma of Meckel's diverticulum. American Journal of Gastroenterology 81: 288–291

Nobles E R 1971 Jejunal diverticula. Archives of Surgery 102: 172–174

Ottinger L W, Carter E L 1975 Obstruction of the ileum by a jejunal diverticular enterolith. Gastroenterology 68: 1596–1597

Palvio D H, Kristensen E S, Falk E 1985 Intestinal ischaemia due to vascular elastosis caused by metastasizing carcinoid tumour of Meckel's diverticulum. Diseases of Colon and Rectum 28: 746–748

Parulekar S G 1972 Diverticulum of terminal ileum and its complications. Radiology 103: 283–287

Payne-James J J, Law N W, Watkins R M 1985 Carcinoid tumour arising in Meckel's diverticulum. Postgraduate Medical Journal 61: 1009–1011

Payson B A, Schneider K M, Victor M B 1956 Strangulation of a Meckel's diverticulum in a femoral hernia (Littré's). Annals of Surgery 144: 277–281

Petrokubi R J, Baum S, Rohrer G U 1978 Cimetidine administration resulting in improved pertechnetate imaging of Meckel's diverticulum. Clinical Nuclear Medicine 3: 385–388

Phillips J H C 1953 Jejunal diverticulitis. Some clinical aspects. British Journal of Surgery 40: 350–354

Quint K M 1986 Primary Crohn's disease of a Meckel's diverticulum. Journal of Clinical Gastroenterology 8: 187–188

Rankin F W, Martin W J 1934 Diverticular of the small bowel. Annals of Surgery 100: 1123–1135

Rhodes I M, Middleton P, Jewell D P 1979 The lactulose hydrogen breath test as a diagnostic test for small bowel bacterial overgrowth. Scandinavian Journal of Gastroenterology 14: 333–336

Rosedale R S, Lawrence H R 1936 Jejuno-ileal diverticulosis. American Journal of Surgery 34: 369–373

Rosswick R P 1965 Perforation of Meckel's diverticulum by foreign body. Postgraduate Medical Journal 41: 105–107

Rutherford R B, Akers D R 1966 Meckel's diverticulum — a review of 148 paediatric patients with special reference to the pattern of bleeding and to mesodiverticular bands. Surgery 59: 618–626

Saadia R, Decker G A 1986 Leiomyosarcoma of Meckel's diverticulum: a case report and review of the literature. Journal of Surgical Oncology 32: 86–88

Salomonowitz E, Wittich G, Hajek P et al 1983 Detection of intestinal diverticula by double contrast small bowel enema: differentiation from other intestinal diverticula. Gastrointestinal Radiology 8: 271–278

Sayfan J, Borowsky A, Halevy A, et al 1985 Volvulus due to a tumour of Meckel's diverticulum. Journal of Clinical Gastroenterology 7: 314–317

Schuffler M D, Rohrmann C A, Chaffe R A et al 1981 Chronic intestinal pseudo-obstruction. Medicine 60: 173–190

Seagram C G F, Louch R E, Stephens A et al 1968 Meckel's diverticulum: a 10 year review of 218 cases. Canadian Journal of Surgery 2: 369–373

Sfakianakis G N, Conway J J 1981 Detection of ectopic gastric mucosa in Meckel's diverticulum and in other aberrations by scintigraphy. II. Indications and methods — a 10 year experience. Journal of Nuclear Medicine 22: 732–738

Sfakianakis G N, Haase G M 1982 Abdominal scintigraphy for ectopic gastric mucosa: a retrospective analysis of 143 studies. American Journal of Radiology 138: 7–12

Shackelford R T, Marcus W Y 1960 Jejunal diverticula — a cause of gastrointestinal haemorrhage. A report of three cases and review of the literature. Annals of Surgery 151: 930–938

Shinya H, McSherry C 1982 Endoscopy of the small bowel. Surgical Clinics of North America 62: 821–824

Silcock A Q 1885 Epithelioma of ascending colon, entero-colitis, and congenital duodenal septum with internal diverticulum. Transcripts of the Pathological Society of London 36: 207

Simms M H, Corkery J J 1980 Meckel's diverticulum: Its association with congenital malformation and the significance of atypical morphology. British Journal of Surgery 67: 216–219

Smith J S 1976 Jejunal diverticula — subtle cause of acute abdomen. Pennsylvania Medicine 79: 60–63

Soderlund S 1959 Meckel's diverticulum: a clinical and histological study. Acta Chirurgica Scandinavica 248: 1–233

Solomons D, Halford M E H 1964 Crohn's disease of Meckel's diverticulum occurring in a case of jejunal diverticulosis. British Journal of Surgery 51: 910–913

Soltero M J, Bill A H 1976 The natural history of Meckel's diverticulum and the relation to incidental removal. American Journal of Surgery 132: 168–171

Sonnenfeld T, Alveryd A, Nyberg B 1986 Jejunal diverticula causing massive haemorrhage. Acta Chirurgica Scandinavica 530: 101–102

Soofi R, Abouchedid C 1986 Intussusception of small bowel secondary to jejunal diverticulosis. New England Journal of Medicine 83: 309–312

Stebbings W S L, Thompson J P S 1985 Perforated duodenal diverticulum: a report of two cases. Postgraduate Medical Journal 61: 839–840

Stewart I C 1985 Neurovascular hamartoma in a Meckel's diverticulum. British Journal of Clinical Practice 39: 411–412

Svanes K, Halvorsen J F 1975 Enterolith obstruction of the ileum as a complication of jejunal diverticulosis. Acta Chirurgica Scandinavica 141: 816–819

Tabaqchali S, Booth C C 1970 Bacteria and the small intestine. In: Card W I, Creane B (eds) Modern trends in gastroenterology Vol 4. Butterworths, London, p. 143

Taylor M T 1969 Massive haemorrhage from jejunal diverticula. American Journal of Surgery 118: 117–129

Thomas C S, Tinsley E A, Brockman S K 1967 Jejunal diverticula as a source of massive upper gastrointestinal bleeding. Archives of Surgery 95: 89–92

Thomas W E G, Williamson R C N 1985a Non-specific small bowel ulceration. Postgraduate Medical Journal 61: 587–591

Thomas W E G, Williamson R C N 1985b Enteric ulceration and its complications. World Journal of Surgery 9: 876–886

Traill M A 1968 Dual carcinoids in a Meckel's diverticulum. Medical Journal of Australia 2: 67–68

Weinstein E C, Cain J C, Remine W M 1962 Meckel's diverticulum. Journal of the American Medical Association 182: 251–253

Weitzner S 1969 Carcinoid of Meckel's diverticulum. Report of a case and review of the literature. Cancer 23: 1436–1440

Wells H R 1967 Massive bleeding from jejunal diverticula. American Surgeon 33: 663–665

Welsh R I H 1966 Jejunal diverticula. Journal of the Royal College of Surgeons of Edinburgh 11: 232–234

Wilk P J, Mollura J, Danese C A 1973 Jaundice and pancreatitis caused by duodenal diverticulum. American Journal of Gastroenterology 60: 273–279

Williams R S 1981 Management of Meckel's diverticulum. British Journal of Surgery 68: 477–480

Williamson R C N, Cooper M J, Thomas W E G 1984 Intussusception of invaginated Meckel's diverticulum. Journal of the Royal Society of Medicine 77: 652–655

Winzelberg G G 1983 Scintigraphic detection of gastrointestinal bleeding: a review of current methods. American Journal of Gastroenterology 78: 324–327

Winzelberg G G, McKusick K A, Froelich J W et al 1982 Detection of gastrointestinal bleeding with 99m Tc labelled red blood cells. Seminars in Nuclear Medicine 12: 139–146

Wolfe R D, Pearl M J 1972 Acute perforation of duodenal diverticulum with roentgenographic demonstration of localised retroperitoneal emphysema. Radiology 104: 301–302

Yamaguchi M, Takeuchi S, Awazu S 1978 Meckel's diverticulum. Investigation of 600 patients in Japanese literature. American Journal of Surgery 136: 247–249

14 *Colonic perforation*

D. J. SCHOETZ, JR.

Perforation of the colon or rectum represents a potentially lethal condition, and despite the various causes of colorectal perforation, death usually results from sepsis caused by the egress of colorectal contents through the bowel perforation. Because approximately half of the dry weight of stool is bacteria, both aerobic and anaerobic microbial infectious complications represent the major cause of morbidity and mortality after this event.

Diverse disease processes may result in perforation of either the colon or rectum, for example, inflammatory processes: diverticulitis, ulcerative colitis, and Crohn's disease; malignant and benign tumours; vascular processes, such as ischaemic colitis; mechanical processes: volvulus, obstruction, pseudo-obstruction, or stercoral and iatrogenic injuries; and penetrating or blunt trauma or trauma caused by foreign bodies. Management is dictated in part by whether the site of perforation is the primary disease process or the colon proximal to an obstructing lesion. In some instances, perforation affects bowel that was healthy until the penetrating event occurred, as in trauma and iatrogenic injuries. This factor also enters into evaluation of potential therapeutic options.

The ultimate resolution of the perforation is also affected by the anatomical site of the lesion. Intra-abdominal colonic perforation is accompanied by localized or generalized peritonitis with the subsequent potential risk of intra-abdominal abscess. Rectal perforation, on the other hand, presents a different challenge: because of the extraperitoneal position of the rectum, sepsis is confined to the perirectal and retroperitoneal spaces. The relative inaccessibility of the rectum to surgical repair necessitates an indirect approach to rectal injuries in many patients.

Because the goal of treating patients with colorectal perforation is to control infection and prevent continued bacterial contamination regardless of primary disease process, basic principles must be adhered to in all instances. Before the specific causes and management of patients with colorectal perforation are reviewed, these basic principles will be discussed.

Basic principles of management

Assessment

Most often colorectal perforation represents an acute event that was not anticipated. Initial evaluation of the patient should include a comprehensive history, whenever possible, to elucidate the potential cause. Physical examination must be tailored to the situation but should include a thorough abdominal and digital rectal examination. Laboratory investigations are those that assist in preparation of the patient for emergency operation and should include haematocrit, white blood cell count, serum electrolytes, and assessment of renal function. Liver function tests may help in formulating a differential diagnosis but, for the most part, will not alter the initial approach to the patient. Radiographic examinations should, in most instances, be kept simple; they will serve as a baseline for postoperative management more than assist in decisions regarding the advisability of operation.

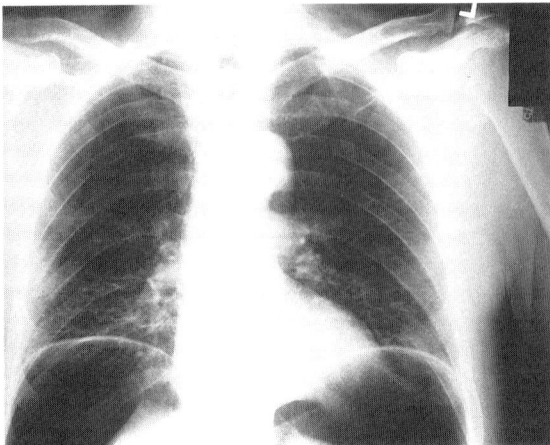

Fig. 14.1 Massive pneumoperitoneum caused by colonic perforation.

Chest radiography with the patient upright may show pneumoperitoneum (Fig. 14.1), and plain radiographs of the abdomen may demonstrate air in the perirectal planes when rectal perforation is present. Furthermore, in colonic obstruction, plain films of the abdomen are utilized to

demonstrate caecal size (Fig. 14.2), which may require intervention to prevent colonic perforation. Contrast radiography and other methods of diagnostic imaging may be appropriate in selected instances as determined by the clinical setting. Finally, electrocardiography should be performed in all patients undergoing abdominal exploration.

Peritonitis

Peritonitis presents an enormous physiological insult that requires vigorous attempts to optimize the patient's physiological status before, during, and after operation. Vigorous fluid replacement with both crystalloid and colloid solutions is necessitated by the outpouring of fluids from the inflamed peritoneal surface as well as by the accompanying sequestration of fluid in the small bowel affected by paralytic ileus. Adequate fluid replacement is indicated by a stable cardiovascular system and satisfactory urine output. Associated electrolyte abnormalities should be corrected; however, operation should not be delayed excessively because of inconsequential alterations in serum electrolytes. Cardiovascular collapse may result from the combination of sepsis and hypovolaemia, and haemodynamic problems may be compounded by pre-existing diseases of the cardiovascular system. Aggressive haemodynamic monitoring using a Swan-Ganz catheter and appropriate pharmacological support with vasopressors in the perioperative period will be required in some instances.

Nasogastric intubation is a traditional adjunct to the management of patients with intestinal perforation, and in colonic obstruction it will delay progressive colonic distension. It is unlikely that a nasogastric tube will be of appreciable benefit in patients undergoing emergency operation except to decompress the stomach of its contents before induction of anaesthesia. In most instances, the nasogastric tube can be removed during or shortly after the operation.

Perforation of the colon and rectum releases intestinal bacteria into the peritoneal cavity or perirectal tissues. Because of the acute nature of the event, it is rare to have had the opportunity to cleanse the colon mechanically before onset of

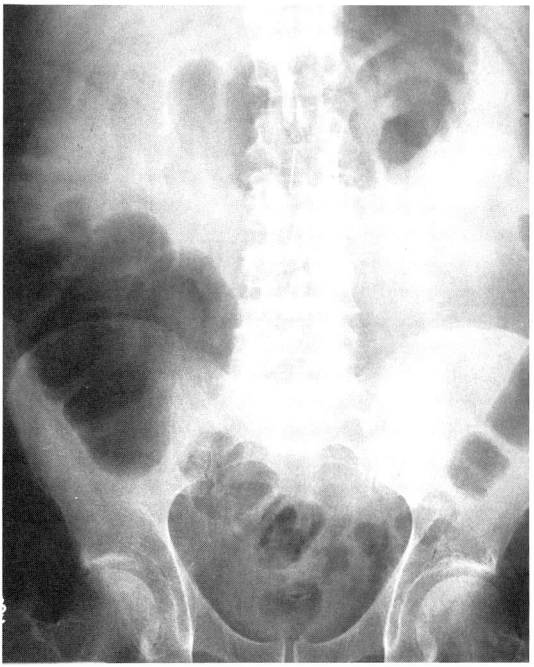

Fig. 14.2 Obstructing sigmoid neoplasm causing 140 mm caecal distension.

the condition. Consequently, broad-spectrum parenteral antibiotic coverage is mandatory once the diagnosis is suspected. Antibiotics should be directed at aerobic coliform bacteria as well as anaerobes (Hau et al 1979, Dunn & Simmons 1984). Current practice favours administration of an aminoglycoside and a specific antianaerobic agent, such as metronidazole or clindamycin. Duration of antibiotic therapy after operation remains controversial; in the presence of established bacterial infection, 7–10 ten days of antibiotic coverage are required.

During operation but after the technical aspects of the procedure have been concluded, copious peritoneal irrigation with saline solution should be performed to dilute the number of bacteria present. Earlier concerns that such a vigorous regimen might contaminate the peritoneal cavity are refuted by the demonstration that contaminated material will circulate throughout the entire peritoneal cavity even in the absence of such manouvres (Hau et al 1979). Drains should be reserved for specific indications, such as an already established abscess cavity or a prophylactic presacral drain for extraperitoneal rectal perforation. Skin wounds may be closed primarily, as long as the surgeon accepts the 30–40% incidence of wound infection that accompanies widely contaminated wounds; alternatively, the wound may be closed by delayed primary closure after 5–7 days or allowed to heal by secondary intention.

Causes and management of colonic perforation

Diverticulitis

Acquired colonic diverticular disease is an affliction of western civilization about which little was known before the 20th century. Pathologically, acquired diverticula are outpouchings of the mucosa of the colon into and ultimately through the colonic musculature. These diverticula almost universally affect the sigmoid colon with variable proximal extension of the disease. Furthermore, acute colonic complications are predominant in the sigmoid colon (Hackford & Veidenheimer 1985).

The cause of acquired diverticula is not known although it is speculated that a primary motility disorder aggravated by relative fibre deficiency results in herniation of the mucosa through anatomical weaknesses in the wall of the colon.

Diverticulitis represents an infectious complication resulting from inspissation of faecal material in the neck of the diverticulum with resultant bacterial proliferation. Consequently, acute diverticulitis is a pericolic infection. Complicated diverticulitis is represented by localized perforation with abscess, generalized peritonitis from uncontrolled perforation, or development of a fistula as a result of extension of an abscess into an adjacent organ. Diverticulitis is the most common cause of perforation of the colon. In a series by Eng and associates (1977), perforation with either generalized peritonitis or localized abscess was the indication for operation in 46 (73%) of 63 patients with diverticulitis.

Clearly, the extent of contamination varies from minimal, as found in a small pericolic abscess contained within the mesentery, to massive with free diffusing faecal peritonitis. The surgical approach must vary depending on the severity of the primary disease process as well as on the general condition of the patient. In fact, it is likely that many patients with small pericolic abscesses will not require surgery in the acute setting; rather, they will respond to bowel rest and parenteral antibiotics and the acute episode will resolve. On the other hand, persistent peritoneal soiling from either rupture of an abscess into the peritoneal cavity or uncontrolled perforation necessitates urgent operative intervention under the most adverse circumstances (Krukowski & Matheson 1984).

Historically, diverticulitis has been treated with multistage operative procedures, the first being the establishment of a proximal diverting colostomy and drainage of the associated pelvic infection (Smithwick 1942). Persistence of sepsis, despite this approach, resulted in the suggestion by Madden & Tan (1961) that the most appropriate management for a patient with perforated diverticulitis would include resection of the perforated segment at the time of initial operation. Since then, emphasis has increasingly been placed on primary resection.

Surgical techniques available for treatment of

patients with perforated diverticulitis are proximal colostomy with drainage or resection of primary disease followed by one of the following: Hartmann closure and end colostomy, end colostomy and mucous fistula, anastomosis with proximal colostomy, or primary anastomosis. Because of the frequent inability to exteriorize the distal segment, the option of end colostomy and mucous fistula is least often available.

In a series from the Lahey Clinic (Hackford et al 1985), complicated diverticulitis was treated by resection with primary anastomosis in 86/140 patients (61.4%). Primary resection represents a particularly attractive alternative in patients with localized pericolic abscesses and phlegmon in which the inflammatory process can be excised totally. In our experience, this operation was attended by a 1% mortality rate and an 18% morbidity rate. Resection with reanastomosis and proximal colostomy is the preferred approach for patients with extensive localized abscess. Finally, resection with performance of a Hartmann procedure or mucous fistula is the choice for patients with generalized peritonitis or purulent peritonitis resulting from rupture of the abscess. The cumulative mortality rate of patients treated with the classic three-stage procedure was 14% and the major morbidity rate was 24%, which compared unfavourably with both primary anastomosis and a two-stage approach.

Other authors (Auguste & Wise 1981, Rodkey & Welch 1984, Underwood & Marks 1984, Nagorney et al 1985) have supported resection of the diseased segment as critical in diminishing morbidity and mortality. Reanastomosis at the time of original resection should be dictated by the degree of peritoneal contamination (Auguste & Wise 1981). Advanced degrees of peritonitis are treated safely by delayed anastomosis, necessitating a two-stage approach.

Inflammatory bowel disease

Colonic perforation is observed in both acute ulcerative colitis and Crohn's colitis. In a series from Mt. Sinai Hospital (Greenstein & Aufses 1985), the incidence of perforation in ulcerative colitis was 4.7% compared with 2% in Crohn's disease.

Toxic dilatation of the colon preceded perforation in 36% of patients with ulcerative colitis whereas perforated colonic Crohn's disease was usually not associated with dilatation of the colon. Furthermore, free colonic perforation without distension has been observed repeatedly in patients with ulcerative colitis as well (Greenstein et al 1986).

A patient with toxic colitis (whether Crohn's disease or ulcerative colitis) typically presents with a relatively short history of inflammatory bowel disease. In fact, 2–5% of patients with toxic colitis present initially with this severe form of the disease. The hallmark of the clinical presentation is that of toxicity: fever, tachycardia, abdominal pain with or without tenderness, and leucocytosis. An abrupt alteration in bowel habits, most often with diminution in diarrhoea, may herald the onset of an episode of toxic colitis. In some instances, the patient has recently undergone a barium enema examination that resulted in clinical deterioration. With a distended abdomen, radiographic studies will usually reveal a dilated transverse colon. Abdominal examination at the time of presentation may also detect signs of peritonitis, indicating the need for urgent surgical intervention.

In the absence of peritonitis and radiographic evidence of pneumoperitoneum, the patient with toxic colitis should not initially be operated on. Fluid replacement, intravenously administered broad-spectrum antibiotics, and, when the diagnosis of colitis has previously been established, parenteral corticosteroids are initial therapeutic measures. Narcotics and antidiarrhoeal medications should be avoided because they may contribute to colonic ileus with progressive distension. If the diagnosis of colitis has not been established previously, proctoscopic examination and stool cultures with testing for amoeba should be performed before beginning corticosteroid therapy. Our policy has been not to perform colonoscopic decompression because of the risk of perforation.

When these emergency measures have been applied, frequent clinical examination (including measurement of pulse, blood pressure, and temperature) and abdominal examination remain the most important determinants of whether operative intervention is required. Repetitive plain film radiography of the abdomen may lull the physician into a false sense of security because clinical deterioration can occur in the absence of radiographic signs of progressive dilatation of the colon. When the patient's condition deteriorates or does not respond while under observation for 24–48 h, operation is obligatory to prevent colonic perforation.

Operative techniques

The preferred operative technique is the performance of abdominal colectomy with end ileostomy and either Hartmann closure of the rectal stump or a mucous fistula when the distal bowel is unable to be sutured or stapled safely. Although single-stage proctocolectomy has some appeal as the definitive operation at this point, the patient is usually systemically ill, and complications associated with proctocolectomy occur more often than after subtotal colectomy (Fazio 1980).

Another operative option that has been suggested (Turnbull et al 1971) is loop ileostomy and 'blow-hole' colostomy for sealed perforation of the colon observed at exploration. The impetus for the development of this procedure by Turnbull and associates was their observation that subtotal colectomy in this specific circumstance resulted in widespread faecal contamination of the peritoneal cavity, with increased mortality. The negative aspect of this operation is the persistence of the severely diseased colon in the peritoneal cavity after performance of the two stomas. In the Cleveland Clinic series (Turnbull et al 1971), the operative mortality rate from the decompression and diversion procedure was 7.8% in comparison with 11.5% after subtotal colectomy. However, some patients required reoperation during the same hospitalization period after decompression and diversion because of persistent toxicity. Careful surgical technique and broad-spectrum antibiotics should permit performance of subtotal colectomy with ileostomy in virtually all patients. Preservation of the rectum in patients with ulcerative colitis enables subsequent consideration of the ileoanal reservoir as well as an ileorectal anastomosis in patients with Crohn's disease.

Perforated colon carcinoma

Colonic perforation associated with carcinoma of the colon may occur under two circumstances. The first, and most common, is perforation occurring remote from the primary tumour as a result of obstruction with resultant proximal distension. In a review of previously published major series of perforated colon carcinoma by Sugarbaker (1981), the cumulative 5-year survival rate for free perforation proximal to an obstructing lesion was less than 35%. Less commonly, the perforation is at the site of the tumour itself, and, despite conceivably curative resection, the 5-year survival rate for this particular circumstance is even less than that for perforation resulting from obstruction, possibly because of peritoneal implantation of viable cancer cells from within the bowel at the time of perforation.

The survival rate for patients with localized perforation with pericolic abscess or contiguous organ involvement with formation of a fistula is not so bad. In the Lahey Clinic experience (de Leon et al 1987), as long as curative resection with en bloc resection of the involved adjacent organs was performed, the survival rate (adjusted for Dukes' stage) was equivalent to that for patients who did not have localized perforation or fistula. This finding agrees with other published series (Sugarbaker 1981).

When a carcinoma has perforated freely into the peritoneal cavity at the site of the tumour, the involved segment should be resected. Re-establishment of the integrity of the gastrointestinal tract should be performed for right-sided lesions at the original operation. Left-sided perforations and localized perforations should be managed in a manner similar to perforated diverticulitis as described previously.

Ischaemic colitis

Ischaemic colitis represents a spectrum of diseases ranging from reversible non-transmural mucosal ischaemia to gangrene with perforation. Boley et al (1978) estimated that gangrenous ischaemic colitis is present in approximately 15% of patients with ischaemic colitis; these patients present acutely as abdominal catastrophes and are most often operated on with a preoperative diagnosis of perforated diverticulitis. Classically, these are older people with a history of atherosclerotic and cardiac disease who present in circulatory collapse with either localized or generalized peritonitis. Unlike patients with the reversible form of the disease, which is characterized by crampy abdominal pain and bloody diarrhoea, most patients with gangrenous ischaemic colitis do not have a history of haematochezia. While the majority of patients have involvement of the region of the splenic flexure, the gangrenous segment may be anywhere in the colon, including the rectum. After appropriate procedures, the ischaemic segment is resected, usually with the construction of an end colostomy and either a mucous fistula or Hartmann procedure.

Persistent segmental ischaemic colitis, characterized by tenderness and bloody diarrhoea without definite evidence of perforation, may also be observed. In these instances, adequate preoperative mechanical preparation of the colon should permit segmental resection of the involved bowel with primary anastomosis.

Visceral angiography has not proved to be beneficial in the diagnosis of ischaemic colitis (Williams & Wittenberg 1975). When the diagnosis of ischaemic colitis is suspected, the appropriate investigations of the patient (based on clinical presentation and in the absence of peritoneal signs) are: flexible sigmoidoscopy to determine the distal extent of the ischaemic segment, and barium contrast radiography. Appropriate treatment in the initial stages of ischaemic colitis not associated with transmural necrosis is bowel rest and broad-spectrum antibiotics with careful clinical examination. Development of peritonitis requires operative intervention.

Mechanical perforation

Volvulus

Volvulus of the colon is an unusual disease that may be accompanied by colonic perforation. Sigmoid volvulus is the most common type, with caecal volvulus the second most common. Regard-

less of the site of the volvulus, the anatomical conditions necessary for its development are redundancy of the involved colonic segment with a relative lack of fixation and a narrow mesentery (Ballantyne 1982b).

Characteristically, the patient with sigmoid volvulus presents with left lower quadrant abdominal pain, abdominal distension, and obstipation. Similar episodes may have occurred previously. Abdominal examination reveals a distended tympanitic abdomen with variable degrees of tenderness. Flat plate radiography of the abdomen demonstrates the characteristic air-filled sigmoid colon extending toward the right upper quadrant with proximal colonic distension. Barium enema examination will confirm the diagnosis (Fig. 14.3). In the absence of peritoneal irritation, the initial approach to the patient should be non-operative, with an attempt made at sigmoidoscopic decompression of the sigmoid colon and insertion of a rectal tube. A collective review by Ballantyne (1982a) indicated successful sigmoidoscopic decompression in 75% of patients. Recently, the colonoscope has been used successfully to achieve acute decompression (Starling 1979). When endoscopic decompression fails, a hydrostatic barium enema study can successfully reduce the incidence

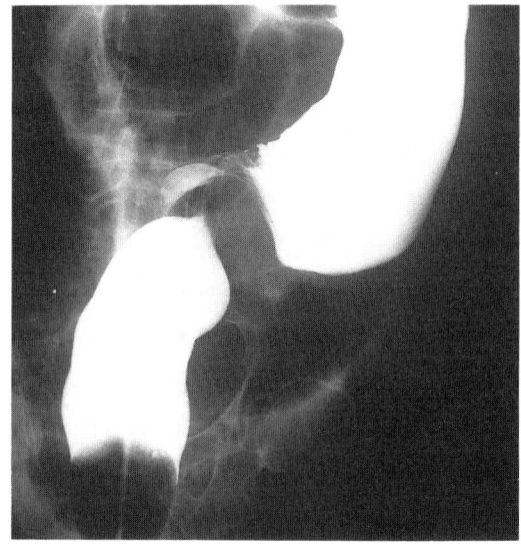

Fig. 14.3 Barium enema examination of sigmoid volvulus demonstrating the characteristic twisted tapering distal to a barium-filled colon.

of sigmoid volvulus by 50% (Ballantyne 1982a).

When both these measures are unsuccessful or when the patient has clinical or radiographic signs of impending or frank perforation, operative intervention is required. Although derotation of the sigmoid colon has successfully been applied in instances in which no gangrene or perforation of the colon was present, sigmoid resection remains the definitive treatment. Again, re-establishment of colonic integrity by anastomosis must depend on local conditions. Operative morbidity and mortality are appreciably higher in patients having perforation or gangrene of the sigmoid colon at the time of exploration.

When volvulus is present, caecal volvulus is the diagnosis 25–40% of the time. The characteristic presentation of caecal volvulus is different from that of sigmoid volvulus: small bowel obstruction is present with crampy abdominal pain, nausea, vomiting, and obstipation. Physical examination demonstrates an air-filled mass arising in the right lower quadrant and extending toward the left

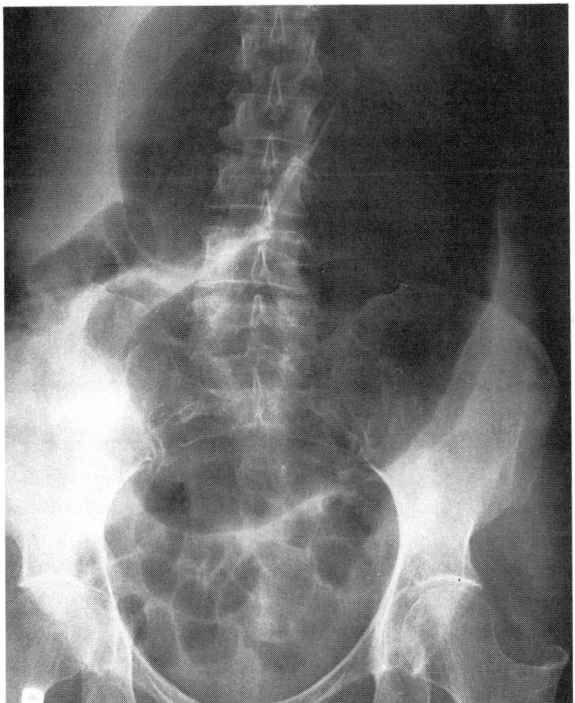

Fig. 14.4 Caecal volvulus demonstrating massive caecal distension with concomitant small bowel obstruction.

upper quadrant. Plain film and abdominal radiography will confirm the diagnosis (Fig.14.4). With absence of peritoneal irritation, an attempt at colonoscopic decompression of the caecal volvulus is warranted (Orchard et al 1984). In fact, colonoscopic decompression has supplanted the current practice of radiographic decompression using a hydrostatic barium enema.

Failure to decompress the volvulus mandates operative intervention. Colonoscopic decompression should not be attempted in patients with signs of peritoneal irritation or perforation. In the presence of perforation of the caecum or gangrene as a result of vascular compromise at the time of exploration, the appropriate operation is resection with primary ileocolonic anastomosis (O'Mara et al 1979).

Obstruction

Large bowel obstruction from any cause can result in perforation proximal to the obstructing lesion because of increased intraluminal pressure. Causes of colonic obstruction, in descending order of frequency, are carcinoma, diverticulitis, and volvulus. The development of frank caecal perforation should be anticipated from plain radiography; a transverse diameter of the caecum greater than 90 mm on a film with the patient in the prone position continues to be a reliable sign of impending caecal rupture in actue colonic obstruction (Lowman & Davis 1956). In cases where caecal perforation has already occurred at the time of exploration for large bowel obstruction, the risk of death from the operation is twice as great, whatever the cause of the obstruction (Jackson 1982).

Proper operative treatment is dependent on the status of the caecum. When the caecum has ruptured, when gangrene is present with impending rupture, or when an obstructing left-sided colonic lesion is found, most surgeons advocate performance of subtotal colectomy to include both the caecum and the obstructing process with primary ileocolic anastomosis. On the other hand, when the caecum does not exhibit signs of impending rupture, resection of the obstructing lesion with performance of an end colostomy and either a

Hartmann procedure or a mucous fistula represents the traditional approach. Recently, the application of on-table colonic lavage with primary anastomosis has been shown to be a safe alternative, even in the presence of colonic obstruction with formed stool in the colon (Radcliffe & Dudley 1983). This technique clearly offers the advantage of eliminating a second procedure to re-anastomose the colon and avoids the potentially poor functional result of subtotal colectomy with ileocolic anastomosis in an elderly patient.

Pseudo-obstruction

Pseudo-obstruction of the colon (Ogilvie's syndrome) is acute colonic distension without mechanical obstruction. Many patients have associated underlying illnesses that might predispose them to the development of colonic ileus (Søreide et al 1977). The clinical presentation is similar to that of mechanical obstruction of the colon with progressive abdominal distension and obstipation. Plain film radiography of the abdomen demonstrates colonic distension indistinguishable from mechanical obstruction. It is incumbent on the examiner to exclude the presence of a mechanically obstructing lesion by the performance of a barium enema study. Perforation of the caecum has been reported in 21% of patients despite the absence of mechanical obstruction (Søreide et al 1977). Tenderness over the distended caecum warrants serious consideration of operative intervention.

The appropriate use of therapeutic colonoscopy as the primary treatment of patients with acute pseudo-obstruction in the absence of peritoneal irritation has been documented (Strodel et al 1983, Bode et al 1984). Initial decompression is successful in approximately two-thirds of patients. When distension recurs, a second colonoscopy cures an additional 10–15%. In the remainder, operation is required. Tube caecostomy is the preferred operative therapy in the absence of extensive gangrenous changes of the right colon (Melzig & Terz 1978).

Stercoral perforation of the colon is a rare clinical entity. Erosion and pressure necrosis from inspissated or impacted stool in a previously healthy portion of the colon is seen in patients with chronic constipation and often affects the sigmoid colon (Carter & Kirkpatrick 1973). An even smaller group of patients with perforation related to chronic constipation includes some with longitudinal antimesenteric sigmoid disruption without stercoral ulceration (Huttunen et al 1975). In these patients perforation is believed to have resulted from increased intracolonic pressure in previously normal colon. In true stercoral perforation, a faecalith corresponding in size to the perforation itself will be found at the time of exploration. Appropriate surgical treatment of both stercoral and idiopathic colonic perforation requires resection of the affected segment with subsequent reanastomosis preceded by on-table lavage or end colostomy.

Iatrogenic perforation

Iatrogenic perforations of the colon and rectum are often a result of endoscopic manipulation. Mucosal lacerations of the rectum resulting from use of thermometers and enema tips are rarely transmural, and these mucosal injuries heal promptly without noticeable clinical effect.

Proctosigmoidoscopy with the rigid instrument is an extremely safe invasive investigative procedure with reported incidences of perforation of 0.01–0.02% (Nelson et al 1982). Perforation during insertion of the rigid instrument is always a technical failure and can be avoided by visualization of the lumen before advancement and by discontinuation of the examination if the patient experiences excessive discomfort. Performance of snare polypectomy above the peritoneal reflection increases the risk of perforation, which is usually recognized immediately and requires urgent operative intervention to close the perforation.

Endoscopy. The advent of flexible endoscopic procedures, including flexible fibroptic sigmoidoscopy and colonoscopy, has resulted in a recognized incidence of colonic perforation during both diagnostic and therapeutic procedures. Smith & Nivatvongs (1975) reported an incidence of perforation in 0.09% in more than 5200 examinations of patients undergoing diagnostic colonoscopy. The addition of snare polypectomy to the colonoscopic procedure doubles the risk of perforation. Perforation may be caused during diagnostic colonoscopy by the tip itself and the deflection bend and shaft of the instrument. Perforation caused by the tip of the colonoscope is usually recognized immediately and is oversewn without colostomy because the colon will have been cleansed mechanically before the procedure. Diagnosis of perforation caused by the deflection bend in the shaft of the instrument itself is frequently delayed until peritoneal signs are evident. In these instances, resection of the involved segment, with or without the performance of a colostomy, may be required (Coller 1985). Similar observations of the time course of perforation after colonoscopic polypectomy show that the diagnosis may not be apparent until necrosis at the polypectomy site results in progressive peritoneal findings.

Gas explosion. Explosion of combustible colonic gases is fortunately rare. This dramatic event has been documented (Coller 1985) during examinations with both rigid and flexible colonoscopes and usually involves ignition of methane or hydrogen. Complete preparation of the bowel using enemas and avoiding the use of mannitol is advised to diminish the concentration of both hydrogen and methane. In addition, carbon dioxide rather than oxygen insufflation should be considered for patients in whom preparation has been less than ideal, because carbon dioxide will not support combustion (Coller 1985). Explosive injury to the colon associated with electrosurgical procedures has usually resulted in multiple longitudinal lacerations caused by the burst effect and has required resection of a long involved segment.

Barium enema. Perforation during the performance of a barium enema study is also rare. Possible mechanisms include intramural injection of barium into the extraperitoneal rectal wall, rupture of the balloon catheter as a result of excessive distension, perforation through a sigmoidoscopic biopsy site, and rupture by hydrostatic pressure (Seaman & Wells 1965). Intramural injection of barium results in the formation of a barium granuloma. Excision of the granuloma is necessitated only by persistent symptoms of pain and bleeding (Weitzner & Law 1972). Transmural perforation of the extraperitoneal rectum, demonstrated fluoroscopically at the time of examination or by the postevacuation film, necessitates admission to hospital with a period of bowel rest and administration of broad-spectrum parenteral antibiotics. In most circumstances this is sufficient, and proximal faecal diversion because of persistent sepsis is not required. Intraperitoneal rupture during barium enema is an acute surgical emergency necessitating prompt laparotomy with vigorous peritoneal toilet to remove as much barium as possible because the combination of barium and stool results in a particularly noxious peritonitis (Hardy et al 1983).

Trauma

Principles and management of patients with a traumatic colorectal injury have resulted from military experience. These traditional treatment regimens evolved in the setting of wounds inflicted by high-velocity missiles and delay in surgical treatment caused by delay in evacuation of casualties. Consequently, individuals with wartime injuries of the colon and rectum presented with established faecal contamination and multiple injuries with an appreciable amount of tissue trauma as a consequence of the nature of the wounding agent. Observations of civilian injuries to the colon and rectum caused by both low-velocity gunshot wounds and stab wounds indicate that treatment of non-military colonic injuries may be altered appreciably and still be successful.

Penetrating injuries to the colon include gunshot wounds and stab wounds. In gunshot wounds, knowledge of the calibre of gun involved is important. Occasionally, high-velocity gunshot wounds are seen in civilian practice, most often caused by hunting rifles. The approach to high-velocity gunshot wounds of the colon should adhere to the military principles of debridement or resection with creation of a stoma. Only low-velocity gunshot wounds should be considered for one of the alternative methods of treatment, such as exterioration as a colostomy, exteriorized primary repair, primary repair, primary repair with proximal colostomy, resection without anastomosis, or resection with anastomosis with or without colostomy. Beall and associates (1971) were one of the first groups to suggest that in instances of minimal faecal contamination, primary repair could be accomplished with acceptable morbidity and mortality. This observation has been substantiated by other authors in major urban trauma centres (Bartizal et al 1974, LoCicero et al 1975).

Primary repair techniques

Exteriorization as a colostomy, the traditional wartime approach to colonic perforation, was replaced by primary repair with exteriorization of the repaired colon by Kirkpatrick (1977). This particular method of treatment is available for all sites of the colon that can be mobilized to the skin and supported with a rod to permit continued observation. When the bowel wound heals, the colon can be returned to the peritoneal cavity before the patient's discharge. The success rate in achieving primary healing is about 75%, but in the remaining 25% of patients the primarily repaired colon breaks down, requiring resultant colostomy with closure at a later date. Careful attention to care of the exteriorized segment with utilization of moist dressings is necessary to optimize healing and minimize breakdown.

Emphasis is increasingly being placed on primary repair of colonic injuries. Consideration for primary repair requires the absence of serious preoperative hypotension and minimal faecal contamination, with prompt exploration within 8 h of the time of colonic injury (Stone & Fabian 1979). Under these specific circumstances, primary repair without faecal diversion is a safe operative technique that provides early results as good as those of other forms of treatment and superior results when the need for a subsequent operation to close the colostomy and re-establish intestinal continuity is considered.

Controversy continues regarding the relative safety of primary repair in right-sided and left-sided colonic injuries. Careful examination of this issue indicates that primary repair is equally safe for right-sided and left-sided injuries provided the degree of faecal contamination and associated injury as well as the overall condition of the patient is favourable (Flint et al 1981).

Resection is reserved for patients with extensive tissue destruction, large associated mesenteric haematomas, or injury to the mesenteric vasculature. In most instances, resection will be accompanied by creation of an end colostomy and mucous fistula because of the degree of tissue destruction and faecal contamination.

Laparotomy. While few would deny that gunshot wounds to the abdomen always require exploration, a policy of selective laparotomy for stab wounds has evolved (Nance et al 1974). In the absence of clinical or radiographic signs of violation of the peritoneal cavity, including significant hypotension, peritonitis, blood in the nasogastric aspirate or bladder, or free air on radiography of the chest in the upright position, repeated clinical examinations, with operation dictated by the development of clinical signs of peritoneal irritation, will avoid unnecessary laparotomy in most instances. Furthermore, delay in the performance of laparotomy does not result in increased morbidity. When a colonic injury is found, it is approached similarly to gunshot wounds as outlined earlier.

Blunt injuries

Blunt injury to the colon is unusual. Mechanisms of blunt injury to the colon include crush injuries and deceleration injuries. In crush injury, appreciable tissue necrosis and associated mesenteric bleeding often necessitate resection without anastomosis. Deceleration injuries associated with the use of lap-type seat belts have been reported (Towne & Coe 1971). Delay in diagnosis is typical, and associated contused tissue with advanced faecal contamination and established infection again mandate resection without anastomosis in most patients.

Rectal injuries

Injuries to the rectum represent a specific subset of colorectal perforations managed in a specialized fashion. Causes of perforations of the rectum include gunshot wound, crush injuries from pelvic trauma, impalements from straddle injuries, and sexual injuries to the rectum. Management of patients with perforating rectal trauma evolved during the Vietnam war to include proximal end colostomy, repair of the rectum when possible, extensive presacral drainage, and, recently, washout of the distal segment to prevent continued faecal contamination (Lavenson & Cohen 1971). The addition of rectal washout resulted in a striking diminution in late septic complications and mortality.

After the patient's condition has been stabilized, the initial approach to diagnosis in a patient who has experienced a potentially traumatic injury to the rectum should include proctosigmoidoscopy. Minor lacerations without transmural injury may be managed safely by local repair and broad-spectrum antibiotics without faecal diversion.

When examination demonstrates a penetrating injury with involvement of the sphincter, attempts should be made to reapproximate the divided edges of the sphincter if possible. Even when total restoration of sphincter competence is not successful, subsequent formal repair of the sphincter under cover of a protecting colostomy will be facilitated.

Blunt injuries resulting from pelvic crush are associated with an appreciably higher mortality than are injuries from a penetrating wound. The majority of patients with blunt injuries to the rectum will have rectal bleeding, requiring sigmoidoscopy to establish the diagnosis (Brunner & Shatney 1987). Performance of colostomy with mucous fistula, distal washout, and broad-spectrum antibiotics will control faecal contamination. Insertion of presacral drains may be impossible because of the presence of a large pelvic haematoma, the result of the injury itself. Delay in diagnosis with subsequent infection of the pelvic haematoma is a potentially lethal situation.

Changing sexual practices have resulted in increased experience with rectal perforation caused by foreign bodies inserted for sexual stimulation. The nature of these foreign bodies is limited more by the size of the anus than the imagination of the inserter. Similarly, extraction methods of these foreign bodies require ingenuity on the part of the treating physician (Barone et al 1976).

A reasonably simple approach to colorectal foreign bodies has been suggested by Eftaiha et al (1977) in that the objects are classified as low-lying or high-lying. The low-lying objects can be classified further into sharp, rounded, and glass.

Anaesthesia is required for extraction of most rectal foreign bodies, and, after extraction of the object, careful proctosigmoidoscopic examination is performed to exclude the presence of perforation. For high-lying foreign bodies, laparotomy may be required. Patients who present with lower abdominal tenderness should be prepared for laparotomy. In the absence of perforation, the first manoeuvre during laparotomy should be to attempt to manipulate the object distally for extraction by the perineal operator. When perforation is apparent, resection with end colostomy and distal washout is the preferred method of treatment.

REFERENCES

Auguste L J, Wise L 1981 Surgical management of perforated diverticulitis. American Journal of Surgery 141: 122–127

Ballantyne G H 1982a Review of sigmoid volvulus: history and results of treatment. Diseases of the Colon and Rectum 25: 494–501

Ballantyne G H 1982b Review of sigmoid volvulus: clinical patterns and pathogenesis. Diseases of the Colon and Rectum 25: 823–830

Barone J E, Sohn N, Nealon T F Jr 1976 Perforations and foreign bodies of the rectum: report of 28 cases. Annals of Surgery 184: 601–604

Bartizal J F, Boyd D R, Folk F A, Smith D, Lescher T C, Freeark R J 1974 A critical review of management of 392 colonic and rectal injuries. Diseases of the Colon and Rectum 17: 313–318

Beall A C Jr, Bricker D L, Alessi F J, Whisennand H H, DeBakey M E 1971 Surgical considerations in the management of civilian colon injuries. Annals of Surgery 173: 971–978

Bode W E, Beart R W Jr, Spencer R J, Culp C E, Wolff B G, Taylor B M 1984 Colonoscopic decompression for acute pseudo-obstruction of the colon (Ogilvie's syndrome): report of 22 cases and review of literature. American Journal of Surgery 147: 243–245

Boley S J, Brandt L J, Veith F J 1978 Ischemic disorders of the intestines. Current Problems in Surgery 15: 1–85

Brunner R G, Shatney C H 1987 Diagnostic and therapeutic aspects of rectal trauma: blunt versus penetrating. American Surgeon 53: 215–219

Carter D C, Kirkpatrick J R 1973 Stercoral perforation of the sigmoid colon. British Journal of Surgery 60: 61–63

Coller J A 1985 Complications of endoscopy of the colon and rectum. In: Ferrari B T, Ray J E, Gathright J B (eds) Complications of colon and rectal surgery: prevention and management. Saunders, Philadelphia de Leon M L, Schoetz D J Jr, Coller J A, Veidenheimer M C 1987 Colorectal cancer: Lahey Clinic experience, 1972–1976. An analysis of prognostic indicators. Diseases of the Colon and Rectum 30: 237–242

Dunn D L, Simmons R L 1984 The role of anaerobic bacteria in intra-abdominal infections. Reviews of Infectious Diseases 6 (suppl l): S139–S146

Eftaiha M, Hambrick E, Abcarian H 1977 Principles of management of colorectal foreign bodies. Archives of Surgery 112: 691–695

Eng K, Ranson J H C, Localio S A 1977 Resection of the perforated segment: a significant advance in treatment of diverticulitis with free perforation or abscess. American Journal of Surgery 133: 67–72

Fazio V W 1980 Toxic megacolon in ulcerative colitis and Crohn's colitis. Clinics in Gastroenterology 9: 389–407

Flint L M, Vitale G C, Richardson J D, Polk H C Jr 1981 The injured colon: relationships of management to complications. Annals of Surgery 193: 619–623

Greenstein A J, Aufses A H Jr 1985 Differences in pathogenesis, incidence and outcome of perforation in inflammatory bowel disease. Surgery, Gynecology and Obstetrics 160: 63–69

Greenstein A J, Barth J A, Sachar D B, Aufses A H Jr 1986 Free colonic perforation without dilatation in ulcerative colitis. American Journal of Surgery 152: 272–275

Hackford A W, Veidenheimer M C 1985 Diverticular disease of the colon: current concepts and management. Surgical Clinics of North America 65: 347–363

Hackford A W, Schoetz D J Jr, Coller J A, Veidenheimer M C 1985 Surgical management of complicated diverticulitis: the Lahey Clinic experience, 1967–1982. Diseases of the Colon and Rectum 28: 317–321

Hardy T G, Hartmann R F, Aguilar P S, Stewart W R C 1983 Survival after colonic perforation during barium-enema examination: modified radical surgical debridement. Diseases of the Colon and Rectum 26: 116–118

Hau T, Ahrenholz D H, Simmons R L 1979 Secondary bacterial peritonitis: the biologic basis of treatment. Current Problems in Surgery 16: 1–65

Huttunen R, Heikkinen E, Larmi T K I 1975 Stercoraceous and idiopathic perforations of the colon. Surgery Gynecology and Obstetrics 140: 756–760

Jackson B R 1982 The diagnosis of colonic obstruction. Diseases of the Colon and Rectum 25: 603–609

Kirkpatrick J R 1977 The exteriorized anastomosis: its role in surgery of the colon. Surgery 82: 362–365

Krukowski Z H, Matheson N A 1984 Emergency surgery for diverticular disease complicated by generalized and faecal peritonitis: a review. British Journal of Surgery 71: 921–927

Lavenson G S Jr, Cohen A 1971 Management of rectal injuries. American Journal of Surgery 122: 226–230

LoCicero J III, Tajima T, Drapanas T 1975 A half-century of experience in the management of colon injuries: changing concepts. Journal of Trauma 15: 575–579

Lowman R M, Davis L 1956 An evaluation of cecal size in impending perforation of the cecum. Surgery, Gynecology and Obstetrics 103: 711–718

Madden J L, Tan P Y 1961 Primary resection and anastomosis in the treatment of perforated lesions of the colon, with abscess or diffusing peritonitis. Surgery, Gynecology and Obstetrics 113: 646–650

Melzig E P, Terz J J 1978 Pseudo-obstruction of the colon. Archives of Surgery 113: 1186–1190

Nagorney D M, Adson M A, Pemberton J H 1985 Sigmoid diverticulitis with perforation and generalized peritonitis. Diseases of the Colon and Rectum 28: 71–75

Nance F C, Wennar M H, Johnson L W, Ingram J C Jr, Cohn I Jr 1974 Surgical judgment in the management of penetrating wounds of the abdomen: experience with 2212 patients. Annals of Surgery 179: 639–646

Nelson R L, Abcarian H, Prasad M L 1982 Iatrogenic perforation of the colon and rectum. Diseases of the Colon and Rectum 25: 305–308

O'Mara C S, Wilson T H Jr, Stonesifer G L, Cameron J L 1979 Cecal volvulus: analysis of 50 patients with long-term follow-up. Annals of Surgery 189: 724–731

Orchard J L, Mehta R, Khan A H 1984 The use of colonoscopy in the treatment of colonic volvulus: three cases and review of the literature. American Journal of Gastroenterology 79: 864–867

Radcliffe A G, Dudley H A F 1983 Intraoperative antegrade irrigation of the large intestine. Surgery, Gynecology and Obstetrics 156: 721–723

Rodkey G V, Welch C E 1984 Changing patterns in the surgical treatment of diverticular disease. Annals of Surgery 200: 466–478

Seaman W B, Wells J 1965 Complications of the barium enema. Gastroenterology 48: 728–737

Smith L E, Nivatvongs S 1975 Complications in colonoscopy. Diseases of the Colon and Rectum 18: 214–220

Smithwick R H 1942 Experiences with surgical management of diverticulitis of the sigmoid. Annals of Surgery 115: 969–985

Søreide O, Bjerkeset T, Fossdal J E 1977 Pseudo-obstruction of the colon (Ogilvie's syndrome): a genuine clinical condition? Diseases of the Colon and Rectum 20: 487–491

Starling J R 1979 Initial treatment of sigmoid volvulus by colonoscopy. Annals of Surgery 190: 36–39

Stone H H, Fabian T C 1979 Management of perforating colon trauma: randomization between primary closure and exteriorization. Annals of Surgery 190: 430–436

Strodel W E, Nostrant T T, Eckhauser F E, Dent T L 1983 Therapeutic and diagnostic colonoscopy in nonobstructive colonic dilatation. Annals of Surgery 197: 416–421

Sugarbaker P H 1981 Carcinoma of the colon: prognosis and operative choice. Current Problems in Surgery 18: 753–826

Towne J B, Coe J D 1971 Seat belt trauma of the colon. American Journal of Surgery 122: 683–685

Turnbull R B Jr, Hawk W A, Weakley F L 1971 Surgical treatment of toxic megacolon: ileostomy and colostomy to prepare patients for colectomy. American Journal of Surgery 122: 325–331

Underwood J W, Marks C G 1984 The septic complications of sigmoid diverticular disease. British Journal of Surgery 71: 209–211

Weitzner S, Law D H 1972 Barium granuloma of the rectum. Digestive Diseases 17: 17–22

Williams L F Jr, Wittenberg J 1975 Ischemic colitis: an useful clinical diagnosis, but is it ischemic? Annals of Surgery 182: 439–448

15 Manifestations of appendicitis

M. J. COOPER

Appendicitis is a common surgical problem in developed countries. One in five males and one in six females are likely to have the diagnosis made during life (Ludbrook & Spears 1965); the maximum risk is during adolescence, when there is a 1% chance every year. Although appendicitis itself has existed for millennia, having even been found in an Egyptian mummy (Bett 1934), it has been epidemic only during the 20th century. Indeed, there is now evidence that as we move to the end of this century the incidence is declining (Noer 1976). For the population at large appendicitis is so common that it may seem to represent a disease of little significance. Yet to the surgeon this small organ of unknown purpose continues to provide a diagnostic challenge and represent a potent source of morbidity and mortality to the patient.

Historical perspective

Berengario Da Carpi (1521) is credited with the first anatomical description of the appendix, although it is clearly visible but undescribed in the earlier drawings of Leonardo da Vinci (McMurrich 1930). Little has been added since its variable position was well described by Morgagni (1719). The disease itself was first described in 1711 by Lorenz Heister (Major 1965) who performed an autopsy on an executed criminal. His observations he felt could 'stand as a proof of the possibility of inflammation arising, and abscess forming in the appendicula'.

Heister's description was largely ignored for 150 years. Although Louyer-Villermay (1824) described gangrenous appendicitis, the 19th cen-

tury was the time of the typhlitis–perityphlitis controversy. The European establishment was influenced by the views of Baron Dupuytren (1833), who taught that the disease was due to the weight of faeces in the ascending colon. The change in opinion was to come from Fitz in America. In 1886 he read a classic paper describing the clinical and pathological features of appendicitis and advocating early operation.

Appendicectomy was first undertaken in 1753 when Claudius Amyand (1736) discovered an appendix perforated by a pin in an inguinoscrotal hernia. The patient, an 11-year-old boy, recovered after an appendicectomy. Occasional reports of surgical treatment appeared over the years (Hancock 1848, Hall 1886, Sands 1888) until Fitz (1886) and Parker (1867) popularized early operation in the USA in the 1880s. The most famous appendicectomy and the one that made the disease fashionable in Europe was performed in 1902. Treves (Stevenson 1962) operated on King Edward VII only two days before his planned coronation. Although this procedure had been delayed for many days it revived interest and early operation soon became the norm.

Aetiology and pathogenesis

Many studies have been undertaken to explain the cause of appendicitis, yet none is entirely satisfactory. It has been shown that the appendix is a secretory organ producing mucus both at rest and in response to chyme in the lumen (Wangensteen & Bowers 1937). It is also known to contain a large number of lymphoid follicles, and in this respect it may act like the tonsil and protect the gut from injurious antigens in the luminal contents. Of the many aetiological theories proposed only two seem important, obstruction and infection.

Since the appendix is a narrow organ its lumen can easily be obstructed, and this can lead to distension and susceptibility to colonization. Faecaliths and lymphoid hyperplasia are probably the commonest causes of obstruction though tumours and a variety of foreign bodies (Balch & Silver 1971) have also been implicated. In a comparative study of the appendix at laparotomy, faecaliths were found to be more common in Canada than in South Africa and were more likely to be found in patients undergoing surgery for appendicitis (Jones et al 1985). Much of the work on obstruction has been undertaken in experimental animals (Piepar et al 1982). The major objections to this theory as a cause in man are that pathologists do not always find evidence of obstruction and that appendiceal pressures have been measured at operation and are not always raised (Arnbjornsson & Bengmark 1984). Many studies have considered the role of dietary fibre, since this is largely a disease of the developed world. Although this theory is initially attractive, the decline in appendicitis started well before the resumption of fibre intake and was not affected by world wars, which profoundly changed diets (Heaton 1987).

The final event in appendicitis is invasion of the appendicular wall by organisms from the enteric flora. Bohrod (1946) argued that infection was actually the initiating event, leading to lymphoid hyperplasia and luminal obstruction. Since children and young adults have the most lymphoid tissue in relation to luminal size, this theory might explain the age pattern at presentation. Such infection could be enteric or could be carried by the blood from distant sites; indeed clusters of cases have been reported (Martin & Gustafson 1985). Barker (1986) has documented the rise in cases in the UK with the implementation of the public health reforms. The consequent reduction in exposure of young children to enteric pathogens has reduced the mortality from diarrhoeal disease. However, he suggests that the response when it does occur in later life is manifest as acute appendicitis.

Obstruction without infection may lead to the development of a mucocoele, and some patients give a history of chronic pain or previous attacks. There is considerable argument as to whether a truly chronic form exists (Morson & Dawson 1979); nevertheless, some patients with right iliac fossa pain are relieved by removal of a histologically normal appendix (Morson & Dawson 1979, Schisgall 1980). More commonly, secondary infection intervenes, leading to vascular damage, gangrene and perforation (Lindgren & Aho 1969).

Clinical features

Acute appendicitis can occur at any age, having been reported both in premature infants (Coetzee 1958, Ayalon et al 1979) and the very old. It appears to be a declining epidemic in western nations (Noer 1976) and remains uncommon in underdeveloped nations (Burkitt 1971). There seems to be a familial tendency both to the disease (Andersson et al 1979) and to the retrocaecal position (Budd & Fouty 1977). The retrocaecal position of the appendix does not alter the course of the disease (Grunditz et al 1983), but it does affect the clinical features. The rare retroileal appendicitis may lead to small bowel or ureteric obstruction and present late in the course of the disease. Though often atypical, the symptoms and signs have a clear pattern that has been established for 150 years (Bright & Addison 1839).

The prodromal features are those of anorexia, nausea and a low-grade fever. The pain starts periumbilically and moves to the right iliac fossa when the serosa becomes inflamed; its precise location will depend on the site of the appendix. The temperature is raised but rarely by more than 1°C, unless perforation has occurred. There is localized tenderness and guarding over the appendix: classically over McBurney's point (McBurney 1889). In early cases rectal examination will only reveal tenderness if the appendix lies in the pelvis. Once perforation ensues the physical signs change, with the development of either an appendix mass or generalized peritonitis.

None of the physical signs are specific to acute appendicitis, and the list of differential diagnoses is impressive (Table 15.1). A careful history and a

Table 15.1 Differential diagnosis of acute appendicitis

Supradiaphragmatic	*Pelvis*
Tonsillitis	Salpingitis
Pneumonia	Ectopic pregnancy
Pleurisy	Ruptured ovarian follicle
	Twisted ovarian cyst
Upper abdomen	
Perforated ulcer	*Retroperitoneum*
Cholecystitis	Ureteric colic
Cyclical vomiting	Pyelonephritis
	Acute pancreatitis
Lower abdomen	
Enterocolitis	*Systemic*
Intestinal obstruction	Herpes
Caecal carcinoma	Spinal disease
Torsion appendix epiploica	Diabetes mellitus
Tuberculosis	Tabetic crisis
Yersinial infection	Porphyria
Perforated lymphoma	Henoch-Schönlein purpura
Mesenteric lymphadenitis	
Crohn's disease	
Meckel's diverticulitis	
Typhoid perforation	
Amoebiasis	
Caecal diverticulum	

thorough examination will narrow the list of differential diagnoses, but a period of observation may help in the difficult case. A multivariate analysis has found seven factors of value in discrimination: sex, age, duration of symptoms, genitourinary symptoms, involuntary muscle spasm in the right lower quadrant, right-sided rectal mass, and white cell count (Teicher et al 1983).

Most diagnostic problems arise in women of child-bearing age and are related to gynaecological disease, giving a diagnostic accuracy in this group as low as 55–68% (Gilmore et al 1975, Jess et al 1981). Some studies have suggested that the incidence of true appendicitis might be related to phases of the menstrual cycle (Arnbjornsson 1983). However, two further studies have since refuted this claim (Robinson & Burch 1984, Bongard et al 1985). Menstrual history may still be important as more cases of pelvic inflammatory disease present early in the cycle (Bongard et al 1985). There appears to be no evidence that taking the contraceptive pill alters the presentation of appendicitis (Bongard et al 1985, Arnbjornsson 1984). Many of the other disorders merit surgical exploration in any case. Moreover, there is a group of patients with 'non-specific abdominal pain' who will benefit from laparotomy and removal of a histologically normal appendix.

Special investigations

Although the diagnosis of acute appendicitis is essentially clinical, certain investigations can help in the complicated case.

White cell count

A neutrophil leucocytosis ($>12\times10^9/l$) develops in about 75% of patients. Nevertheless a normal value does not preclude the diagnosis.

Mid-stream urine

Examination of the urine is a routine part of the investigation of abdominal pain and may reveal a significant urinary infection. Pyuria or microscopic haematuria occur in 30% of acute appendicitis patients, particularly if the appendix is adherent to the bladder or ureter. Operation is clearly justified, therefore, if appendicitis cannot be ruled out in patients with urinary symptoms.

Serum amylase estimation

This has become a routine part of the investigation of central abdominal pain, high levels ($>1,200$ iu/l) usually being considered diagnostic of acute pancreatitis. Lower levels of hyperamylasaemia have been reported in appendicular peritonitis but may be seen even before the appendix has perforated (Burnett & Ness 1955, Abruzzo et al 1958). Care must be taken in evaluating a finding of elevated amylase as it can lead to a delay in diagnosis and unnecessary rupture (Swensson & Maull 1981). Laparotomy is certainly indicated if diagnostic doubt persists, since it does not worsen the prognosis of acute pancreatitis (Trapnell & Anderson 1967).

Radiology

A plain abdominal X-ray is seldom performed in patients with appendicitis, so there are few reports of its usefulness. Faecoliths were first described radiologically in 1906 (Weisflog), and although their relevance was soon doubted (Strom 1921–22) they remain a common finding (in about 7% of patients with acute appendicitis) (Morson & Dawson 1979). Pneumoperitoneum is a rare finding, with only 40 published cases (Saebo 1978). Also uncommon is the finding of a gas-filled appendix (Killen & Brooks 1965). The possible findings on plain abdominal X-ray (Brooks & Killen 1965) are given below, but the sensitivity of this investigation remains low and such films are rarely indicated.

Radiological signs of acute appendicitis

Air/fluid levels in RIF
Increased soft tissue density
Appendicolith
Gas-filled appendix
Caecal deformity
Localised adynamic ileus
Altered flank stripe
Altered psoas outline
Extraluminal gas

Recently there has been some interest in the use of barium enema to improve diagnostic accuracy, particularly in children. Some features are thought to be 'pathognomonic' of appendicitis (Schey 1973), but there are many false positives (Fedyshin et al 1984). Barium enema is an uncomfortable and invasive procedure that is of potential value in differentiating carcinoma of the caecum from an appendiceal mass. As a primary diagnostic examination, though, it is generally superfluous, and irradiation should be avoided in children (Berry & Malt 1984). Schisgall (1983) has recommended a delayed film after the oral ingestion of barium to avoid the problems of an enema. However, it is probable that careful clinical observation during this 12-hour period might be just as valuable.

Ultrasound was initially used to exclude gynaecological pathology rather than as a positive diagnostic tool. However, the advent of real-time imaging has permitted recognition of normal bowel patterns and characterization of appendicitis. The main feature is dilatation of the appendiceal lumen with surrounding zones of increased and then decreased reflectivity. Other occasional findings are faecoliths, caecal thickening and periappendiceal fluid. Two recent European studies have shown that it is possible to achieve a sensitivity of 83–89% with a specificity of 94–100% (Pwylaert 1986, Karstrup et al 1986). Compression may be required to visualize the appendix but is apparently not too uncomfortable if applied slowly (Pwylaert 1986). In dedicated hands, therefore, ultrasound can achieve a high degree of accuracy in the diagnosis of acute appendicitis. It is unlikely that a skilled 24-hour service is available in most hospitals, and it remains a fact that as the percentage of normal appendices removed decreases the perforation rate rises. For the time being the major use of ultrasound will be the measurement of appendiceal masses and it will not affect the treatment of true appendicitis.

Other radiological techniques such as scintiscanning for pus with gallium or indium are occasionally useful, while excretion urography can demonstrate partial obstruction of the ureter in retroileal appendicitis.

Laparoscopy

Early operation is the correct policy in acute appendicitis, but it does prove to be unnecessary in 20% of cases (Gilmore et al 1975). Laparoscopy is a well-established gynaecological tool which has been advocated to reduce this negative appendicectomy rate. Several studies have shown that up to 37% of women may be saved from an unnecessary appendicectomy by laparoscopy (Leape & Ramenofsky 1980, Deutsch et al 1982). In expert hands laparoscopy is undoubtedly safer than a negative appendicectomy (Deutsch et al 1982). It may be indicated in women of child-bearing age, but the consensus is that 'considered as a diagnostic test, appendectomy is probably more cost-effective and certainly more reliable than laparoscopy' (Way et al 1982).

Computer-aided diagnosis

It is apparent that laboratory and radiological investigations do not appreciably help the clinician and attempts have thus been made to make better use of the clinical information available. Computer programmes have now been written that use Bayesian algorithms to increase the accuracy of diagnosis. De Dombal and his colleagues (1974) reported a drop in the rates of both perforation and negative laparotomy during a study of 552 patients with abdominal pain. A similar study from Augusta, Georgia also reported a 92% diagnostic accuracy using a programme that can be made to run on a programmable pocket calculator (Edwards & Davies 1984). This points out that the data base matrix may need to be varied from hospital to hospital, but that it is easy to use and does not delay the clinical process. The technique works best if observer variation can be minimized, something that requires training. It is for the latter reason that computer diagnosis is not yet a totally reliable tool, but it certainly does have potential for answering the question 'appendicitis or not-appendicitis'.

Treatment

As soon as the clinical diagnosis has been reached appendicectomy should be performed. The operative approach is well described in all text books of operative surgery and is basically unchanged from McBurney's description in 1894 (Sands 1888), although many surgeons now employ a more transverse skin incision (Battle 1897, Davis 1906). The stump is usually ligated and then inverted by a purse string. There seem to be few problems with these techniques, although Kelly (1905) felt that they should be avoided. There are, however, several circumstances that make management more difficult or controversial.

Appendix mass and abscess

Although early operation is the norm, 2–3% of patients continue to present late in the course of their disease with tachycardia, pyrexia and a mass in the right iliac fossa. Since appendicitis is such a common problem this in itself is a frequent occurrence. The underlying lesion may be either an inflammatory phlegmon or a true abscess. It has been recognized since the beginning of the century that an appendix mass often resolves with conservative therapy (Ochsner 1902, Sherren 1905). Improvements in intravenous fluid management

have led to an almost negligible mortality rate (Arnheim & Neuhof 1940). However, the introduction of antibiotics prompted Fields et al (1957) to suggest a policy of early operation.

Modern conservative management consists of bed rest, intravenous fluids, analgesia and antibiotics. The size of the mass should be documented on the patient's abdomen or measured by ultrasound. Enlargement of the mass accompanied by a swinging pyrexia, rising leucocytosis or deteriorating general condition indicates suppuration. Appendix abscess requires prompt surgical drainage, which can often be achieved without entering the peritoneal cavity. The appendix itself should only be removed if it is reasonably visible and the procedure is likely to be straightforward.

Advocates of this conservative approach claim that immediate appendicectomy will convert a localized problem into generalized peritonitis, that the friable oedematous bowel is more easily damaged, and that incorrect assessment may lead to unnecessary resections in the mistaken belief that a neoplasm is present, or alternatively overlooked (Jordan et al 1981). Others claim that immediate appendicectomy is a safe operation with a morbidity rate no higher than that for perforated appendicitis (Fields et al 1957, Gastrin & Josephson 1969). Total hospital stay is also likely to be reduced, particularly if an interval appendicectomy is planned (Jordan et al 1981, Foran et al 1978). Whatever course of action is taken it is essential to exclude the possibility of an obstructing colonic carcinoma, particularly in patients over 40 years of age. In patients with a mass barium enema is thus indicated, since palpation of the caecum may be very difficult. As many as 3% of patients over 40 years of age with appendicitis will have an obstructing neoplasm (Collins 1961, Peltokallio 1966). Indeed, many authors feel that appendicectomy in any patient over 40 years should include a full laparotomy and that the conventional incision is inadequate (Sumpio et al 1986).

Interval appendicectomy

The concept that once the appendix had been inflamed it should be removed led to the introduction of interval appendicectomy by Murphy in 1904. This established dogma has recently been challenged by those who feel that conservative treatment of an appendix mass by observation or drainage should not automatically lead to appendicectomy.

The operation itself is not without risks and has been reported to have a complication rate as high as 30% (Skoubo-Kristensen & Hvid 1983, Bradley & Isaacs 1978, Paull & Bloom 1982). However, many of these cases may have been treated without the use of prophylactic antibiotics and rates as low as 5% are certainly possible (Janik et al 1980). This figure has to be set against the likely recurrence rate of acute appendicitis over the subsequent years. Long-term follow-up series are few, but the recurrence rate is probably in the order of 10–20 per cent (Bradley & Isaacs 1978, Paull & Bloom 1982, Mosegaard & Nielsen 1979, Hoffmann et al 1984). In the elderly or unfit patient appendicectomy can be deferred, although a coexistent neoplasm must be excluded. In the young the position is more contentious, but at this age the balance is still in favour of appendicectomy.

Children

Much of the morbidity and mortality of acute appendicitis occurs at the extremes of age. Approximately 20% of all patients will present before their 15th birthday (Fock et al 1969), but appendicitis is rare below the age of 2 years. At this age history-taking and examination may be difficult and there may also be parental delay in referral. These factors result in a 30–40% perforation rate (Fock et al 1969, Ladd 1938, Schwartz et al 1983, Jackson 1963, Harrison et al 1984), and since the infant omentum is deficient the disease is more dangerous at this age. The high incidence of perforation in small children does not seem to have changed during this century, although the use of intravenous fluids and antibiotics has all but eliminated the risk of death (Fock et al 1969, Ladd 1938). In babies the problem is particularly acute, 75% of appendices being perforated on admission (Fields et al 1957, Fields & Cole 1967). The only way to reduce the morbidity rate further is by

earlier treatment and hence earlier diagnosis. We must continue to educate the public and primary care physicians that acute appendicitis remains an important surgical emergency, and that delay and difficulty in diagnosis are major factors contributing to death (Pledger et al 1987). Unless there is an obvious mass, adequate fluid replacement and early operation must be the norm (Pledger et al 1987, Bennion & Thompson 1987).

The elderly

Approximately 5% of all patients with appendicitis are over 60 years of age. Here again there is a high incidence of perforation (>50%) on presentation (Owens & Hamit 1978, Ryden et al 1983, Burns et al 1985). There is now general agreement that symptoms in the elderly are identical to those in younger patients, but the physical signs are more diffuse (Burns et al 1985, Peltokallio & Jauhiainen 1970) and there are more alternative diagnoses. The main reason for the high perforation rate is delay, some of which is due to lack of recognition by physicians (Burns et al 1985). Nevertheless, in 20–30% of cases the pathophysiological process is very rapid and rupture follows a very short history, possibly because of atheroma in the appendicular artery and early vascular occlusion (Ryden et al 1983, Burns et al 1985, Peltokallio & Jauhiainen 1970). The risk of complications and death remains high in the elderly, mainly as a result of concomitant medical conditions present in nearly 60% of cases (Peltokallio & Jauhiainen 1970). The complication rate can only be reduced by decreasing the delay between onset and operation.

Pregnancy

Appendicitis will complicate about 1 in 1000 pregnancies (DeVore 1980). The problems are: difficulty in diagnosis owing to an abnormal position of the appendix, and fear of inducing abortion. From the third month of pregnancy the appendix rises and moves laterally, to lie near the costal margin by the eighth month. The risk of abortion is slight providing perforation has not occurred. Early operation should therefore be undertaken if there is any diagnostic doubt. Once perforation occurs, there is a real risk of death for both the fetus (10–35%) and the mother (2%) (Masters et al 1984, Punnonen et al 1979, Cunningham & McCubbin 1975). Again the delay is largely due to late presentation. Babler's statement of 1908 bears repitition: 'The mortality of appendicitis complicating pregnancy and the puerperium is the mortality of delay'.

Crohn's disease

Since Crohn's disease can present with right iliac fossa pain, it is not surprising that from time to time every surgeon will discover an inflamed length of terminal ileum whilst operating for appendicitis. A degree of uncertainty still exists as to what the correct operative approach should be in these circumstances. Some patients have other reasons for inflammation of the terminal ileum, such as yersinial infection; biopsy and culture of a mesenteric node should therefore be performed. To alleviate future doubts about right iliac fossa pain, it is generally considered that appendicectomy is safe if the caecum is not involved by presumed Crohn's disease. This dictum would seem to hold true as long as symptoms have been present for less than a week (Simonowitz et al 1982). After this time the diagnosis of appendicitis must be dubious and the fistula rate is high. Some authors (Fonkálsrud et al 1982) believe that established Crohn's disease rules out the possibility of acute appendicitis and that the complication rate is so high that appendicectomy is contra-indicated. Fistulas certainly do follow laparotomy in Crohn's disease, but these seldom develop from the appendix stump. Appendicectomy should therefore be performed during an operation for patients with an acute history of pain in the right iliac fossa and appropriate physical signs, even if they are known or suspected to have Crohn's disease.

Incidental appendicectomy

Both general surgeons and gynaecologists have incidentally removed the appendix during other operations to prevent the patient later developing appendicitis (Strom et al 1983, Walters 1977). This procedure appears to be safe, conveying no increase in infection rate (Strom et al 1983), but the possibility of contamination should always be considered, especially if access is poor. A recent study (Morris et al 1987) has shown a non-statistical increase in wound infections during staging laparotomy after incidental appendicectomy. The practice would not seem to be advisable in immunocompromised or splenectomized patients. Attack rates drop steeply between adolescence and age 50 years. It is estimated that 6000 appendicectomies would need to be performed in adults to avoid one case of appendicitis at age 75 years. Berry and Malt (1984) feel that incidental appendicectomy is a dubious practice over 30 years of age, and it is certainly contra-indicated in patients over 65 (Nockerts et al 1980). However, there may be other indications during certain procedures. Westermann et al (1986) reported their experience during 223 extensive gynaecological procedures. Thirty-four appendices were histologically abnormal, including those in 15 patients with either endometriosis or metastatic carcinoma whose appendices appeared macroscopically normal. This total included one patient undergoing a second-look procedure whose only positive biopsy was from the appendix. Their experience suggests that incidental appendicectomy is a safe and often useful procedure for reasons other than pure prevention of possible appendicitis.

Complications (Table 15.2)

Mortality

If perforation has not occurred then death from appendicectomy is extremely uncommon. As we have already seen, perforation is more common at the extremes of life, and it is in these groups that death may still occur (Fields & Cole 1967, Pledger et al 1987, Ryden et al 1983, Burns et al 1985, Peltokallio & Jauhiainen 1970). The annual number of deaths in children in England and Wales has declined from 500 in the 1930s to 45 in the 1960s and to 8 in the 1980s (Pledger et al 1987). In 1961 Truelsen noted a decline in mortality for

Table 15.2 Complications of appendicectomy

Immediate	Delayed
Wound infection	Right inguinal hernia
Intra-abdominal abscess	Infertility
Haemorrhage: intraperitoneal	Adhesions
into wound	
into bowel	
Stump intussusception	
Faecal fistula	

both uncomplicated (from 2.6% to 0.5%) and perforated appendicitis (from 14.1% to 2.6%). He attributed this drop to better fluid and electrolyte management rather than to antibiotics, which makes the review of Pledger et al (1987) somewhat disheartening. They reported 35 deaths in children in England and Wales between 1980 and 1984. Although the major cause of death was delay in diagnosis, lack of adequate fluid replacement contributed to one third of the deaths. They note that children with peritonitis have an increased need for fluid replacement.

In the elderly deaths still occur, but here coexistent medical conditions and sepsis are more important (Burns et al 1985), although these are rarely a problem prior to perforation. Mortality at the Massachusetts General Hospital dropped from 26% in 1886 to 0.8% in 1984 (Berry & Malt 1984), but there is no room for complacency. Deaths will continue to occur, especially in the very young and old, until all patients come to operation before the appendix has perforated.

Infection

The wound is the commonest site of post-appendicectomy infection. The incidence of wound infection varies from 2% in non-perforated appendicitis (Nystrom 1979, Simonowitz & White 1979) to 3% in appendix abscess (Nystrom 1979, Simonowitz & White 1979, Schultz et al 1983). Delay in diagnosis and operation is thus the most important determinant, and these factors are also responsible for the development of intra-abdominal abscess. The second commonest site for infection is the pelvis, where sepsis occurs in up to 18% of patients (Finne 1978). The usual presentation is the onset of diarrhoea 5–10 days after appendicectomy. A boggy mass can then be felt, and often drained, transrectally (Finne 1978). Stump abscess following invagination is uncommon (Sinha 1977, Thomas 1974), and a faecal fistula rarely results. In the pre-antibiotic era one-third of pyogenic liver abscesses were secondary to appendicitis (Oschner et al 1938), but this and the associated problem of portal thrombophlebitis are uncommon (Wintch et al 1982).

As the appendicitis progresses bacterial migration occurs through the wall. In early appendicitis aerobic infection is common, whilst a mixed growth of aerobes and anaerobes predominates later (Lau et al 1984b). Overall bacteriological swabs usually produce a mixed growth with a predominance of anaerobes (Ochsner et al 1938, Brook 1980, Leigh et al 1974). Antibacterial agents were first shown to reduce mortality in the 1940s (Ravdin et al 1940), and the introduction of prophylaxis in the 1970s has reduced the wound infection rate towards zero (Kortelainen et al 1982) and has become standard practice. There are numerous trials of antibiotic prophylaxis in acute appendicitis, but as the infection rate is now low they are unlikely to show drug X to be superior to drug Y. The ideal choice at present would seem to be a single preoperative dose of metronidazole (Kortelainen et al 1982), with the addition of an aerobicide if the appendix is found to be perforated or gangrenous at operation (Berne et al 1982). If single agent therapy is essential, then moxalactam (Lau et al 1984a) or Imipenem (Heseltine et al 1986) would appear to be effective. There is no doubt that antibiotics are effective both medically and financially (Gill et al 1986).

The surgical treatment of an established abscess is drainage, but should drains be used in other cases? This problem has been well aired in the surgical literature since 1880 and was reviewed by Warren (1939). His conclusion that morbidity and mortality rates were lower if drains were not used is reinforced by the increased incidence of abscess and faecal fistula formation in their presence (Haller et al 1973, Stone et al 1978). Many surgeons confronted with a perforated appendix and contamination still continue to pack the wound (Burns et al 1985), although Pettigrew (1981) has demonstrated that delayed primary closure does not reduce the incidence of wound infection.

Infertility

Adhesions consequent upon pelvic sepsis are a major cause of infertility. Although infertility has never been related to appendiceal perforation alone, it is twice as common in women who subsequently develop a pelvic abscess (Wiig et al 1979). Despite the high negative appendicectomy rate, this fact alone might justify a liberal policy of operation in young women.

Stump problems

Haemorrhage may occur from the invaginated stump but should be prevented by previous ligature (Sinha 1977). Ileocolic intussusception is rare and may necessitate a right hemicolectomy (Wolfson et al 1984). Faecal fistula complicates <1% of operations and may also require ileocaecal resection, if it does not close spontaneously.

Right inguinal hernia

Denervation of the transversalis muscle guarding the deep ring has been widely reported to lead to inguinal hernia formation after appendicectomy (Arnbjornsson 1982a, 1982b), although not all authors agree (Leech et al 1972).

Malignancy

The commonest tumour of the appendix is a carcinoid, which as an incidental finding after appendicectomy usually requires no further action.

Adenocarcinomas are unusual but do require reoperation and a right hemicolectomy (Simonowitz & White 1979, Gilhome et al 1984). There is no relationship between appendicectomy and an increased tendency to develop general (Cooperman 1983) or colorectal (Moertel et al 1974) neoplasms, despite previous claims (McVay 1964).

Negative appendicectomy

Around 20% of all operations for appendicitis will reveal a normal appendix. Although half of these patients have another lesion that requires operation, others do not and may suffer unnecessary complications (Lau et al 1984a, Bell et al 1982). The financial loss to the patient may be considerable and the negative operation is not without complications (Lau et al 1984a). Clearly if the patient's condition is satisfactory a period of observation is justified, but delay must not lead to perforation, since this single event is responsible for most of the morbidity and mortality of appendicitis. Careful clinical evaluation can reduce, but will not eliminate, the incidence of negative appendicectomies.

Conclusion

Appendicitis treated prior to perforation is a benign disease with a low complication rate. Once perforation does occur serious sequelae will ensue. A high degree of diagnostic skill is required to keep both the perforation rate and the incidence of negative appendicectomy low.

REFERENCES

Abruzzo J L, Homa M, Houck J C, Coffey R J 1958 Significance of the serum amylase determination. Annals of Surgery 147: 921–930

Amyand C 1736 Of an inguinal rupture, with a pin in the appendix caeci, incrusted with stone; and some observations on wounds in the guts. Philosophical Transactions of the Royal Society of London 39: 329–342

Andersson N, Griffiths H, Murphy J et al 1979 Is appendicitis familial? British Medical Journal ii: 697–698

Arnbjornsson E 1982a Development of right inguinal hernia

after appendectomy. American Journal of Surgery 143: 174–175

Arnbjornsson E 1982b A neuromuscular basis for the development of right inguinal hernia after appendectomy. American Journal of Surgery 143: 367–369

Arnbjornsson E 1983 Acute appendicitis risk in various phases of the menstrual cycle. Acta Chirurgica Scandinavica 149: 603–605

Arnbjornsson E 1984 The influence of oral contraceptives on the frequency of acute appendicitis in different phases of the menstrual cycle. Surgery Gynecology and Obstetrics 158: 464–466

Arnbjornsson E, Bengmark S 1984 Role of obstruction in the pathogenesis of acute appendicitis. American Journal of Surgery 147: 390–392

Arnheim E E, Neuhof H 1940 The severer forms of acute appendicitis with special reference to the treatment of appendiceal abscess. Surgery Gynecology and Obstetrics 70: 42–47

Ayalon A, Mogilner M, Cohen O, Luttwak Z, Schiller M 1979 Acute appendicitis in a premature baby. Acta Chirurgica Scandinavica 145: 285 286

Babler E A 1908 Perforative appendicitis complicating pregnancy. Journal of the American Medical Association 51: 1310–1314

Balch C M, Silver D 1971 Foreign bodies in the appendix. Archives of Surgery 102: 14–20

Barker D 1986 Epidemiology of appendicitis. In: The aetiology of acute appendicitis (MRC Scientific report No 7) Medical Research Council, London, pp 3–9

Battle W H 1897 A contribution to the surgical treatment of diseases of the appendix vermiformis. British Medical Journal i: 965–967

Bell M J, Bower R J, Ternberg J L 1982 Appendectomy in childhood. Analysis of 105 negative explorations. American Journal of Surgery 144: 335–337

Bennion R S, Thompson J E 1987 Early appendectomy for perforated appendicitis in children should not be abandoned. Surgery Gynecology and Obstetrics 165: 95–100

Berne T V, Yellin A W, Appleman M D, Heseltine P N R 1982 Antibiotic management of surgically treated gangrenous or perforated appendicitis. American Journal of Surgery 144: 8–13

Berry J, Malt R A 1984 Appendicitis near its centenary. Annals of Surgery 200: 567–575

Bett W R 1934 Appendicitis. In: Bett W R (ed) A short history of some common disease. Oxford University Press, London pp 162–171

Bohrod M G 1946 The pathogenesis of acute appendicitis. American Journal of Clinical Pathology 16: 752–760

Bongard F, Landers D V, Lewis F 1985 Differential diagnosis of appendicitis and pelvic inflammatory disease. American Journal of Surgery 150: 90–96

Bradley E L, Isaacs J 1978 Appendiceal abscess revisited. Archives of Surgery 113: 130–132

Bright R, Addison T 1839 Elements of the practice of medicine. Longmans Green, London

Brook I 1980 Bacterial studies of peritoneal cavity and postoperative surgical wound drainage following perforated appendix in children. Annals of Surgery 192: 208–212

Brooks D W, Killen D A 1965 Roentgenographic findings in acute appendicitis. Surgery 57: 377–384

Budd D C, Fouty W J 1977 Familial retrocaecal appendicitis. American Journal of Surgery 133: 670–671

Burkitt D P 1971 The aetiology of appendicitis. British Journal of Surgery 58: 695–699

Burnett W, Ness T D 1955 Serum amylase and acute abdominal disease. British Medical Journal ii: 770–772

Burns R P, Cochran J L, Russel W L 1985 Appendicitis in mature patients. Annals of Surgery 201: 695–704

Coetzee T 1958 Acute appendicitis in an infant. South African Medical Journal 382: 890–891

Collins D C 1961 Left-sided colonic lesions masquerading as acute appendicitis. American Journal of Gastroenterology 36: 521–524

Cooperman M 1983 Complications of appendectomy. Surgical Clinics of North America 63: 1233–1247

Cunningham F G, McCubbin J H 1975 Appendicitis complicating pregnancy. Obstetrics and Gynecology 45: 415–420

Da Carpi B 1521 Commentaria, in Williams R G 1983 A history of appendicitis. Annals of Surgery 197: 495–506

Davis G G 1906 A transverse incision for the removal of the appendix. Annals of Surgery 43: 106–110

De Dombal F T, Leaper D J, Horrocks J C, Staniland J R, McCann A P 1974 Human and computer aided diagnosis of abdominal pain. British Medical Journal i: 376–380

Deutsch A A, Zelikovsky A, Reiss R 1982 Laparoscopy in the prevention of unnecessary appendicectomies: a prospective study. British Journal of Surgery 69: 336–337

DeVore G R 1980 Acute abdominal pain in the pregnant patient due to pancreatitis, acute appendicitis, cholecystitis, or peptic ulcer disease. Clinical Perinatology 7: 349–369

Dupuytren G 1833 Des abcès de la fosse iliaque droite. Leçons Chirurgiques 3: 330–332

Edwards F H, Davies R S 1984 Use of a Bayesian algorithm in the computer-assisted diagnosis of appendicitis. Surgery Gynecology and Obstetrics 158: 219–222

Fedyshin P, Kelvin F M, Rice R P 1984 Nonspecificity of barium enema findings in acute appendicitis. American Journal of Roentgenology 143: 99–102

Fields I A, Cole N M 1967 Acute appendicitis in infants 36 months of age or younger. American Journal of Surgery 113: 269–275

Fields I A, Naiditch M J, Rothman P E 1957 Acute appendicitis in infants. American Journal of Diseases of Children 93: 287–301

Finne C O 1978 Transrectal drainage of pelvic abscesses. Diseases of the Colon and Rectum 23: 293–297

Fitz R H 1886 Perforating inflammation of the vermiform appendix. American Journal of Medical Sciences 92: 321–346

Fock G, Gastrin U, Josephson S 1969 Appendiceal peritonitis in children. Acta Chirurgica Scandinavica 135: 534–538

Fonkalsrud E W, Ament M E, Fleisher D 1982 Management of the appendix in young patients with Crohn's disease. Archives of Surgery 117: 11–14

Foran B, Berne T V, Rosoff L 1978 Management of the appendiceal mass. Archives of Surgery 113: 1144–1145

Gastrin U, Josephson S 1969 Appendiceal abscess — acute appendectomy or conservative treatment. Acta Chirurgica Scandinavica 135: 539–542

Gilhome R W, Johnston D H, Clarke J, Kyle J 1984 Primary adenocarcinoma of the vermiform appendix: report of a series of ten cases, and review of the literature. British Journal of Surgery 71: 553–555

Gill M A, Chenella F C, Heseltine P N R et al 1986 Cost analysis of antibiotics in the management of perforated or gangrenous appendicitis. American Journal of Surgery 151: 200–204

Gilmore O J A, Brodribb A J B M, Browett J P et al 1975 Appendicitis and mimicking conditions. Lancet ii: 421–424

Grundtiz T, Ryden C I, Janzon L 1983 Does the retrocecal position influence the course of acute appendicitis. Acta Chirurgica Scandinavica 149: 707–710

Hall R J 1886 Suppurative peritonitis due to ulceration and supuration of the vermiform appendix. New York Medical Journal 43: 662–663

Haller J A, Shaker I J, Donahoo J S, Schnaufer L, White J J 1973 Peritoneal drainage versus non-drainage for generalized peritonitis from ruptured appendicitis in children: a prospective study. Annals of Surgery 177: 595–600

Hancock H 1848 Disease of the appendix caeci cured by operation. Lancet ii: 380–381

Harrison M W, Lindner D J, Campbell J R, Campbell T J 1984 Acute appendicitis in children: factors affecting morbidity. American Journal of Surgery 147: 605–610

Heaton K W 1987 Aetiology of acute appendicitis. British Medical Journal 294: 1632–1633

Heseltine P N R, Yellin A E, Appleman M D et al 1986 Imipenam therapy for perforated and gangrenous appendicitis. Surgery Gynecology and Obstetrics 162: 43–48

Hoffmann J, Lindhard A, Jensen H E 1984 Appendix mass: conservative management without interval appendectomy. American Journal of Surgery 148: 379–382

Jackson R H 1963 Parents, family doctors and acute appendicitis in childhood. British Medical Journal ii: 277–281

Janik J S, Ein S H, Shandling B, Simpson J S, Stephens C A 1980 Non surgical management of appendiceal mass in late presenting children. Journal of Pediatric Surgery 15: 574–576

Jess P, Bjerregaard B, Brynitz S 1981 Acute appendicitis; prospective trial concerning diagnostic accuracy and complications. American Journal of Surgery 141: 232–234

Jones B A, Demetriades D, Segal I, Burkitt D P 1985 The prevalence of appendiceal fecaliths in patients with and without appendicitis. Annals of Surgery 202: 80–82

Jordan J S, Kovalcik P J, Schwab C W 1981 Appendicitis with a palpable mass. Annals of Surgery 193: 227–229

Karstrup S, Torp-Pedersen S, Roikjaer A 1986 Ultrasonic visualisation of the inflamed appendix. British Journal of Radiology 59: 985–986

Kelly H A 1905 In: The vermiform appendix and its diseases. Saunders, Philadelphia

Killen D A, Brooks D W 1965 Gas filled appendix: a roentgenographic sign of acute appendicitis. Annals of Surgery 161: 474–478

Kortelainen P, Huttunen R, Kairaluoma M I, Mokka R E M, Laitmen S, Larmi T K I 1982 Single-dose intrarectal metronidazole prophylaxis against wound infection after appendectomy. American Journal of Surgery 143: 244–245

Ladd W E 1938 Immediate or deferred surgery for general peritonitis associated with appendicitis in children. New England Journal of Medicine 219: 329–333

Lau W, Fan S, Yiu T, Chu K W, Wong S H 1984a Negative findings at appendectomy. American Journal of Surgery 148: 375–378

Lau W Y, Teoh-Chan C H, Fan S T, Yam W C, Lau K F, Wong S M 1984b The bacteriology and septic complication of patients with appendicitis. Annals of Surgery 200: 576–581

Leape L L, Ramenofsky M L 1980 Laparoscopy for questionable appendicitis: Can it reduce the negative appendectomy rate? Annals of Surgery 191: 410–413

Leech P, Waddel G, Main R 1972 The incidence of right inguinal hernia following appendectomy. British Journal of Surgery 59: 623

Leigh D A, Simmons K, Norman E 1974 Bacterial flora of the appendix fossa in appendicitis and postoperative wound infection. Journal of Clinical Pathology 27: 997–1000

Lindgren I, Aho A J 1969 Microangiographic investigations on acute appendicitis. Acta Chirurgica Scandinavica 135: 77–82

Louyer-Villermay J B 1824 Observations pour servir à l'histoire des inflammations de l'appendice du caecum. Archives of General Medicine, Paris 5: 246–250

Ludbrook J, Spears G F S 1965 The risk of developing appendicitis. British Journal of Surgery 52: 856–858

McBurney C 1889 Experience with early operative interference in cases of disease of the vermiform appendix. New York Medical Journal 50: 676–684

McMurrich J P 1930 Leonardo da Vinci the anatomist. Williams & Wilkins, Baltimore p 291

McVay J R 1964 The appendix in relation to neoplastic disease. Cancer 17: 929–939

Major R H 1965 Classic descriptions of disease. C C Thomas, Springfield Ill, pp 648–650

Martin D L, Gustafson T L 1985 A cluster of true appendicitis cases. American Journal of Surgery 150: 554–557

Masters K, Levine B A, Gaskill H V, Sirinek K R 1984 Diagnosing appendicitis during pregnancy. American Journal of Surgery 148: 768–771

Moertel C, Nobrega F T, Elveback L R, Wentz D R 1974 A prospective study of appendicectomy and predisposition to cancer. Surgery, Gynecology and Obstetrics 138: 549–553

Morgagni G B 1719 Adversaria anatomica tertia pp 24–28, in Williams R G 1983 A history of appendicitis. Annals of Surgery 197: 495–506

Morris D M, Cocker D D, Coleman J J, Wiernik P H, Elias E G 1987 Effect of incidental appendectomy on the development of wound infection in patients undergoing staging laparotomy for Hodgkin's disease. American Journal of Surgery 153: 226–229

Morson B C, Dawson I M P 1979 Inflammatory disorders. In: Gastrointestinal pathology. Blackwell Scientific, London pp 455–465

Mosegaard A, Nielsen O S 1979 Interval appendectomy. Acta Chirurgica Scandinavica 145: 109–111

Murphy J B 1904 Two-thousand operations for appendicitis with deductions from his personal experience. American Journal of Medical Sciences 128: 187–197

Nockerts S R, Detmer D E, Fryback D G 1980 Incidental appendectomy in the elderly? No. Surgery 88: 301–306

Noer T 1976 Decreasing incidence of acute appendicitis. Acta Chirurgica Scandinavica 141: 431–432

Nystrom P O 1979 Contamination with enterobacteria and postoperative wound infection after appendicectomy. Acta Chirurgica Scandinavica 145: 411–413

Ochsner A J 1902 In: A handbook of appendicitis. G P Gerhardt, Chicago

Ochsner A M, DeBakey M, Murray S 1938 Pyogenic abscess of the liver. American Journal of Surgery 40: 292

Owens B J, Hamit H F 1978 Appendicitis in the elderly. Annals of Surgery 187: 392–396

Parker W 1867 An operation for abscess of the appendix veriformis caeci. Medical Record New York 2: 25–27

Paull D L, Bloom G P 1982 Appendiceal abscess. Archives of Surgery 117: 1017–1019

Peltokallio P 1966 Acute appendicitis associated with carcinoma of the colon. Diseases of the Colon and Rectum 9: 453–456

Peltokallio P, Jauhiainen K 1970 Acute appendicitis in the aged patient. Archives of Surgery 100: 140–143

Pettigrew R A 1981 Delayed primary wound closure in gangrenous and perforated appendicitis. British Journal of Surgery 68: 635–638

Piepar R, Kager L, Tidefeldt U 1982 Obstruction of appendix vermiformis causing acute appendicitis. Acta Chirurgica Scandinavica 148: 63–67

Pledger H G, Fahy L T, Mowrik G A, Bush G H 1987 Deaths in children with a diagnosis of acute appendicitis in England and Wales. British Medical Journal 295: 1233–1235

Punnonen R, Aho A J, Gronroos M, Liukko P 1979 Appendicetomy during pregnancy. Acta Chirurgica Scandinavica 145: 555–558

Pwylaert J B C M 1986 Acute appendicitis: ultrasound evaluation using graded compression. Radiology 158: 355–360

Ravdin I S, Rhoads J E, Lockwood J S 1940 The use of sulfanilamide in the treatment of peritonitis associated with appendicitis. Annals of Surgery 111: 53–63

Robinson J A, Burch B H 1984 An assessment of the value of the menstrual history in differentiating acute appendicitis from pelvic inflammatory disease. Surgery Gynecology and Obstetrics 159: 149–152

Ryden C I, Grunditz T, Janzon L 1983 Acute appendicitis in patients above and below 60 years of age. Acta Chirurgica Scandinavica 149: 165–170

Saebo A 1978 Pneumoperitoneum associated with perforated appendicitis. Acta Chirurgica Scandinavica 144: 115–117

Sands H B 1888 An account of a case in which recovery took place after laparotomy had been performed for septic peritonitis due to a perforation of the vermiform appendix with remarks upon this and allied diseases. New York Medical Journal 147: 197–205

Schey W I 1973 Use of barium in the diagnosis of appendicitis in children. American Journal of Roentgenology 118: 95–103

Schisgall R M 1980 Appendiceal colic in childhood. The role of inspissated casts of stool within the appendix. Annals of Surgery 192: 687–693

Schisgall R M 1983 Use of barium swallow in the diagnosis of acute appendicitis. American Journal of Surgery 146: 663–667

Schultz A, Jorgensen P M, Jorgensen S P 1983 Septic complications after appendicectomy for perforated appendicitis. Acta Chirurgica Scandinavica 149: 517–520

Schwartz M Z, Tapper D, Solenberger R I 1983 Management of perforated appendicitis in children. The controversy continues. Annals of Surgery 197: 407–411

Sherren J 1905 The causation and treatment of appendicitis. Practitioner 74: 833–844

Simonowitz D A, White T T 1979 Post operative complications of appendectomy. Clinical Gastroenterology 8: 429–441

Simonowitz D A, Rusch V W, Stevenson J K 1982 Natural history of incidental appendectomy in patients with Crohn's disease who required subsequent bowel resection.

American Journal of Surgery 143: 171–173

Sinha A P 1977 Appendicectomy: an assessment of the advisability of stump invagination. British Journal of Surgery 64: 499–500

Skoubo-Kristensen E, Hvid I 1983 The appendiceal mass. Results of conservative management. Annals of Surgery 196: 584–587

Stevenson S R 1962 In: Famous illnesses in history. Eyre, London, pp 32–43

Stone H H, Hooper C A, Millikan W J 1978 Abdominal drainage following appendectomy and cholecystectomy. Annals of Surgery 187: 606–612

Strom P R, Turkleson M L, Stone H H 1983 Safety of incidental appendectomy. American Journal of Surgery 145: 819–822

Strom S 1921–22 In: On the roentgen diagnostics of changes in the appendix and caecum. Acta Radiologica 1: 133–136

Sumpio B E, Ballantyne G H, Zdon M J, Modlin I M 1986 Perforated appendicitis and obstructing colonic carcinoma in the elderly. Diseases of the Colon and Rectum 29: 668–670

Swensson E E, Maull K I 1981 Clinical significance of elevated serum and urine amylase levels in patients with appendicitis. American Journal of Surgery 142: 667–670

Teicher I, Landa B, Cohen M, Kabnick L S, Wise L 1983 Scoring system to aid in diagnoses of appendicitis. Annals of Surgery 198: 753–759

Thomas M P 1974 Burst stump abscess following appendicectomy: a report of four cases. New Zealand Journal of Surgery 44: 47–49

Trapnell J E, Anderson M C 1967 Role of early laparotomy in acute pancreatitis. Annals of Surgery 165: 49–55

Truelsen F 1961 Comments on the treatment of acute appendicitis. Acta Chirurgica Scandinavica Suppl 283: 275–281

Walters E G 1977 Elective appendectomy with abdominal and pelvic surgery. Obstetrics and Gynecology 50: 511–517

Warren R 1939 Primary closure of peritoneum in acute appendicitis with perforation. Annals of Surgery 110: 222–230

Way C W V, Murphy J R, Dunn E L, Elerding S C 1982 A feasibility study of computer aided diagnosis in appendicitis. Surgery Gynecology and Obstetrics 155: 685–688

Wangensteen O H, Bowers W F 1937 Significance of the obstructive factor in the genesis of acute appendicitis. Archives of Surgery 34: 496–526

Weisflog 1906 Zur rontgenographischen Diagnose der Enterolithen des Processus vermiformis. Fortschritte auf dem Gebiete der Röntgenstrahlen 10: 217–219

Westermann C, Mann W J, Chumas J 1986 Routine appendectomy in extensive gynaecological operations. Surgery Gynecology and Obstetrics 162: 307–312

Wiig J N, Janssen C W, Fuglesang P et al 1979 Infertility as a complication of perforated appendicitis. Acta Chirurgica Scandinavica 145: 409–410

Winch R W, Reines H D, Rambo W M 1982 Liver abscess: a changing entity. American Journal of Surgery 48: 11–15

Wolfson S, Shachor D, Freund U 1984 Ileocolic intussusception in an adult. A postoperative complication of appendectomy. Diseases of the Colon and Rectum 27: 265–266

16 *Gynaecological causes of the acute abdomen*

M. E. SETCHELL and P. L. CASS

The gynaecological causes of an acute abdominal crisis discussed in this chapter are important for a number of reasons. Firstly, some of the conditions are potentially fatal and require prompt diagnosis and treatment to save life. Secondly, gynaecological causes of the acute abdomen are often difficult to differentiate from surgical causes; just as the gynaecologist needs knowledge of related surgical conditions, so the surgeon needs to be aware of the gynaecological problems which he or she may encounter. Paterson-Brown et al (1988) showed that 13% of patients admitted by a surgical unit with acute abdominal pain had pain of gynaecological origin. Thirdly, the pelvic organs are delicate, and their proper function is of immeasurable importance to women. It is no exaggeration to say that injudicious or inappropriate surgery may ruin a woman's health, reproductive capacity, marriage and happiness.

Disorders of the uterus, ovaries or Fallopian tubes may be responsible for acute abdominal pain, and vaginal examination is an obligatory part of the examination of a woman presenting with acute abdominal pain. Certain investigations are particularly helpful as diagnostic aids in acute gynaecological conditions.

Diagnostic aids

Pelvic ultrasound

Ultrasonic scanning of the pelvis has added a whole dimension to the diagnosis of the acute gynaecological abdomen. This examination is increasingly available in casualty departments, and the development of transvaginal scanning means that the acutely ill patient can be scanned without the need for filling the bladder. Ovarian cysts and tumours, uterine enlargement, and early pregnancy, whether intrauterine or extrauterine, may be confidently diagnosed.

Rapid Beta HCG testing

Human chorionic gonadotrophin (HCG) is produced by the trophoblast, and the beta sub-unit can be detected as early as 7 days after conception. Ectopic pregnancy and pain associated with early pregnancy can be diagnosed much earlier nowadays because of the advent of sensitive and rapid beta HCG assays, which may be done either on blood or urine. A positive beta HCG and an ultrasonic scan that fails to demonstrate an intrauterine pregnancy are almost diagnostic of ectopic pregnancy.

White blood count

A raised white blood count may occur in acute pelvic inflammatory disease, or following abortion, and may be a helpful supportive test.

Radiography

Radiography has little place in the diagnosis of acute gynaecological emergencies, but it may be useful to rule out intestinal causes of pain and renal calculi.

Laparoscopy

Laparoscopy has a most useful part to play in the diagnosis of acute pain in young women. It may preclude the need for laparotomy or guide the surgeon to the diagnosis and prevent the need for a large 'exploratory laparotomy' incision. Laparoscopy is a skilled procedure, which should not be undertaken unless the surgeon is trained and has the opportunity to maintain his or her skills. Most gynaecological surgeons are pleased to help their surgical colleagues with this procedure, even in male patients. Laparoscopy is contraindicated in the presence of intestinal obstruction or ileus, or in generalized peritonitis, and caution should be exercised if the patient has had previous abdominal surgery.

Ovarian causes of acute abdominal pain

The ovary is an organ that undergoes dramatic cyclical physiological changes, and disturbances of its physiology, as well as pathological conditions, may give rise to acute abdominal pain. At the beginning of a menstrual cycle a cohort of ovarian follicles begins to develop. By about the eighth day of the cycle one (or occasionally two) of the follicles has become dominant and is destined to ovulate. Prior to ovulation a ripe Graafian follicle is 20–30 mm in diameter. Many women are aware of ovulation because the release of the oocyte and follicular fluid is accompanied by a transient abdominal pain (Mittelschmerz). Following ovulation, the granulosa cells undergo the process of luteinization and the corpus luteum is formed. Various disturbances of physiology may give rise to pain.

Multiple follicular development

Multiple follicles may develop, as in polycystic ovary syndrome or in hyperstimulation from gonadotrophin therapy. Pain is not usually severe in these circumstances unless gross hyperstimulation and cyst formation is produced. In the fully blown 'hyperstimulation syndrome' which may occur with gonadotrophin treatment, large ovarian cysts develop, together with ascites, pleural effusions, electrolyte disturbances and hypoproteinaemia. Conservative supportive management is appropriate, and surgical intervention is rarely required.

Follicular rupture and haemorrhage

Occasionally the follicle rupture is accompanied by quite marked haemorrhage from the follicle wall, producing intra-abdominal bleeding sufficient to cause severe pain, with physical signs of intraperitoneal haemorrhage. This is a kind of exaggerated Mittelschmerz, but there may be confusion with the diagnosis of ectopic pregnancy if a large ovarian bleed has occurred.

Follicular/corpus luteum cyst formation

Sometimes a Graafian follicle fails to rupture and goes on growing to 50–60 mm in diameter. The unruptured follicle produces oestrogen and delays menstruation so that pregnancy may be suspected. Eventually the cyst either ruptures or regresses over the course of 2–3 months.

After ovulation there is always some haemorrhage into the follicle, and if this is excessive a corpus luteum cyst may develop either in a cycle associated with pregnancy or in a cycle associated with delayed menstruation. Again the cyst is not likely to be more than 50–60 mm in diameter, but the occurrence of lower abdominal pain and delayed menstruation will cause diagnostic confusion.

Ultrasonic scans and laparoscopy may be helpful in the diagnosis, but essentially the management of small cysts is conservative and expectant. If laparotomy has been undertaken because of the severity of pain, simple puncturing of the follicular cyst or oversewing of a haemorrhagic cyst is all that is required. Many a healthy ovary has been removed or damaged in a young woman explored for suspected appendicitis, and the right ovary is more vulnerable than the left to such attack.

Ovarian neoplasm

Truly neoplastic cysts of the ovary may give rise to acute pain, but usually only when they have undergone a complication such as torsion, haemorrhage, rupture or infection.

Torsion

Torsion of an ovarian cyst results in the acute onset of severe abdominal pain, usually accompanied by vomiting. The pain is constant, often localized to one iliac fossa. Abdominal and vaginal tenderness are present, often precluding precise definition of the margins of the tumour. The presence of a cyst/tumour may be confirmed by ultrasound, or the outline of the cyst may be visible on plain abdominal X-ray, particularly if there is any calcification such as teeth in a dermoid cyst or *Psammoma* bodies in a malignant tumour.

Laparotomy should be arranged early, as it may be possible to save the ovary if infarction has not occurred. The incision will depend on the size of the cyst: as a general guide, if the cyst is larger than a pregnancy at 14 weeks (the size of a grapefruit), a midline or paramedian incision is preferred, but if it is smaller, and there is no particular suggestion of malignancy, a transverse suprapubic incision is satisfactory. If the patient is a young woman, an attempt should be made to untwist the cyst; if colour reverts to normal within 10 minutes, the cyst may be enucleated and the remaining ovarian tissue refashioned. It is important to use fine non-absorbable sutures on the surface of the ovary (such as 4/0 Prolene), and to pay meticulous attention to haemostasis in order to avoid adhesion formation. Infarction, suspicion of malignancy or torsion in a perimenopausal woman are indications for oophorectomy. If malignancy is suspected (contralateral ovarian tumour, considerable ascites, warty excrescences on the ovarian surface, fixity, omental or peritoneal deposits), hysterectomy and removal of the other ovary should be performed. If there is any doubt a gynaecological opinion should be sought. It is important to stage ovarian malignancy at laparotomy, and this includes taking peritoneal washings for cytology, inspecting and taking smears from the subdiaphragmatic peritoneum, palpating and if necessary biopsying para-aortic nodes, as well as carrying out a thorough laparotomy. The possibility of the ovarian tumour being a secondary malignancy should not be overlooked (Shepherd & Monaghan 1985).

Rupture

Rupture of an ovarian cyst presents as acute abdominal pain, usually generalized with symptoms and signs of peritonism. Ultrasound or radiography may indicate the presence of some free fluid, but neither are likely to identify the ruptured ovarian cyst, and laparoscopy or laparotomy will usually be carried out before a precise diagnosis is made. Sometimes it will be possible to enucleate the ovarian cyst, but often it may be necessary to remove the whole ovary. Decisions about removal of the other ovary and uterus will depend upon age of the patient and suspicion of malignancy. Rupture of an endometriotic (chocolate) cyst is not uncommon, and dark brown (chocolate) material will be disseminated throughout the pelvis and abdomen. It is important to mop out as much chocolate material as possible, as it may contain endometrial cells which can implant widely. There may be dense adhesions if the endometriosis is long established, making operation difficult. Having dealt with the ruptured cyst by enucleation or oophorectomy and mopped out the chocolate material, it is often best to be conservative, as modern hormone preparations may be given postoperatively with considerable improvement in the residual endometriosis. It is particularly important to preserve ovarian tissue now that in-vitro fertilisation and other methods of assisted reproduction are available to treat the infertility associated with this condition.

If a ruptured cyst has the characteristics of a malignant cyst, pelvic clearance is advisable, with careful inspection of the rest of the abdomen, biopsy of any suspicious nodules and omentectomy if the omentum appears to be involved. Subsequent chemotherapy or radiotherapy is likely to be necessary if there has been spillage of malignant cells.

Tubal causes of abdominal pain

Ectopic pregnancy

Ectopic pregnancy is a gestation outside the uterine cavity. Ninety-five per cent occur in the Fallopian tube, and most of these are in the ampullary portion. Less common sites are the isthmic and fimbrial portions of the tube, and rarely implantation occurs in the uterine cornu, cervix, ovary or elsewhere in the peritoneal cavity.

In England and Wales in the years 1982–1984, 13 women died from ectopic pregnancy. The main cause of death was delay in diagnosis and subsequent operation (HMSO 1989). The effects on further childbearing are serious, the risks of a repeat ectopic pregnancy, sterility and abortion being high. Seventy percent of women having a first ectopic do not subsequently produce a living child, and up to 30% will have a further ectopic pregnancy.

It is wise to assume that any woman of childbearing age presenting with amenorrhoea, irregular bleeding or pelvic pain is pregnant until proved otherwise, and all these pregnancies are potentially ectopic.

Incidence

There is considerable variation in the incidence of ectopic pregnancy in different countries. The incidence in the UK is of the order of 1:300 mature intrauterine pregnancies, although in the West Indies an incidence of 1:28 live births has been reported (Douglas 1963).

Aetiology

Pelvic inflammatory disease and associated tubal damage are widely regarded to be the most important aetiological factors in ectopic gestation. The incidence of pelvic inflammation has risen sharply over the last 20 years, and this probably accounts for the rise in the incidence of ectopic pregnancy. Tubal infection may damage both cilial function, vital in transporting the ovum, and tubal peristalsis.

Some forms of contraception have been associated with an increased incidence of ectopic gestation. If a woman conceives with an intrauterine contraceptive device in situ there is a high incidence of ectopic gestation, and this risk increases with prolonged use of an intrauterine contraceptive device (IUD). Using oral progestogen as the only means of contraception may carry an increased risk of ectopic pregnancy, probably due to delayed tubal motility as a result of progesterone action on smooth muscle.

The incidence of ectopic pregnancy is also raised if conception follows sterilization by tubal ligation, reversal of sterilization, tubal surgery, in-vitro fertilization (IVF) and other methods of assisted reproduction. Transperitoneal migration of the ovum into the contralateral tube may result in an ectopic pregnancy, as may implantation in a congenital tubal diverticulum.

Diagnosis

The Confidential Report (HMSO 1989) demonstrates the importance of diagnosis being made early and treatment instituted as soon as possible. An incorrect diagnosis is initially made in 25–50% of cases, and the time between initial consultation and surgery exceeds 48 hours in 40–50% cases; it is longer than 1 week in 20–25% of cases (Kadar 1983). The two common types of ectopic pregnancy present very differently. Frank rupture of the Fallopian tube produces acute intraperitoneal haemorrhage and shock, and the accompanying classical symptoms and signs should lead to the diagnosis. A leaking ectopic pregnancy may be much more difficult to diagnose, especially when the woman has a history of irregular menses, appears well and has minimal symptoms. The cardinal symptoms are abdominal pain, secondary amenorrhoea and abnormal vaginal bleeding, and the cardinal signs are adnexal tenderness and cervical excitation. Ninety-five percent of patients complain of abdominal pain, 75% give a history of amenorrhoea and/or abnormal vaginal bleeding, and 10–15% have syncope, shoulder tip pain, or bowel abnormalities (notably tenesmus); shock is present in 10–15% of cases.

An adnexal mass can be felt in 30–50% of patients, although vaginal examination is best performed where facilities for rapid resuscitation and operation are available, in case the examination ruptures the ectopic, leading to sudden collapse. Most cases of ectopic pregnancy will not be diagnosed early without the aid of special investigations, and several valuable aids to diagnosis are now available.

Until recently pregnancy tests as an aid to diagnosis were notoriously inaccurate. However, with the advent of extremely sensitive immuno-enzymetric assays for the beta-subunit of HCG, this investigation has an important place in diagnosis. A negative serum beta-HCG virtually discounts pregnancy of whatever nature from the differential diagnosis. A positive beta-HCG, with the exception of rare germ cell tumours, confirms that the woman is pregnant but gives no indication as to the site or the viability of the pregnancy.

The finding of a positive beta-HCG necessitates locating the intrauterine or extrauterine site of the pregnancy. Abdominal ultrasound is useful when it demonstrates an intrauterine pregnancy, as the incidence of pregnancies which are both intrauterine and ectopic is very rare (1:30 000). However, unless a fetus or fetal heart is demonstrated lying outside the uterine cavity ultrasonographers will rarely commit themselves to a positive diagnosis of ectopic pregnancy. With the advent of transvaginal ultrasound scanning, giving excellent resolution, visualization of the pelvis is far better and may provide the diagnosis without resorting to diagnostic laparoscopy.

Diagnostic laparoscopy has become the outstanding diagnostic tool in recent years. It has completely altered the management of suspected ectopic pregnancy by giving a first-hand view of the pelvis and hence eliminating diagnostic error. It has replaced culdocentesis and diagnostic laparotomy. Although the laparoscope has to be used with caution and restraint, it obviates the need for laparotomy in one third of suspected ectopic pregnancies.

Treatment

A ruptured ectopic pregnancy presents either as an acute massive intraperitoneal haemorrhage or as slow recurrent bleeding from an extrauterine pregnancy, with the formation of a pelvic haematocoele and an intra-abdominal collection of blood. In the former the main requirement is to secure haemostasis by immediate laparotomy. Although adequate amounts of blood should be crossmatched, Group O rhesus-negative blood is used in extremis, and one should not await full resuscitation or attempt to achieve a normal blood pressure prior to surgery. Once haemorrhage is controlled by clamping of the bleeding vessels, then formal resuscitation and an adequate assessment can be made.

Most tubal pregnancies occur in the third decade of life, and over half of these women will probably wish to conceive again. Although the primary role of surgery in cases of ectopic pregnancy is to arrest or prevent haemorrhage, one has to consider ways to improve the subsequent live birth rate and reduce the recurrent ectopic pregnancy rate.

Salpingectomy is the recognized treatment for ruptured ectopic pregnancy and is still the method used in over 80% of cases. There is no justification for removing the ipsilateral ovary, and doing so may be detrimental to the woman if she ever requires assisted reproductive techniques, i.e. IVF. There is little place for conservative surgery in cases of frank rupture, but early diagnosis of an unruptured ectopic pregnancy may allow a more conservative approach.

Approximately 90% of tubal pregnancies are located in the distal two-thirds of the Fallopian tube and can be removed without sacrificing the tube. Conservative operations have been performed for many years, but the fear of subsequent postoperative haemorrhage, recurrent ectopic pregnancy in the conserved tube and the subsequent low rate of intrauterine pregnancies have restricted their acceptance. There is conflicting evidence as to whether there is any benefit to be gained from conservative tubal surgery as opposed to salpingectomy.

Patency rates of Fallopian tubes following linear salpingostomy for ectopic pregnancy vary between 75 and 100%, and tubal function after linear salpingostomy has been clearly demonstrated by patients with only one tube having successful pregnancies. Although there is no evidence to suggest that tubal conservation improves the live birth rate after an ectopic pregnancy, neither is there any evidence to suggest that it increases the rate of recurrent ectopic pregnancy (DeCherney & Kase 1979). Linear salpingostomy is the operation of choice for unruptured ectopic pregnancies and is best performed by using needle diathermy on the antimesenteric border of the tube over the site of the pregnancy. The products of conception are then extruded. Haemorrhage at the implantation site can be controlled by digital pressure, and the incision is closed with fine Prolene sutures or left to heal by secondary intention. Haemostasis is achieved by either point diathermy or a fine continuous locked haemostatic suture of absorbable material along the incision edges.

Ampullary and fimbrial pregnancies may be manually 'milked' out of the tube, but trophoblastic tissue may be left in situ with the danger of secondary haemorrhage. Any contralateral tubal pathology found at the time of operation is best left to be corrected at a later date if and when the need arises.

Linear salpingostomy may also be performed via the laparoscope and the tubal incision left open. Alternatively the pregnancy may be aspirated from the fimbrial end of the tube. The results obtained are just as good as those of laparotomy and reduce patient morbidity and hospitalization time. The conservative methods of treatment of ectopic pregnancy require experience and expertise, and the occasional operator is probably wiser to opt for salpingectomy in most cases.

A nonsurgical method of treatment of ectopic pregnancy has recently been described by Sauer et al (1987). Patients with unruptured ectopic pregnancies diagnosed at laparoscopy were treated with intramuscular methotrexate for a week. Seventy-five percent of the patients treated were subsequently shown to have tubal patency.

Pelvic infection

Acute pelvic infection is a common cause of acute abdominal pain in women. It usually results from ascending infection from the lower genital tract and involves the endometrium, Fallopian tubes and ovaries. It may occur as a result of sexual transmission, in the puerperium or following abortion. Minor gynaecological procedures (e.g. D & C, insertion of IUD or hysterosalpingography) carried out in the presence of lower genital tract infection may cause ascending infection and salpingitis. Secondary infection from appendicitis, diverticulitis or other primary intestinal sepsis may also occur.

Acute salpingitis

Salpingitis is almost invariably bilateral and causes lower abdominal pain and acute dyspareunia, usually associated with a purulent vaginal discharge and pyrexia. Sometimes there is vomiting and diarrhoea. Most cases (if not associated with recent pregnancy) result from sexually transmitted infection, and the risk of ascending infection is increased if the woman is an IUD user. Unilateral salpingitis is unusual unless the woman has had a previous salpingectomy (e.g. for ectopic pregnancy).

The physical signs include systemic illness with pyrexia and tachycardia, abdominal tenderness, guarding and rebound, and on pelvic examination there is cervical excitation pain and tenderness in the fornices, possibly with palpable adnexal masses due to a pus-filled tube or tubo-ovarian mass.

It is important to take cervical, urethral and vaginal swabs, as high vaginal swabs alone will frequently fail to grow the relevant organism. There may be a raised leucocyte count and a raised ESR. The important differential diagnoses are appendicitis, ectopic pregnancy and ovarian cyst accidents. Laparoscopy may be necessary to make a diagnosis, in which case swollen, inflamed tubes are seen, often with pus dripping from the fimbrial ends. If possible a sample of the pus should be obtained at laparoscopy by needle aspiration for microbiological culture (Table 16.1). In later or

Table 16.1 Organisms in acute salpingitis

Organism	Estimated incidence, %
Neisseria gonorrhoea	30–50
Chlamydia trachomatis	40–60
Bacteroides fragilis	0–10
Haemophilus influenzae	0–10
Mycoplasma hominis and *genitalium*	?
Escherichia coli	0–10

recurrent cases, a closed pyosalpinx or tubo-ovarian abscess may be seen, or there may be a pelvic abscess in the pouch of Douglas. In such circumstances there may be considerable omental and small bowel adhesions preventing adequate visualization. Sometimes acute salpingitis will be discovered at laparotomy undertaken for another suspected diagnosis. After taking microbiological specimens (including anaerobic and *Chlamydia* culture) the abdomen should be closed. If an abscess is present however it should be drained through a separate incision. Often an inflammatory mass will be found that has not yet progressed to abscess formation. Rarely it may be appropriate to remove tube and ovary if the abscess or inflammatory mass is easily separable, particularly if the infection is recurrent or future fertility is not desired. The decision to remove the uterus or ovaries should not be undertaken without careful thought and prior discussion with the patient.

A curious presentation of pelvic inflammatory disease is the FitzHugh-Curtis syndrome, which presents with right upper quadrant pain mimicking acute cholecystitis. Findings at operation are a normal gallbladder but fine fibrinous adhesions between the liver and anterior abdominal wall (perihepatitis), in addition to signs of pelvic inflammation. This syndrome is associated with either *Neisseria* or *Chlamydia* pelvic infection, and treatment is with the appropriate antibiotics.

It is important to treat salpingitis aggressively with antibiotics in order to prevent permanent tubal damage and sterility. Westrom et al (1979) have shown that a single attack of salpingitis is associated with a 10–20% incidence of sterility, whilst a second increases the incidence to 25% and a third attack to 60%. It would be reasonable to start antimicrobial therapy with erythromycin or tetracycline (or amoxycillin) and metronidazole until results of culture are available. If *Gonococcus* is cultured or suspected, penicillin or ampicillin may be preferred. There is often a mixed infection of aerobes and anaerobes, hence the need for combination chemotherapy. Quite often cultures are negative, and in such cases continuation of the chosen antibiotic depends upon clinical response. In severe infections with systemic illness or signs of peritonitis, intravenous antibiotics and fluids will be required. It is important to continue anti-biotics for 14 days, but if there is failure to improve clinically laparoscopy should be carried out, and if a mass develops laparotomy may be necessary. If the woman has an IUD it should be removed once antibiotics have been given for 24 hours.

A ruptured pyosalpinx or tubo-ovarian abscess results in an acutely ill patient, often with signs of shock, peritonitis and bacteraemia. Such patients will require intensive fluid therapy and antibiotics, in addition to laparotomy and drainage of pus.

Torsion of the Fallopian tube

Torsion of the Fallopian tube may occur with or without the ovary. The torsion may be partial and self-correcting, but then tends to recur. Patients are usually children or adolescents, complaining of severe lower abdominal pain to one or other side of the midline. Torsion may cause vomiting and occasionally bladder and bowel irritability.

When the condition is associated with tubal abnormality it usually follows a hydrosalpinx. Torsion of the tube also inevitably occurs when there is torsion of a paraovarian (fimbrial) cyst, because the tube is tightly stretched over the wall of the cyst.

Treatment is by laparotomy. If the tube is normal and still viable, it is possible to conserve it and stabilize it with a suture. When the tube is beyond recovery, salpingectomy is carried out.

Fibroid complications

Leiomyomas are extremely common benign uterine tumours, principally found in the reproductive years. They are present in about 20% of women over 30 years of age and are more common in black women. Even very large tumours are frequently asymptomatic, but occasionally fibroids do produce acute abdominal pain.

Red degeneration

This is a form of necrobiosis which begins as a venous infarction but eventually progresses to necrosis. It is particularly liable to occur in a fibroid which is growing rapidly, as may occur in pregnancy or on hormonal therapy. There is severe lower abdominal pain over the site of the fibroid, and a tender uterine mass is palpable. If the fibroid is large, a mild pyrexia and leucocytosis may occur. Management is essentially conservative with analgesics and supportive measures. It is particularly important not to attempt to remove fibroids in pregnancy as catastrophic haemorrhage and abortion is likely. The pain will subside once the infarction process is complete.

Torsion

A pedunculated submucous poylpoid fibroid may undergo torsion, producing acute pain, often with vomiting and systemic illness. If a pedunculated fibroid has a long stalk, the fibroid may be quite distant from the uterus, leading to confusion with an ovarian cyst; the diagnosis may not be confirmed until laparotomy. Simple ligation and excision is all that is required, unless there are multiple fibroids producing other symptoms such as menorrhagia, when myomectomy or hysterectomy may be considered. A submucous polypoid fibroid may be extruded through the cervix, often accompanied by severe colicky pain and heavy bleeding. In such circumstances the fibroid may be excised vaginally.

Impaction

A posterior wall fibroid may cause acute retroversion of the uterus and if large enough become impacted in the pelvis, leading to acute retention of urine because of pressure at the bladder neck. The bladder will be palpable as a cystic abdominopelvic mass, and vaginal examination will reveal a pelvis filled by the fibroid uterus. Treatment is to catheterize the patient, and when the bladder is empty to attempt to dislodge the uterus by bimanual manipulation. Myomectomy or hysterectomy is likely to be necessary in due course. Occasionally a calcified fibroid in an elderly patient may behave in a similar fashion.

IUD problems

Problems with an intrauterine contraceptive device may be a cause of acute abdominal pain. An IUD may be expelled by painful uterine contractions, usually shortly after insertion or during menstruation. Perforation of the uterus by an IUD can cause severe pelvic pain. The perforation will have been initiated at the time of insertion. Uterine contractions then result in further propulsion of the device through the uterine wall, causing severe pain until the device becomes an intra-abdominal foreign body. Once in the abdominal cavity an IUD rarely causes problems, although intestinal obstruction has been reported as a result of a band of adhesions. Finally, an IUD may be associated with acute pelvic infection.

It is important in taking a gynaecological history to enquire into the method of contraception and to remember that ectopic pregnancy not infrequently occurs in the presence of an IUD.

Menstrual pain

Dysmenorrhoea may be of such severity as to present as an acute abdominal emergency. It may be either the primary spasmodic type, in young women, or in older women secondary congestive dysmenorrhoea associated with pelvic inflammatory disease or endometriosis. Many women have retrograde menstruation, and on occasion this may be sufficient to cause severe abdominal pain with peritonism.

Surgical complications of gynaecological surgery

Complications of gynaecological surgery may occasionally present to the general surgeon, or his or her opinion may be sought by the gynaecologist in treating them. Even when the greatest care is taken with laparoscopy or laparotomy, there may occasionally be inadvertent damage to abdominal structures which may not have been noticed at the time. Other gynaecological procedures that can very occasionally result in damage to bowel or even the ureter are suction termination of pregnancy and less commonly, dilatation and curettage.

Vascular damage

Laparoscopy has been known to result in damage to omental vessels, iliac vessels, aorta and inferior vena cava, resulting in major intra-abdominal haemorrhage and shock. Hysterectomy and other pelvic operations may lead to primary or reactionary haemorrhage requiring the assistance of general or vascular surgeons. If haemorrhage cannot be arrested, occasionally it may be necessary to ligate the internal iliac arteries.

Intestinal injury

Dilatation and curettage of the uterus and vaginal termination of pregnancy may result in uterine perforation and damage to small or large bowel. If this is not immediately recognized, the patient will develop acute abdominal pain and peritonitis within 24 h of the operation.

Laparoscopy may result in intestinal damage, either from perforation with the Verre's needle or the laparoscopic trocar, or from diathermy procedures. Perforation from the Verre's needle will often seal spontaneously unless a postoperative ileus causes intestinal distension, but other injuries will lead to escape of bowel contents and peritonitis.

Rarely, intestinal damage may be caused during a gynaecological laparotomy. All these causes of intestinal injury will require laparotomy and repair of the viscus with or without defunctioning colostomy.

Urinary tract damage

At hysterectomy, the ureter is at risk of injury either at the pelvic brim or close to the cervix. The ureter may be severed, clamped, devascularized or caught in a ligature. Injury may occur less commonly at laparoscopy or termination of pregnancy. Failure to recognise the injury will lead to an immediate urinary leak, a urinary peritonitis or a fistula at a later stage. The bladder may similarly be damaged and the injury not observed until some days postoperatively. Cystoscopy, intravenous urography and other imaging techniques may be necessary to localize the site of urinary tract damage, and surgical repair is likely to be necessary.

REFERENCES

DeCherney A H, Kase N 1979 The conservative surgical management of unruptured ectopic pregnancy. Obstetrics and Gynecology 54: 451

Douglas C P 1963 Tubal ectopic pregnancy. British Medical Journal i: 638

HMSO 1989 Report on confidential enquiries into maternal deaths in England and Wales 1982–1984. HMSO, London

Kadar N 1983. Ectopic pregnancy In: Studd J (ed) Progress in obstetrics and gynaecology 3. Churchill Livingstone, Edinburgh, pp 305–323

Paterson-Brown S, Eckersley J R T, Dudley H A F 1988 The gynaecological profile of acute general surgery. Journal of the Royal College of Surgeons of Edinburgh. 33: 13–15

Sauer M V, Gorrill M J, Rodi I A et al 1987 Non surgical management of unruptured ectopic pregnancy: an extended clinical trial. Fertility and Sterility 48(5): 752–755

Shepherd J, Monaghan J 1985 Clinical gynaecological oncology. Blackwell, Oxford

Sweet R L, Mills J, Hadley K et al 1979 Use of laparoscopy to determine microbiologic aetiology of acute salpingitis. American Journal of Obstetrics and Gynecology 134: 68–74

Westrom L, Iosif S, Svensson L et al 1979 Infertility after acute salpingitis: results of treatment with different antibiotics. Current Therapeutic Research and Clinical Experiment 26 (suppl): 752–759

17 *Mesenteric ischaemia*

L. W. OTTINGER

Mesenteric infarction is a frequent postmortem finding. Such injuries are almost always the result of terminal and even agonal failure of intestinal perfusion. As an indication for urgent laparotomy, mesenteric infarction is rather uncommon. In the practice of an usual abdominal surgeon, less than 5% of operations will be done for this diagnosis. Further, most cases can be expected to have a fatal outcome. Survival rates, though they do vary somewhat depending on the underlying aetiology of infarction, are generally in the range of only 10–20% (Boley et al 1978).

Non-occlusive infarction, in which no underlying artery or vein obstruction can be found, accounts for about a third of all cases diagnosed in living patients (Table 17.1). Next in frequency is superior mesenteric artery occlusion, due in about equal numbers to thrombosis and embolism, with aortic dissections a third, though rare, cause. Then in decreasing order are venous thrombosis, inferior mesenteric artery occlusion and occlusion of peripheral arteries by local processes such as arteritis (Ottinger & Austen 1967).

Except in some cases of acute superior mesenteric artery occlusion, the clinical presentation is notably obscure. The clinical management is further complicated by the need for prompt intervention. Though the rate of progression from mesenteric ischaemia to infarction is variable, early operation can in some cases salvage all or part of the threatened intestine by restoring circulation, and in others can avoid secondary systemic effects by prompt resection of non-viable segments.

This chapter will first discuss general aspects of mesenteric circulation and the response to ischaemia. Next, the clinical presentation and useful diagnostic measures, both before and during the operation, will be described. Finally, management structured on underlying cause of failure of perfusion will be detailed.

Clinical presentation

Mural response to ischaemia

Of the layers of the wall of the intestine, the submucosa is perhaps most sensitive to ischaemic injury. With interruption of arterial flow, changes begin to occur promptly and within half an hour are apparent on gross examination. First oedema is noted; then submucosal haemorrhages become apparent. Associated injury to the mucosa soon results or follows. Mucosal slough leads to intraluminal bleeding. This bleeding, from small vessels and capillaries, is negligible in amount but may lead to clinically important signs. If the viability of the muscular layers is preserved by collateral flow or revascularization, the mucosa will regenerate. This process may take several weeks.

Table 17.1 Aetiology of infarction in 136 consecutive cases in a general hospital (Ottinger & Austen 1967)

Aetiology	No.	%
Non-occlusive	67	49
Embolus	29	22
Arterial thrombosis	22	16
Venous thrombosis	10	7
Aortic dissection	4	3
Arteritis	4	3
Totals	136	100

During it, areas of ulceration and granulation may lead to persistent haemorrhage, sometimes massive. The absorptive capacity of the mucosa is also impaired, and this contributes to diarrhoea, a uniform problem if extensive segments are involved.

The muscularis is less susceptible to ischaemic injury and may be unaffected by failure of perfusion which is severe enough, or lasts long enough, to cause mucosal infarction. When injury does occur, it is usually through the entire thickness, leading to perforation, an event probably hastened by intraluminal enzymes. Perforation of the small intestine may occur within a few hours. It may be preceded by the formation of characteristic foul-smelling, bloody peritoneal fluid. The presence of this fluid invariably indicates at least a short segment of non-viable bowel. Partial-thickness injury, seemingly uncommon, can result in chronic ulceration or the formation of strictures. These segments may require subsequent resection.

The initial response of the muscularis to ischaemia can be a state of spastic contraction. This sometimes causes vomiting, diarrhoea and rectal urgency. Later, loss of tone leads to atony and distension. Pain, so characteristic of ischaemia of the intestine as to be almost invariably present, originates from the muscularis. Being of visceral type, it is poorly localized, cramplike in nature, and may be remarkably severe. It is identical to that seen in chronic intestinal ischaemia, though more severe and persistent. It is to be distinguished from that of peritonitis, a late sign which is of somatic origin.

Ischaemic injury to serosal surfaces is a potent stimulus to exudate and adhesion formation. This process may tend to prevent early peritoneal soilage and general peritonitis, especially in cases of left colon infarction and localized infarction from occlusion of peripheral arteries, as in an arteritis.

Extensive intestinal infarction is associated in some patients with systemic effects. These take the form of metabolic acidosis, sequestration of large volumes of fluid, and the release of vasoactive substances provoking hypotension. These effects have value, albeit late, in diagnosis. They often contribute to a fatal outcome and can be avoided by early intervention.

Collateral perfusion

The major sources of arterial inflow to the intestinal arterial system are the coeliac axis, the superior mesenteric artery, and the inferior mesenteric artery. Oesophageal and rectal vessels of other origin serve as collaterals to this interconnected system. The coeliac axis and the superior mesenteric artery share in the perfusion of the duodenum and, to a lesser extent, the pancreas. The inferior and superior pancreaticoduodenal vessels form interconnecting arcs which become markedly enlarged with occlusion of the coeliac axis. In that these vessels originate from the proximal superior mesenteric artery, they are seldom of use in maintaining flow with acute occlusion of the vessel. Interconnections in the circulation of the pancreas may originate from more distal levels. The superior and inferior mesenteric vessels are interconnected by the marginal artery at the splenic flexure, but these may be quite small. Also, the left branch of the middle colic artery from the superior mesenteric artery and the trunk of the left colic artery from the inferior mesenteric artery often participate in a connection, the arc of Riolan or great meandering vessel. The branches of the major vessels share at least one peripheral connection, the marginal vessel, also with a varying number of connecting vessels proximal to them. All these vessels, as a unit, form a network from oesophagus to anus with three points of major inflow.

The marginal vessel gives rise to short arteries, the vasa recta, that penetrate the muscularis of the intestine. On serosal surfaces and within the bowel itself there are additional interconnecting arcs. These and the associated arterioles have an important role in regulating flow to the bowel and are the site of shunting arterial flow to, or bypassing, the extensive vascular beds of the mucosa. This system is largely oriented circumferentially, with a limited longitudinal component. Thus, intramural collaterals alone can sustain viability over only a centimetre or two in the absence of extramural connecting vessels.

This collateral flow will almost invariably sustain the intestine when gradual occlusion of one, two or even three of the major inflow channels occurs slowly enough to allow enlargement of collateral channels. In addition, it is nearly always sufficient even in the event of sudden termination of coeliac or inferior mesenteric inflow. In most instances of acute occlusion of the main trunk of the superior mesenteric artery, it is not, and damaging ischaemia will ensue, affecting most severely the terminal ileum in most instances. Sudden occlusion of more peripheral vessels will rarely lead to infarction unless they be those of the marginal vessel itself. The collateral flow also gives rise to a graded pattern in infarction with a central area of major injury or infarct, and peripheral areas less affected.

Congenital variations in the arterial supply, such as replaced branches of the coeliac axis originating from the superior mesenteric artery, can alter the collateral pattern but are rarely of clinical importance. More important is the occasional absence of usual collaterals due to atherosclerotic occlusive disease or prior surgical excision.

Venous outflow parallels the arterial supply, major branches collecting to form the portal vein. Collaterals are, if anything, more extensive. With the exception of surgical ligation of the superior mesenteric vein, cases of infarction reflect the propagation of thrombus into an extensive segment of the marginal vessels rather than central occlusion.

Factors other than occlusion influencing mesenteric perfusion

Under usual conditions there is marked variation in arterial flow to the intestine. This is under the regulation of the autonomic nervous system and endogenous hormones and varies with digestion and exercise. Regulation also reflects metabolic and other local stimuli. In pathological states, profound changes in peripheral resistance and hence mural flow may ensue. These may be compensatory for a fall in central perfusing pressure, as in cardiogenic or hypovolaemic shock. Drugs also affect flow: cardiac glycosides and pressor agents can markedly decrease mesenteric perfusion. All these factors can reduce flow below a critical level necessary for viability even in the presence of an anatomically normal mesenteric circulation. In a compromised system, as with chronic atherosclerotic occlusive disease or a ligated inferior mesenteric artery, they may precipitate or cause extension of an ischaemic injury.

Mechanical mural factors may also have the same effect. These include haemorrhage, oedema and bowel distension. As all commonly follow an initial ischaemic injury, they can lead to further infarction and perhaps explain the patchy patterns sometimes noted even with central arterial occlusion.

Clinical course in infarction

A major problem in the diagnosis and management of mesenteric infarction is the variable clinical course, which reflects the extent and severity of the initial insult, variability in adequacy of collateral perfusion or drainage, and a summation of secondary elements further reducing perfusion.

The symptom of pain is perhaps the single unifying element. Pain is present almost always — if not always — though it may be masked by obtundation or other aspects of a complex illness. Second, there is a disturbance in intestinal function with vomiting, diarrhoea, ileus and rectal urgency serving as nonspecific but useful clues. Third is the presence of slow blood loss into the intestinal lumen leading to occult or gross blood in gastric or rectal contents. Fourth, extensive infarcts produce systemic effects with metabolic acidosis, hypovolaemia and shock induced by the release of vasoactive products. Finally, perforation with diffuse peritonitis or abscess formation add additional clinical elements in late stages.

Diagnosis

At presentation

In practice, the early diagnosis of mesenteric ischaemia is elusive. The elements of the clinical course, as described in the preceding section, are so indistinct as to suggest at first almost invariably a somewhat atypical presentation of some more common illness such as pancreatitis, gastroenteritis or diverticulitis. To avoid an error in diagnosis, two points must be emphasized. The first is familiarity with the symptoms, signs and clinical course and an inclination to evaluate patients within this framework. The second is vigorous pursuit of the diagnosis in patients with otherwise unexplained abdominal pain.

The only symptom which occurs frequently is pain. Though it may be indistinct, it is usually severe, more general than local, more aching than burning or piercing and often referred to the mid anterior abdomen. Although typically unremitting, it may wax and wane and even disappear as variations in perfusion occur. Less specifically suggestive of mesenteric ischaemia but of use in diagnosis are disturbances in bowel function such as vomiting, diarrhoea, anorexia and rectal urgency. Other findings that at least alert the observer are a history of peripheral atherosclerotic occlusive disease or arterial emboli, intermittent pain and chronic weight loss suggesting chronic intestinal ischaemia, a hypercoagulable state, a recent myocardial infarction or a recent diagnostic aortic catheterization or operation on the heart, aorta or its branches.

Findings on physical examination are so sparse as to be useful primarily in ruling out other diagnoses. Except with ischaemic injuries to the left colon, signs of peritoneal irritation are found only with advanced infarction. Occult blood in the rectal and gastric contents should be sought, and the presence of peripheral arterial occlusive disease and an abdominal bruit are suggestive findings.

Laboratory tests also are of more use in eliminating other diagnoses than in establishing the diagnosis of infarction. A leucocytosis, sometimes twice the normal or more, is observed in perhaps three-quarters of cases, but in the others the white blood cell count is normal. The serum amylase may also be elevated but will only rarely exceed twice normal levels. This helps to distinguish infarction from acute pancreatitis. Other laboratory data are even less specific and therefore not helpful in a positive sense.

Plain X-ray films of the abdomen may show a pattern of ileus but otherwise do not contribute except in late stages. Then they may show mural or portal venous gas. Again, though, they help indirectly by helping to eliminate conflicting diagnoses such as intestinal obstruction (Tomchik et al 1970).

With increasing sophistication in technique and interpretation, angiographic methods have come to have an important role in the diagnosis and even management of mesenteric ischaemia and infarction (Boley et al 1977). Direct findings establish the diagnosis of occlusion of the major arteries and, equally important, provide the surgeon with useful information to aid in planning revascularization. Indirect findings can suggest the presence of venous and non-occlusive infarction. By direct infusion into the involved vessels, arterial spasm can be relieved with resultant protection of all — or at least the peripheral — segments of the affected bowel. Thrombolytic therapy and mechanical dilatation may also be employed.

The proper use of angiography in management is a difficult issue. Obviously the quality and actual availability of these techniques is a primary consideration. A second is the clinical condition of the patient, as angiography is not always helpful. Sometimes immediate laparotomy must take precedence over diagnostic steps, either because of peritonitis or relative clinical certainty as to the diagnosis and the need for urgent surgical intervention. Except when there is a highly sophisticated unit available, angiography is perhaps most useful in the management of patients without local signs or systemic effects of infarction but with a suggestive history. These patients, especially those with a reconstructable superior mesenteric artery, will have an earlier diagnosis and an easier operation with a preoperative angiogram.

At operation

The diagnosis of mesenteric infarction and its underlying cause presents a distinct series of questions to the operating surgeon. In most cases the general diagnosis is obvious, but this is not always the case. The major exception is in cases of acute occlusion of the superior mesenteric artery. In a few instances the only change in the appearance of the intestine will be decreased or absent pulses. Though the bowel itself may appear pale or avascular, such an appearance is often encountered as the result of vasospasm during laparotomy and is not an obvious clue. The suspected diagnosis of mesenteric ischaemia should not be abandoned without examining the main trunk of the superior mesenteric artery for pulses.

Occasionally, volvulus or hernias can produce segmental intestinal infarction and should be considered in obscure cases. Otherwise, the next step is to seek the specific underlying vascular aetiology.

The pattern of infarction may provide useful clues. Although venous infarction may affect any segment of the large or small intestine and though severity may be patchy within the segment, it is almost invariably only one segment and often the mid small bowel. Superior mesenteric artery occlusion in the absence of alterations in collateral supply usually produces infarction centred in the distal ileum. Non-occlusive infarction tends to be patchy but with circumferential infarcts, and there may be concomitant infarction of other viscera, especially the gallbladder. The usual finding with an arteritis is patchy, noncircumferential infarcts of varying age, some acute and some healing with exudate and adhesions.

When the site of infarction is the colon distal to the splenic flexure, examination of the perfusing or draining vessels has no value because resection is the proper treatment in any case. Otherwise, the superior mesenteric artery in the region of the origin of the middle colic artery, the major branches and the terminal arcades should be carefully palpated. Absence of pulses requires explanation. The venous drainage can be best explored by incising the mesentery of a non-viable segment of the intestine. With venous thrombosis the arteries may be collapsed and in spasm but will still show flow. The veins will be filled with thrombus under pressure.

A final diagnostic problem is whether a given segment of intestine has lost viability and must be resected, can be expected to recover under the conditions prevailing at the end of the operation, or should be the subject of a second-look operation. Haemorrhage into the intestinal wall, leading to discoloration and oedema, obscures the determination of viability. More useful observations relate to loss of muscle tone and surface characteristics. Especially after restoration of arterial perfusion, the decision about viability is

troublesome. Studies show that experienced surgeons are accurate in their assessment, though tending to somewhat overestimate the extent of the actual infarction. The use of intravenously administered fluorescein, and the illumination of the intestine in question by ultraviolet light can enhance the accuracy of the decision, but usually not so much as to alter the clinical management. Pulsatile flow in the intestinal wall may also be assessed with a Doppler ultrasound device, which has some applications, as in evaluation of the sigmoid colon after ligation of the inferior mesenteric artery. Fortunately, the surgeon's impression is accurate enough when such techniques are unavailable (Bulkley et al 1981).

Non-occlusive infarction

Clinical aspects

Non-occlusive infarction is a classification that includes four distinct types. They share a clinical presentation which reflects the fact that, whatever the specific underlying causes, the signs and symptoms are those of an ischaemic or infarcted segment of small or large intestine.

1. The most frequent type is that caused by loss of perfusion due to extramesenteric factors. These include cardiac failure and hypovolaemic or septic shock. A secondary response is contraction of the mesenteric vessels and a further decrease in mesenteric flow. Digitalis preparations and vasoactive drugs, by a direct effect on mesenteric arteries, may further accentuate this decrease in flow. Finally, there is, as demonstrated at times on angiograms, a further locally mediated component of segmental spasm. The clinical setting should suggest the diagnosis when typical symptoms of mesenteric ischaemia are manifest. In fact, these symptoms are likely to be obscured by other elements of the overall course. Although infarction tends to be superficial, it can be transmural and lead to perforation and extensive necrosis with associated metabolic alterations.

2. Next in frequency are cases of non-occlusive infarction without apparent systemic or other underlying cause. These cases present with symptoms of infarction, often quite dramatic in

onset and severity. Segments of either small or large intestine may be involved. The symptoms are pronounced, and the typical history includes early surgical exploration without an accurate preoperative diagnosis. It seems likely that this idiopathic group will be found to include several causes, perhaps some infectious. Some cases have been associated with the use of oral contraceptives. Typically, infarction involves only a single segment of intestine with normal perfusion of adjacent segments. Perforation is common.

3. The third type, a variant of the second, involves a segment of the descending colon, usually just distal to the splenic flexure; categorized separately because its specific presentation, course and management differ from cases involving segments of the small intestine and more proximal colon. This form, sometimes termed ischaemic colitis, is, except for its location, entirely similar to infarction due to acute occlusion of the inferior mesenteric artery; but, unlike this, it rarely, if ever, extends into the lower 20 cm of the rectum, eliminating easy diagnosis with a rigid sigmoidoscope. The pain is both generalized and localized to the region of the infarct, the left lower abdomen. Thus, unlike other types of mesenteric infarction, tenderness over the area of ischaemia is typical. This tenderness perhaps reflects bacterial colitis following early loss of the mucosal barrier to invasion by luminal organisms. Diarrhoea, usually bloody, is a prominent early symptom in most cases. Systemic manifestations are relatively minimal due to the short length of infarction. Submucosal oedema and haemorrhage with resultant thumb-printing are useful components for diagnosis either by colonoscopy or barium enema studies, and are sometimes seen on plain X-ray films (Fig. 17.1). The segment is rapidly walled off by adhesions, and in the somewhat unusual event of full thickness infarction and perforation, this may lead to delay — of even some days — in the presentation of the complications. By contrast, infarcts of the right and transverse colon more resemble lesions of the small intestine with respect to presentation and management. The location of the segment generally affected is in the collateral region of the middle colic and inferior mesenteric vessels. Tenuous marginal vessels in this area may be a contributing cause. A history of a systemic

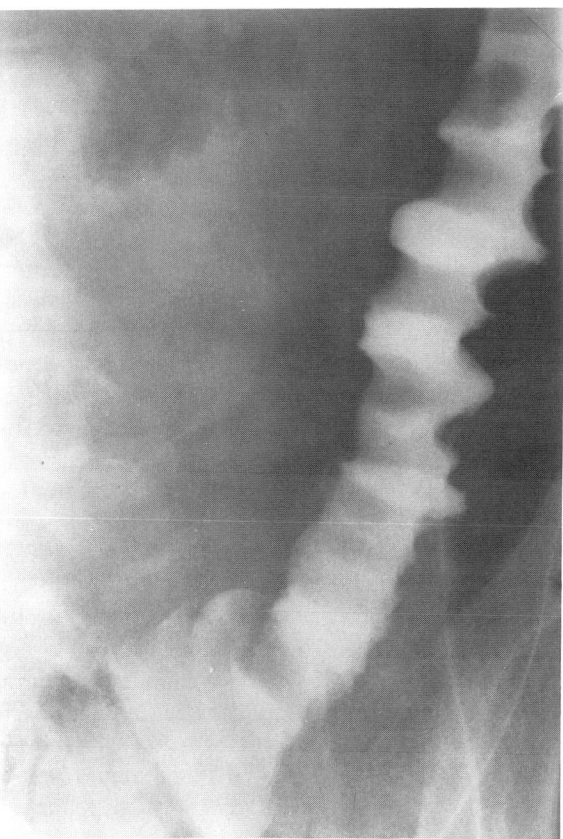

Fig. 17.1 Nodular lesions of the left colon in ischaemic injury shown on a barium contrast study.

cause of decreased perfusion is seldom present.

4. Fourth is a small group of patients with the history of chronic intestinal ischaemia who develop infarction in the distribution of the superior mesenteric artery without acute occlusion. The vessel is chronically occluded or narrowed. The history of chronic ischaemia classically includes postprandial pain, and weight loss due to abstinence from eating; an abdominal bruit completes the triad. Most patients also report nonspecific changes of intestinal function. These include bloating, constipation, cramps and diarrhoea. The clinician more often diagnoses occult malignancy than chronic intestinal ischaemia. When infarction is the central clinical element, whether there has been acute occlusion is unimportant and a course of revascularization is obvious. With a precipitating cause such as cardiac failure, however, the history of chronic ischaemia

may be overlooked. Such patients do not often survive because they require both successful management of the antecedent precipitating cause and revascularization of the intestine.

Nonoperative measures in management

With extramesenteric failure of perfusion, management is obviously directed first at correction of primary causes. This will include whenever possible avoidance of pharmacological agents tending to increase mesenteric vascular resistance. Relief of mesenteric spasm can be achieved by direct infusion into the mesenteric artery, using a catheter placed percutaneously by angiographic techniques, of a drug such as papaverine, which is that most frequently recommended (Renton 1972). Patient selection and management pose formidable problems and have made evaluation of the useful role in actual clinical management difficult to assess. Long-acting or continuous epidural anaesthesia has also been used, although its efficacy in improving mesenteric perfusion in this setting is more theoretical than proven. Angiography also has a role in diagnosis by showing patterns of spasm and vessel contraction and in demonstrating chronic narrowing and occluding lesions at the origin of vessels (Boley et al 1977).

With 'idiopathic' non-occlusive infarction there is little evidence that nonoperative techniques are effective, and in practice the diagnosis will usually be first suspected at the time of laparotomy anyway. In the special case of ischaemia of the left colon this does not apply. Usual steps will then include placing the colon at rest by eliminating oral intake and the use of parenteral antibiotics. Most cases will recover; a few will go on to perforation and require abscess drainage or resection with anastomoses deferred for a second operation.

It is difficult to find rules or principles to apply to cases with a history of chronic intestinal ischaemia and infarction precipitated by an unrelated extramesenteric condition. Percutaneous dilatation of superior mesenteric artery narrowing and anticoagulation to prevent secondary thrombosis have been suggested (Golden et al 1982).

Operative measures in management

With cases in the major category of non-occlusive infarction, namely those with a clinically apparent extra-abdominal cause of failure of perfusion, exploratory operations to establish the diagnosis have no practical application. The diagnosis will be suspected on clinical grounds and an operation can be delayed pending reversal of extramesenteric elements. The appearance of evidence of perforation or systemic changes suggesting extensive infarction will thus serve as the indications for an operation.

In the absence of chronic intestinal ischaemia, resection of infarcted segments is all the surgeon has to offer. Healing of anastomoses under these general conditions is tenuous. Important technical elements are careful handling of bowel, meticulous hand-sewn anastomoses and, perhaps, side-to-side rather than end-to-end anastomosis to avoid further compromise of the circulation at the antimesenteric border by inversion. Even then, the turned-in end may leak. Finally, a second-look operation after the patient is more stable can be used to verify viability or to perform deferred anastomoses.

As has been suggested, operative management of primary non-occlusive infarction of the small intestine and colon proximal to the splenic flexure is more straightforward. Perfusion of adjacent viable segments is normal, and resection with immediate anastomosis is likely to succeed. Depending on the condition of the patient and local factors of contamination and perfusion, construction of a stoma with staged restoration of intestinal continuity should be considered, especially with lesions of the colon. An early second look is not indicated unless the first operation has revealed other doubtful bowel segments besides those resected.

With lesions of the more distal colon, management takes the form of close observation for evidence of perforation. Then, in the absence of generalized peritoneal contamination, simple drainage of the abscess may suffice. Resection of the involved segment is usually preferred. Rarely, a primary anastomosis may be performed. Local factors of contamination and marginal circulation in viable adjacent segments will usually dictate formation of a colostomy and later anastomosis after several weeks have elapsed.

When there is a prior history of chronic intestinal ischaemia, resection alone seldom succeeds. There will be relative ischaemia of long segments of the small bowel and colon which jeopardize healing of anastomoses and lead to other areas of infarction in the postoperative period. To resect all this intestine often precludes long-term recovery, though it may be the only alternative. Theoretically, revascularization of the superior mesenteric artery should precede resection, as in acute occlusion of the superior mesenteric artery. In the presence of an extra-abdominal condition precipitating this form of non-occlusive infarction, this is seldom feasible. When it is, the same techniques including resection after revascularization, and second-look operations should be used.

In all non-occlusive cases, techniques to prevent postoperative embarrassment of mesenteric flow by contraction and spasm can be considered. In addition to epidural anaesthesia and direct perfusion of the superior mesenteric artery by an inlying arterial catheter, mentioned above, the artery can be skeletonized to disrupt the autonomic nerve plexus that surrounds it. Such techniques, it must be admitted, rarely alter the final outcome.

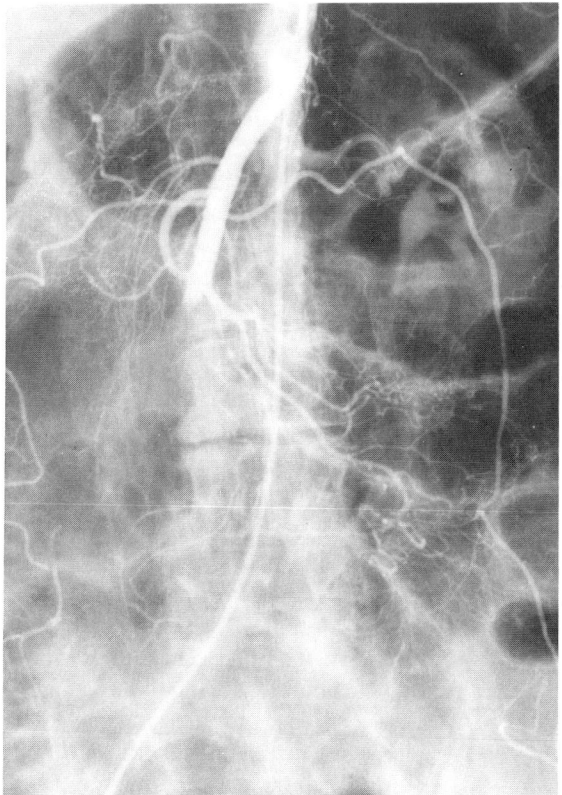

Fig. 17.2 Occlusion of the superior mesenteric artery by an embolus distal to the origin of the middle colic artery. The angiogram was performed by selective transfemoral catheterization of the origin of the artery.

Acute occlusion of the superior mesenteric artery

About 40% of cases of mesenteric infarction coming to operation are due to occlusion of the main trunk of the superior mesenteric artery. They are almost equally divided between those due to emboli and those due to thrombosis. Dissection of the aorta is a third but rare cause.

Emboli most often originate from the heart, with atrial thrombus or mural thrombus following infarction accounting for most. Some have their origin in the aorta itself. This includes cases of plaque disruption following clamping and arterial catheterization. Emboli rarely lodge at the origin of the artery. Most are found at the point of narrowing at the origin of the middle colic artery, sometimes occluding it, or in the main trunk beyond this point (Fig. 17.2). Emboli that lodge more peripherally may result in infarction, but most do not. An unusual exception is with cholesterol emboli, showers of atherosclerotic debris following disruption of a plaque. They may result in patchy infarcts resembling those of arteritis. Some patients with emboli will have a history of a recent myocardial infarction or of other peripheral emboli.

Thrombosis of the superior mesenteric artery almost invariably occurs at the origin of the artery (Ottinger 1978). More peripheral disease leading to occlusion in the mesenteric system is rare. Some patients will have a history of chronic ischaemic symptoms. As might be predicted, patients with thrombosis are on average older, have more extensive infarcts and a higher mortality rate than cases with emboli.

Clinical presentation and diagnosis

In a typical case of mesenteric infarction due to superior mesenteric artery occlusion, symptoms are abrupt in onset, pain is severe, infarction is extensive and only immediate surgical intervention can save the patient. In practice, most cases differ from this pattern. Collateral inflow from the coeliac axis through the duodenal and pancreatic arteries and from the inferior mesenteric artery through marginal and central arcs at the splenic flexure provide at least a potential route for maintaining viability. The degree to which this mechanism is effective influences the clinical course. Further, already marginal flow is eventually reduced by such local factors as arterial spasm and oedema and dilatation of the affected bowel, leading to extension of the ischaemic lesions. Finally, central elements reducing flow can also enter in. These can lead to a stuttering or a crescendo course rather than the typical one, which may occupy several days, sometimes even with asymptomatic periods.

Angiography has a dual role in the management of superior mesenteric artery occlusion. In patients with symptoms that do not suggest rapidly progressing infarction requiring urgent laparotomy or even raise only a question of the diagnosis, angiography cannot only confirm superior mesenteric artery occlusion but also establish the site. By this means cases of thrombosis can be separated from those of embolization. This information is very useful to the surgeon in the execution of a revascularization. The additional possible contributions to management of lysis of thrombus and dilatation of strictures have not been thoroughly evaluated in the clinical setting. Because of the high incidence of infarction and the urgent necessity for its diagnosis, the need for laparotomy favours a more direct approach to restoration of arterial flow.

Surgical management

At exploration, extensive ischaemia is usually apparent. In a few cases, however, the bowel is as yet unaffected, at least on gross examination. The presence of a normal pulse in the main trunk of the artery must be verified before the diagnosis is abandoned. The presence of faint collateral pulses in peripheral vessels can be deceptive. Infarction, when present, is usually centred in the distal ileum. With more extensive involvement, the proximal small bowel and right side of the colon are included. Absence of the inferior mesenteric artery or interruption of marginal vessels by prior surgery may extend the infarct to involve the left colon as well. Exposure of the superior mesenteric artery for inspection and palpation is accomplished by approaching it from the left at the ligament of Treitz. The vein almost invariably is on the right and venous branches are thus avoided. This approach will allow exposure back to the emergence of the vessel beneath the inferior margin of the pancreas, proximal to the origin of the middle colic artery. Presence of a pulse at this proximal level favours an embolus; absence, thrombosis.

Resection without revascularization is the proper approach only for cases of infarction from occlusion of mesenteric artery branches. These infarcts are limited in length, and adjacent segments of bowel are well perfused. Such lesions also are unusual since these peripheral occlusions seldom lend to infarction (Fig. 17.3). More often, a limited infarct will be associated with central occlusion and extensive ischaemia. Resection alone in such cases invariably fails and successful management requires revascularization, then resection, if needed. Extensive resections, even with revascularization, give poor results in older patients. Younger patients can survive with 25 cm or even less of normally functioning small intestine. Parenteral nutrition is sometimes useful in early management after extensive resections (Gusberg & Gump 1974); long-term use is questionable.

Mesenteric embolectomy is not a technically demanding procedure and has a high local success rate. An anterolateral longitudinal incision facilitates closure in a diseased vessel and can also serve as a site of insertion of a bypass graft. Mesenteric vessels are more fragile than those in the extremities and must be handled carefully to avoid iatrogenic injury. The embolus is usually found at or just beyond the middle colic artery

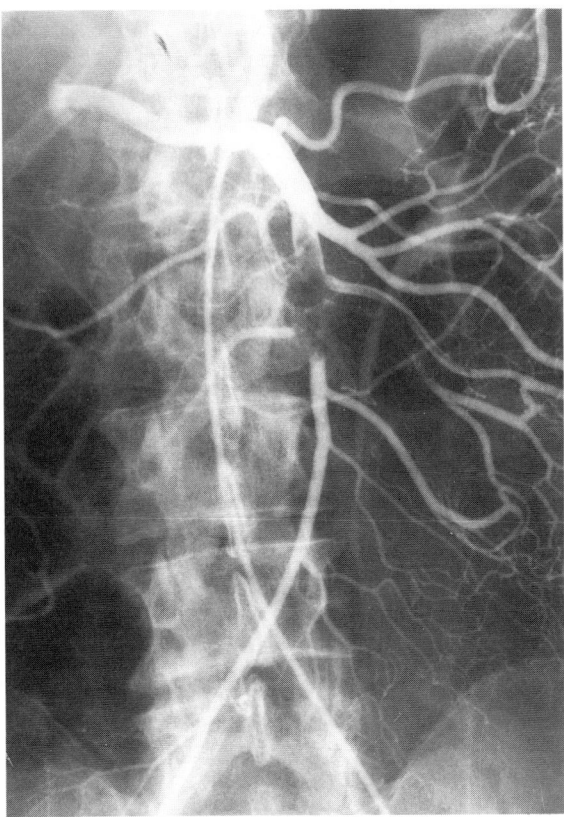

Fig. 17.3 An asymptomatic embolus to the distal main trunk of the superior mesenteric artery. The selective injection shows that the hepatic artery arises from the superior mesenteric artery. The study was performed during investigation of a renal artery embolus (not shown).

origin and is easily dislodged. If this is not the case, thrombosis should be suspected. Distal propagation is ordinarily quite limited and can be removed with a fine balloon embolectomy catheter, being careful not to rupture the vessels. Small peripheral fragments need not be extracted. If the vessel is involved by severe atherosclerotic disease, a patch or even local endarterectomy may be needed to obtain a satisfactory closure. Usually, this is not needed, and a running suture to approximate the edges without eversion will succeed.

Superior mesenteric artery

Revascularization for superior mesenteric artery thrombosis is much more difficult and has a lower technical success rate. As previously noted, oc-

clusion is almost invariably localized to the origin of the vessel. The balloon embolectomy catheter may produce a little blood clot with restoration of only slight inflow. Satisfactory endarterectomy requires visualization of the site and cannot be performed blindly from below. Rather, the origin must be exposed, which usually requires reflecting the spleen and pancreas to the right. Then direct endarterectomy is feasible. This approach has the disadvantage of being at times technically very difficult, especially without more exposure than can be gained through an abdominal incision. An alternative is the placement of a bypass between the aorta or iliac artery and the superior mesenteric artery. A reversed segment of saphenous vein or a prosthetic graft may be utilized, the former being preferable if an intestinal resection is required. The mesenteric anastomosis should be performed first, allowing the proximal small intestine to fall back into place before performing the proximal anastomosis. This will allow proper tailoring of the graft to avoid kinking. The proximal anastomosis may be to a soft area of either iliac artery or abdominal aorta. A more stable reconstruction is a bypass graft from the aorta superior to the coeliac axis to the superior mesenteric artery. Except in thin patients exposure is such a problem that this graft is seldom utilized in revascularization for acute occlusion (Fig. 17.4).

Following revascularization, the intestine should be returned to the abdominal cavity and examination to determine the need for resection deferred for 10–15 min. If the intestine at sites of transection appears viable and the edges bleed, healing of the anastomosis can be expected even in the presence of mucosal infarction. Meticulous technique is important and the formation of stomas rather than anastomosis, especially to the colon, may be used.

Fluorescein injection, described previously, may be used to supplement the surgeon's own observations but is not usually needed.

Second-look operations are used to extend the period of observation. For this purpose, a few hours will suffice. In the setting of arterial revascularization, the approach is not necessary if residual intestine seemed definitely viable at the time of closure. If the surgeon has genuine doubt about some areas, a re-exploration for the purpose

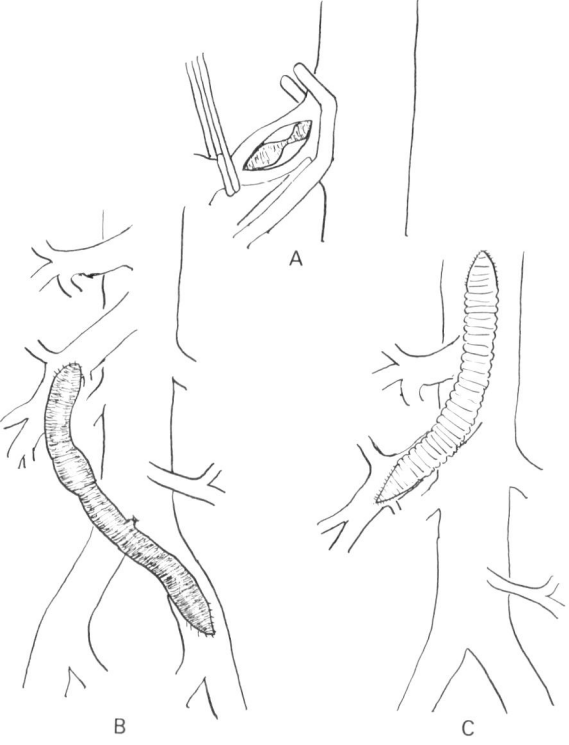

Fig. 17.4 Techniques for superior mesenteric artery with thrombosis at the origin. (A) Endarterectomy. (B) Iliac to mesenteric artery by-pass. (C) Aorta to mesenteric artery by-pass.

of possible further resections is indicated. It must be emphasized, though, that definitely non-viable segments should not be left behind for later resection. Also, the clinical course cannot be used to judge the necessity for an early second look. Finally, the surgeon should anticipate the fact that the patient's general condition may not withstand a second look (Ottinger 1978).

Many patients with mesenteric emboli die from other emboli during their hospitalization, so anticoagulation, beginning in the postoperative period, is essential. Early on the value must be balanced against the risk of inducing bleeding in the operative field. After 24 h this risk decreases markedly. With reconstructions for thromboses, anticoagulation has so little value that the risk of abdominal and retroperitoneal bleeding easily outweighs this.

Complications. Several specific postoperative complications after superior mesenteric artery revascularization deserve mention. Thrombosis or

re-embolization precipitates symptoms identical to those of the original occlusion. In this event, angiography is helpful in the diagnosis, and a repeat revascularization has succeeded. Early bleeding from arterial suture lines is usually a complication of anticoagulation; after a few days, it more likely indicates infection. Intestinal fistulas do not require comment. With regeneration of mucosal surfaces a degree of chronic bleeding and diarrhoea is the rule. With more extensive mural injuries other complications are noted. These include ulceration into larger arteries with even massive haemorrhage. Angiography is helpful in localizing the area of bleeding to facilitate resection. Strictures, diagnosed by barium contrast studies, are a later complication and also require resection.

Finally, a chronic ulcerative process may develop in long segments of the small intestine or colon and dictate a later extensive resection (Fig. 17.5). Parenteral feedings and courses of specific antibiotics have an important role in the management of all these complications.

Aortic dissection with associated occlusion of

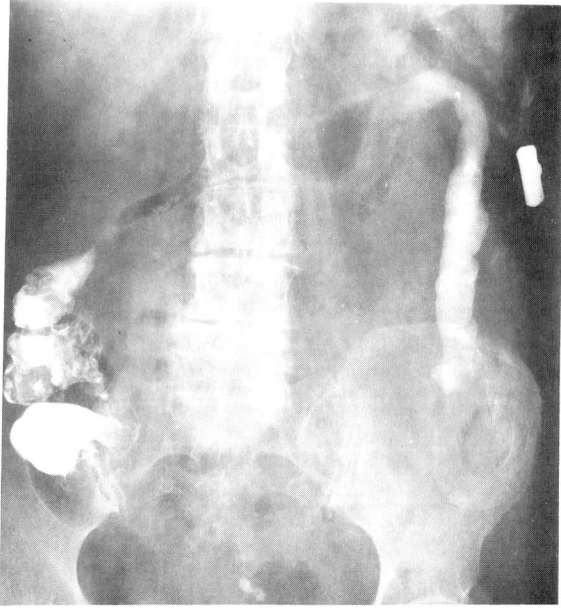

Fig. 17.5 Stricturing and ulceration in the transverse and descending colon 3 months after a superior mesenteric embolectomy. The patient had undergone a previous resection of the rectum for a carcinoma with ligation of the inferior mesenteric artery.

mesenteric vessels and resultant mesenteric infarction is rare. Management of the dissection, either by surgical or medical measures, is a separate issue. Laparotomy is reserved for patients with clinical evidence of extensive infarction or of perforation. The summation of risks usually predicts a fatal outcome.

Despite advances in vascular techniques and patient management, overall mortality rates exceeding 80% are still reported in unselected series of acute superior mesenteric artery occlusion. This reflects the fact that patients are frequently beyond hope at the time of diagnosis. Still, early diagnosis and aggressive revascularization can save many patients.

Acute occlusion of the inferior mesenteric artery

Sudden occlusion of the inferior mesenteric artery by thrombosis or an embolus is rare. Most cases seen in clinical practice are the result of surgical division of the vessel during aortic procedures. In either setting, full thickness infarction has an incidence of only 2–5% (Schroeder et al 1985). This reflects the relatively short length of colon involved and consequently the adequacy of collateral flow from the middle colic artery and branches of the hypogastric arteries. Vascular surgeons are aware of the importance of ligation of the artery at its origin to preserve the continuity of the first branch (the left colic artery) with the main trunk, maintaining collateral inflow from the proximal vasculature. Avoiding mechanical trauma to the sigmoid colon by unnecessary dissection, handling and haematomas is also important. Chronic occlusion of the superior mesenteric artery, usually suggested by the finding of a markedly enlarged inferior mesenteric artery, will require revascularization of the superior mesenteric artery, reimplantation of the inferior mesenteric artery, or both.

Clinical course

Except in the presence of chronic occlusion of the superior mesenteric artery, acute occlusion of the inferior mesenteric artery results in an infarction of limited extent. Systemic effects are therefore minimal. Pain, localized tenderness over the affected bowel, and diarrhoea, often bloody, are the usual symptoms and signs. They may be masked in the early period following aortic reconstruction. Sigmoidoscopy will show patches of friable ischaemic mucosa and later, ulceration. If perforation does not ensue, recovery may take several weeks. Persistent fever and leucocytosis are unfavourable signs.

Management

Revascularization is sometimes possible following surgical ligation but is seldom attempted. Rather, close observation for perforation and prompt management of this complication when it occurs are preferable. Later, resection of strictures may be required. Barium and endoscopic studies should be used to ensure final return of the colon to normal, after eliminating any unsuspected second diagnosis such as carcinoma or chronic inflammatory bowel disease.

Perforation rarely leads to generalized peritonitis. Since it is delayed, formation of a walled-off abscess is the rule. Closed percutaneous radiologically-guided catheter drainage or open surgical drainage can then be used. Early cases are better managed by drainage and resection of the injured colon, construction of a proximal end colostomy, and later restoration of intestinal continuity. The distal end may, during the first operation, be brought out as a mucous fistula but is often so short that it must be closed with local drainage. Protected by its collateral arterial supply, the rectum is seldom so severely injured as to require removal. After aortic reconstruction with placement of a left iliac graft, fear of graft contamination and subsequent graft sepsis may favour early resection of the colon. Such infections in fact are not common.

Venous thrombosis with mesenteric infarction

Venous thrombosis is the underlying cause in about 10% of patients with bowel infarction of vascular origin. There are three general categories of causes, each with a somewhat different management and prognosis (Grendell & Ockner 1982).

Cases of idiopathic thrombosis have the most favourable prognosis. Other than an infrequent history of peripheral thrombophlebitis, associated medical conditions are seldom present.

Second are cases with a predisposing cause for thrombosis. Included are intra-abdominal sepsis, the postoperative state especially following splenectomy and hypercoagulable states including those of neoplasms, polycythaemia and the use of oral contraceptives.

Third are cases associated with cirrhosis and hepatic neoplasms with preceding portal vein thrombosis.

The relative incidence of these types is unknown, but from the surgeon's perspective, most cases are of the idiopathic variety.

Because of the relatively rich venous collateral drainage in the periphery of the mesentery, venous infarction occurs only with propagation of thrombus into the veins in this area. Central thrombosis

alone results in thickening and nodularity in the mesentery, occasionally seen at laparotomy, but without intestinal infarction. Extensive thrombosis results in marked oedema of the mesentery and may result in ascites, usually blood-tinged. Any segment of the small or large bowel may be affected, but the most frequent site of infarction is the middle small bowel.

Clinical course

The mural effects of venous infarction do not differ from those with other causes. The final ischaemic injury may even reflect a component of spasm and thrombosis of the peripheral arterial networks. Pain is a central symptom, probably always present. Signs of intraluminal bleeding with gross or occult blood in gastric or rectal contents are frequent. The symptoms of anorexia, bloating, cramping and constipation all reflect disruption of normal bowel function. Tenderness is frequently

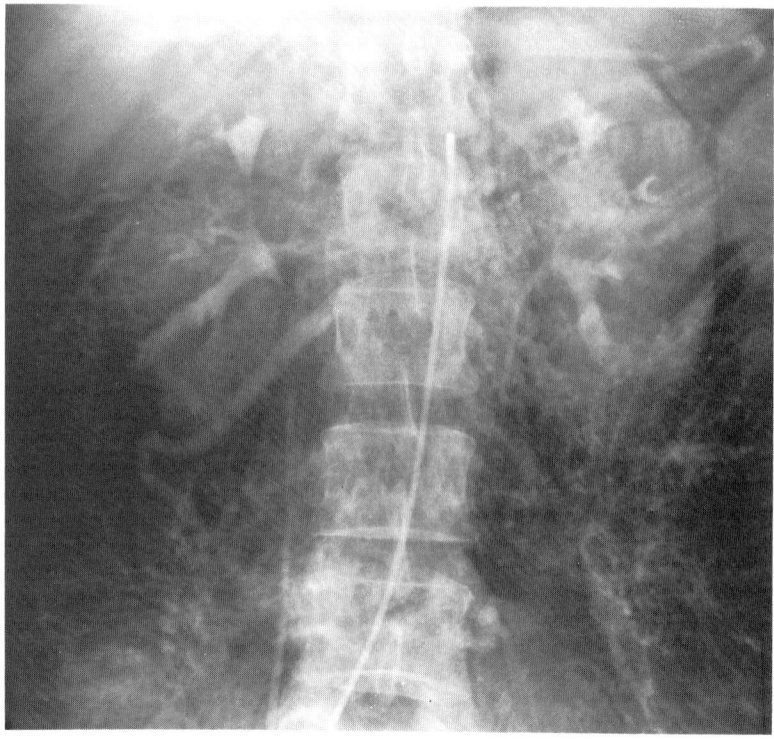

Fig. 17.6   Thrombosis of the superior mesenteric vein. This late frame of a superior mesenteric artery angiogram shows only opacification of a right colic vein. The superior mesenteric vein itself could not be demonstrated.

observed, though peritonitis is present only with perforation.

In some patients, thrombosis proceeds over days or even weeks before infarction. Low-grade fever and malaise are characteristic of this delayed course, but the disease is rare and the symptoms so nonspecific that the underlying cause is not suspected. Aggressive anticoagulation would perhaps control the process before infarction if it were employed. Eventually, infarction alters the clinical course and patients come to exploratory laparotomy with a diagnosis of mesenteric infarction or some other intra-abdominal catastrophe.

Results of laboratory studies resemble those in other forms of infarction, with leucocytosis the only striking finding. Plain X-ray films of the abdomen may show ascites, patterns of ileus or thickened segments of intestine with fluid separation and thumb-printing due to submucosal oedema and haemorrhage. CT scanning has sometimes been shown to demonstrate these thickened loops clearly and may be a very useful diagnostic method. Late studies may demonstrate gas in the bowel wall or portal venous channels. If angiography is performed, two specific observations are of importance. The first is delayed arterial opacification in the affected segment; the second is failure to opacify the venous drainage channels on late films (Fig. 17.6). These latter changes are less subtle because both peripheral and larger, more central, veins are similarly occluded. How often the diagnosis can be established by angiography is not known, but the findings could be quite useful in the early stages, perhaps allowing the prevention of infarction by the use of anticoagulants.

Surgical management

Treatment of infarction involves surgical exploration, often for diagnosis but certainly for management. Operative findings include thickening and nodularity of the mesentery, bloody ascites, often foul-smelling, and haemorrhagic infarction of the intestinal wall. The diagnosis is established by incision of the mesentery, when open arteries with meagre flow and thrombus extruding from veins are found. When feasible, resection should be extended well into adjacent

segments of intestine which appear normal, because the central thrombosis usually extends into these adjacent areas, and subsequent infarction is a complication in up to 60% of resections. Almost always it is the area of the anastomosis rather than a separate segment of intestine that is so affected.

The high incidence of further infarction and resulting anastomotic leak suggests the efficacy of second-look operations. Here, unlike cases of arterial revascularization, timing is a difficult problem. Ongoing venous thrombosis has an unpredictable time course, and further infarction may be delayed for several days. Nevertheless, exploration in 24–36 h does make an important contribution to survival in some cases.

Early postoperative anticoagulation offers theoretical protection against further thrombosis and infarction (Abdu et al 1987). Because of associated bleeding complications, it has been difficult to document its impact on survival. When the use of anticoagulation carries additional risks because of medical contraindications, it is not justified in the early postoperative period. Prolonged anticoagulation for perhaps 3–6 months is probably worthwhile in the absence of contraindications, even though delayed recurrence of infarction is rare.

Surgical thrombectomy has little application in cases of mesenteric infarction. This is because of the peripheral extension of thrombosis. It can perhaps be helpful in earlier stages of the process. Thrombolytic therapy is a promising approach in the absence of infarction.

Mortality rates approach 100% in cases associated with advanced cirrhosis, hepatic tumours, abdominal malignancy and diffuse thrombotic conditions, or other grave underlying causes. The, survival rate of other patients is likely to be 50% or more. Superficial infarction in retained intestine is usually quite limited, so the postoperative course in the absence of further infarction is often quite uncomplicated when compared to that of patients who have undergone arterial revascularization.

Arteritis with mesenteric infarction

Degenerative and thrombotic lesions associated with a wide range of allergic and autoimmune disorders can result in ischaemic injury and infarction of the intestine. In most cases the underlying cause will be known; in a few, only the intestine is affected and the diagnosis will first be suggested by findings at laparotomy. The clinical course reflects the sequential development of small infarcts of varying depth, many of which heal without perforation.

Clinical course

The clinical course may be leisurely or fulminant. Abdominal pain is less striking than with other causes of mesenteric infarction, although it seems invariably present. Disturbances of intestinal function also are noted. Signs of peritoneal irritation are prominent on physical examination. In the absence of prior or obvious involvement of other systems, the diagnosis is not likely to be suspected. If it is, measures of limiting oral intake and the use of parenteral antibiotics should be combined with those more general steps dictated by the primary diagnosis. Then surgical exploration can

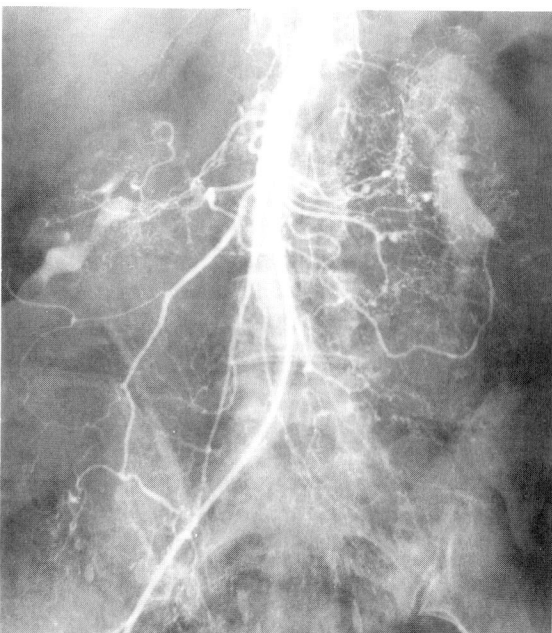

Fig. 17.7 Microaneurysms in the jejunal arteries in a case of mesenteric arteritis. This is a late frame in a selective superior mesenteric artery angiogram.

be reserved for patients who develop evidence of perforation.

In establishing the diagnosis of mesenteric arteritis, angiography is sometimes useful (Fig. 17.7). Studies may show segmental thrombosis, localized spasm and the formation of aneurysms at the site of vessel wall disruption. Occasionally, drugs to combat vasospasm may be directly infused angiographically.

Surgical management

When the underlying diagnosis is not at hand, laparotomy will suggest or confirm it. Characteristic lesions are patchy and not circumferential. Their appearance suggests a variability in age: early lesions are haemorrhagic and oedematous; later ones show serosal exudates and adhesion formation. A specific diagnosis may sometimes be obtained from biopsy of peripheral mesenteric vessels. A more certain one comes from resection of an intestinal segment containing an early lesion with its associated mesentery. Seldom will resection of all lesions be feasible, and this, at any rate, cannot be expected to alter the outcome of what is a systemic rather than local disorder.

When the diagnosis is reasonably certain, either because of prior or concomitant involvement of other system, or angiographic findings, surgical exploration is deferred unless the condition is acutely exacerbated by peritonitis or there are signs of perforation. Upright radiographs of the upper abdomen to demonstrate free gas may provide a useful early clue to perforation. Surgical resection of the perforated segment or segments is then performed. It is often not feasible to resect all involved segments. The choice of immediate anastomosis or the formation of an enteric stoma will depend on the site of the lesion and the extent of peritoneal soilage. In most cases, segments of normally perfused intestine will be available for anastomosis, even with limited resections.

The postoperative course is sometimes complicated by the development of new infarcts and even perforations. The prognosis reflects the course of the underlying disorder more than the surgical management of mesenteric lesions. With the cessation of the formation of new lesions, recovery of the intestine is rapid.

REFERENCES

Abdu R A, Zakhour B J, Dallis D J 1987 Mesenteric
venous thrombosis. Surgery 101: 383–388

Boley S J, Sprayregan S, Siegelman S S, Veith F J 1977
Initial results from an aggressive roentgenological and
surgical approach to acute mesenteric ischemia. Surgery
82: 848–853

Boley S J, Brandt S J, Veith F J 1978 Ischemic disorders of
the intestine. Current Problems in Surgery 15: 1–85

Bulkley G B, Zuidema G D, Hamilton S R, O'Mara C S,
Klacsmann P G, Horn S D 1981 Intraoperative
determination of small intestine viability following
ischemic injury. Annals of Surgery 193: 628–637

Golden D A, Ring E J, McLean G K, Freimann D B 1982
Percutaneous transluminal angioplasty in the treatment of
abdominal angina. American Journal of Roentgenology
139: 247–249

Grendell J H, Ockner R K 1982 Mesenteric venous
thrombosis. Gastroenterology 82: 358–372

Gusberg R, Gump F E 1974 Combined surgical and
nutritional management of patients with acute mesenteric
vascular occlusion. Annals of Surgery 179: 358–361

Ottinger L W 1978 The surgical management of acute
occlusion of the superior mesenteric artery. Annals of
Surgery 188: 721–731

Ottinger L W, Austen W G 1967 A study of 136 patients
with mesenteric infarction. Surgery Gynecology and
Obstetrics 124: 251–261

Renton C J C 1972 Non-occlusive intestinal infarction.
Clinical Gastroenterology 1: 655–673

Schroeder T, Christoffersen J K, Andersen J et al 1985
Ischemic colitis complicating reconstruction of the
abdominal aorta. Surgery Gynecology and Obstetrics
160: 299–303

Tomchik F S, Wittenberg J, Ottinger L W 1970 The
roentgenographic spectrum of bowel infarction. Radiology
96: 249–260

18 Ruptured abdominal aneurysms

R. J. LUSBY and D. HUBER

Despite the shift in recent years towards early intervention in the treatment of asymptomatic abdominal aneurysm disease, this condition still leads to rupture and as such constitutes one of the common major surgical emergencies. The problems facing the emergency room staff are predominantly those of diagnosis and resuscitation, while the surgeon is challenged with a difficult dissection in the presence of haemorrhage and often distorted anatomical landmarks. Complications associated with successful repair include cardiac, renal and respiratory failure as well as distal limb ischaemia of thromboembolic origin. A successful outcome is dependent on early intervention and control of haemorrhage, necessitating the general surgeon as well as the specialized vascular surgeon being familiar with the investigation and management of ruptured intra-abdominal aneurysm.

Abdominal aortic aneurysms

Background to rupture

The natural history of aneurysms is one of rupture. Within the abdomen the infrarenal abdominal aorta and common iliac arteries are most at risk. However, visceral aneurysms and false aneurysms associated with previous vascular surgery may also present as acute ruptures. Unlike many other acute conditions of the abdomen, aneurysms tend to be silent during their formative phase and many remain asymptomatic and unnoticed up to the time of rupture. The finding of incidental aneurysms has become more frequent,

and the early detection of aneurysms has increased, since ultrasound and CT examinations of the abdomen have become almost routine for disorders of the biliary tree, urinary tract, pelvic and back disorders (Fig. 18.1). Expansion of an aneurysm may mimic frank rupture or merely present with low-grade localized tenderness, allowing the diagnosis to be made on physical examination, or, in the more obese patient, following CT or ultrasound scanning.

The risk of rupture of aneurysms is related in part to the transverse diameter of the vessel as well as the dynamic relationship between collagen deposition and breakdown within the vessel wall. Darling (1970) reviewed 16 483 autopsies and found 282 aortic aneurysms. Of those less than 50 mm in size, 18% had ruptured, while 20% of all ruptured aneurysms in the group were 70 mm

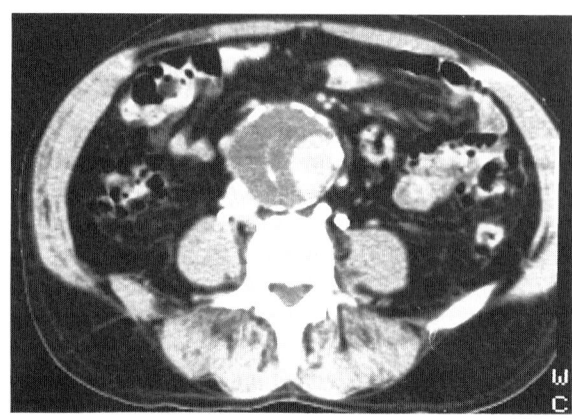

Fig. 18.1 CT scan of abdomen demonstrating a centrally located abdominal aortic aneurysm. The lumen is eccentrically placed while laminated thrombus occupies most of the aneurysm.

or less. In the same series of cases, 4% of ruptures involved the renal arteries and a similar number perforated the duodenum, forming primary aortoenteric fistulas. Many studies have demonstrated that once the diameter rises above 50–70 mm the patients chance of surviving longer than two years is less than 50% (Szilagyi et al 1966, Foster et al 1969, Darling et al 1977). Repeated imaging of aneurysms has indicated an annual growth rate of about 5 mm, but there is a great deal of individual variation in both growth rates and the size at which the aneurysms rupture (Dale & Bernstein 1976).

Cronenwett et al (1985) attempted to define more carefully those patients with small aneurysms who went on to rupture. Obstructive pulmonary disease, aneurysm site and raised diastolic blood pressure were prognostic factors. The rupture rate over the following five years ranged from 2% if none of the factors were present, to 100% if all three were present. Rupture of large aneurysms can follow laparotomy for other primary disease (Swanson et al 1980). The wall of the abdominal aorta, being a biological organ, is constantly laying down and reabsorbing collagen. Following laparotomy the wound-healing process elsewhere appears to influence the deposition reabsorption balance in the aneurysm wall, leading to a net reabsorption of collagen and weakening of the wall. Collagenase activity is at a maximum in the early postoperative period, during which time rupture may occur or the aneurysm can increase in size, enhancing the likelihood of rupture in the near future. Care must be taken in planning abdominal surgery in the presence of a known aortic aneurysm. A decision should be made to repair the aneurysm either before or shortly after the primary problem has been dealt with.

As rupture can best be prevented by elective repair, the crucial question is when to intervene. The decision to operate electively must be based on expected morbidity and mortality rates. In specialist centres a mortality rate of <5% for elective surgery is readily achieved. When weighed against the risks of rupture it is now common to recommend surgery for aneurysms having a diameter greater than 45 mm, or $2\frac{1}{2}$ times the diameter of the normal suprarenal aorta as seen on CT scanning. Aneurysms of less than 50 mm that are tender, that contain large amounts of thrombus, or that are associated with distal embolic events should also be given preferential consideration for early intervention.

Clinical presentation

Symptoms arising from an aortic aneurysm are generally sudden in onset and may be associated with either expansion or frank rupture. At times it is difficult to differentiate between the two conditions, although in the presence of the more stable expanding aneurysm it is possible to undertake some basic investigations. The prognosis of expanding aneurysms is significantly better, with a survival rate approaching that of elective resection. Patients with a ruptured abdominal aortic aneurysm usually complain of sudden onset of tearing back or loin pain, which may be similar to that of renal colic. In Darling's series (1970) back pain was present in 93% of cases, flank pain in 6%. Abdominal pain is a feature in almost half the patients presenting. It may be associated with feeling faint and sweaty and a history of syncope. On examination the patient generally appears shocked, cool and clammy, the pulse feels thready with a decreased volume and there is tachycardia. The blood pressure may be low, and the urine output poor. All is suggestive of a decreased blood volume. Examination can reveal a tense abdominal wall, which may be distended and tender. On deep palpation there is usually a pulsatile tender mass, but this sign is dependent on a reasonable blood pressure: in a contained retroperitoneal rupture this sign may be lost as the flanks fill with blood and no aortic mass is palpable, a trap for the inexperienced house officer. Distal pulses are often present, but this depends on the absence of appreciable peripheral vascular disease. Occasionally there is evidence of distal emboli which have originated from thrombus on the wall of the aneurysm.

Although the above description is typical of the symptoms and signs on presentation of a ruptured abdominal aortic aneurysm, it is well recognized that the presentation varies. The triad of abdominal and/or back pain, hypotension and a pulsatile mass is present in approximately three-quarters of cases. The exact symptoms and signs depend on the site of rupture and in which direction the haematoma has extended. Posterior rupture is the most common and is responsible for the back pain, but it should be remembered that any retroperitoneal structure may be involved. The femoral nerve may become involved (Merchant et al 1981) and present as neuropathy.

Rupture may be associated with thigh ecchymosis (Thompson & Bergan 1987). If the femoral nerve becomes compressed between the psoas and iliacus muscles, there is diminished pinprick sensation over the front of the thigh. A number of authors have reported ruptured aortic aneurysms presenting as an inguinal mass (Khaw et al 1986, Louras & Welch 1984), when most patients were male and had a previous history of an inguinal mass that was reducible. 'Chronic contained' ruptured abdominal aortic aneurysm has been reported by Rosenthal et al (1986) as a definite entity which is diagnosed by CT scan (Fig. 18.2). These aneurysms may present several months after the initial rupture, with confusing abdominal symptoms and signs. The aneurysm is often not palpable due to the organized thrombus alongside the aorta.

In 1831 Syme described an aortic aneurysm rupturing into the vena cava and forming a primary aortocaval fistula. Since then there have been reports of this as a spontaneous event responsible for presentation to the emergency room (Mohr & Smith 1975, Cooperman et al 1977, Johnson & Wood 1978). Most patients present with characteristic features: sudden abdominal or back pain with venous hypertension, oedema and arterial insufficiency (Johnson & Wood 1978). Other presentations include haematuria owing to rupture into either the kidney or ureter (Mercurias-Taylor & Kurer 1986) and spontaneous aortoenteric fistula (Graeber et al 1978).

Aneurysms may become acutely tender and produce signs suggestive of rupture but may not have actually ruptured. They still constitute an emergency, as rupture is both difficult to exclude and likely to be imminent. There is more time to evaluate these patients, and as long as they arrive in the operating theatre before the aneurysm ruptures the mortality rate will be similar to that of an elective procedure. These patients often present with a short history of abdominal pain, which may resemble renal colic, but without gross signs of acute blood loss. A tender pulsatile mass is the usual finding. At operation an acute inflammatory process may be present over part of the aneurysm wall to account for the symptoms, although no evidence of rupture is found.

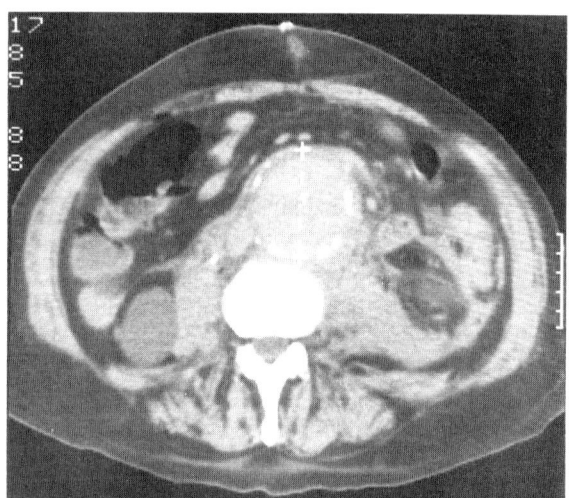

Fig. 18.2 CT scan demonstrating a 58 mm diameter aneurysm with blood tracking laterally from the aneurysm in a contained rupture.

Investigations

In general, rupture of an abdominal aortic aneurysm is a diagnosis made on clinical grounds alone. For this reason as well as the urgency of initiating treatment, no major diagnostic procedures are undertaken unless there is doubt about the diagnosis. When doubt exists, ultrasound imaging in the emergency room may identify the presence of an aneurysm that is clinically impalpable. Alternatively, if CT scanning is readily available, this technique should be performed to aid the diagnosis.

An advantage of CT scanning is the added information regarding surrounding structures. The exact position of the renal vein can be seen on the CT scan, and this may be important in planning the surgical procedure. Senapati et al (1986) point out that CT scans can differentiate ruptured aneurysms from those that are simply expanding (Fig. 18.2). Digital subtraction angiography can be of value in an expanding aneurysm for determining the quality of the proximal and distal vessels (Figs 18.3, 18.4).

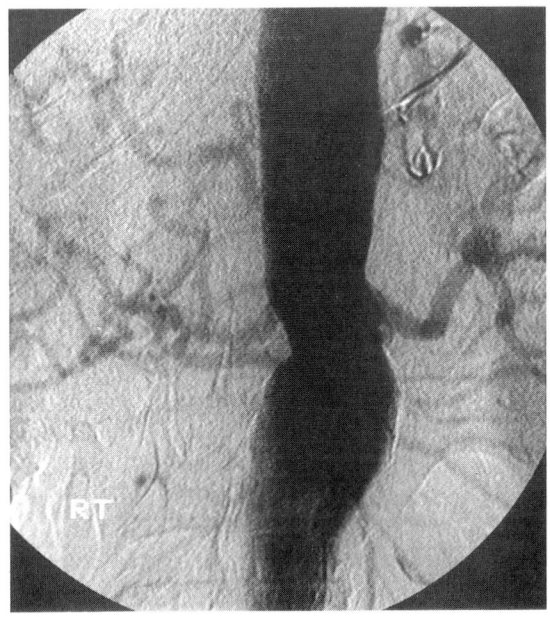

Fig. 18.3 Digital subtraction angiogram showing the 'neck' of an infrarenal aneurysm just below the origin of the renal arteries.

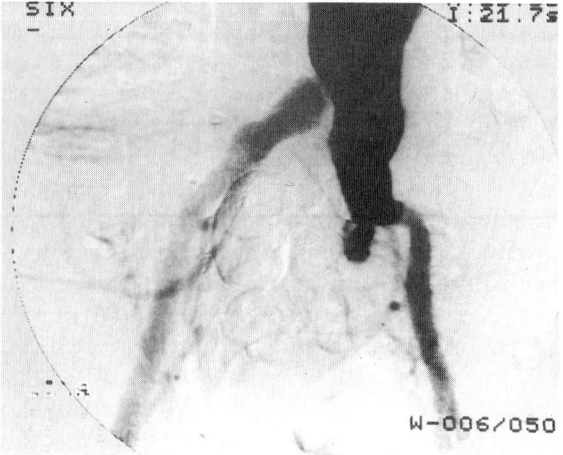

Fig. 18.4 Digital subtraction angiogram showing a large left common iliac aneurysm distal to the aortic aneurysm as well as disease of the right common iliac artery.

Initial management

At least half the patients with ruptured aneurysms present with a blood pressure less than 80 mm Hg. Seventy percent present with symptoms which have lasted more than 6 hours (Garrett & Ilabaca 1982). Immediate and efficient action is essential to achieve a successful outcome. On presentation to the hospital, and while the final diagnosis is being made, two large cannulas should be inserted, preferably one in a central vein, and infusion of crystalloid solutions begun. The amount of fluid given will depend on the blood pressure. In general the aim should be to keep the pressure around 100 mm Hg systolic. This level will be sufficient to ensure adequate perfusion of the renal vasculature. A blood pressure above this level will only encourage further extravasation and hypovolaemia.

The operating theatre and anaesthetic staff should be notified immediately the diagnosis is made, and the patient moved into the operating suite as soon as possible. Initial resuscitation can be carried out in the operating room while the patient is being prepared for surgery. Blood for crossmatch and basic haematological and biochemical studies should be taken, and a urinary catheter inserted. Arrest of haemorrhage is the basic aim of resuscitation, and this can only be effectively achieved by cross-clamping the aorta. Every effort must be made to achieve this end in the shortest possible time. Thereafter such measures as the insertion of arterial pressure and central venous cannulas can be undertaken.

Operative technique

It is important to remember that on induction of anaesthesia the protective effect of the patient's guarding will be absent. The loss of tamponade will result in a fall in blood pressure. For this reason, the time between induction and control of the neck of the aneurysm must be as short as possible.

Immediately on arrival in theatre, the patient is prepared and draped, ensuring that there is access to both femoral arteries. The surgeon must check the available clamps and ensure that there are two sump suckers working. Only then does the anaesthetist induce the patient. A long midline incision is generally used, although some surgeons prefer a transverse incision, the advantage being a lower incidence of postoperative chest complications. Bleeding from the wound edge should be ignored until after the neck of the aneurysm has been clamped and distal vessels controlled. Once the anterior peritoneum has been opened, the transverse colon and small bowel are reflected superiorly and to the patient's right. The precise approach to the aneurysm neck then depends on the extent of the haematoma. On most occasions the neck can be displayed by opening the retroperitoneum through the reflections of the third and fourth parts of the duodenum. Ligation and division of the inferior mesenteric vein above the region of the neck of the aneurysm may help to free the tissues and improve exposure. If possible, remaining clear of the haematoma and dissecting at the top end will be an advantage. This manoeuvre is not always possible, and damage to the gonadal vein, not clearly visualized in the angle between the renal vein on the left and the aneurysm neck, can lead to venous bleeding that is difficult to control. By keeping close to the aortic wall, damage to adjacent veins can be minimized. Following this dissection a finger can be worked around the neck and the clamp applied.

In difficult circumstances a number of techniques are available to control the proximal aorta. A wooden spatula 40 mm in diameter can be used to press the anterior wall of the aorta against the spine in the region of the lesser sac while the lower dissection is taking place. Alternatively, supracoeliac control may be gained by cross-clamping the aorta above the pancreas. The lesser sac is opened and the oesophagus moved to the patient's left. The aorta can then be approached directly without fear of damaging the inferior vena cava. Better access can be achieved by incising the right crus. If this approach is used then the clamp should be moved to an infra-renal position as soon as possible. Thompson et al (1975) suggested the use of Foley catheters inserted into the neck of the aorta while the bleeding is controlled by compression of the neck above. Smaller catheters are used in a similar fashion for the iliac vessels. Once

control has been achieved, the infrarenal neck can be dissected in relative safety.

When the top clamp is in position, the anaesthetist can replace lost volume more rapidly, and attention can be paid to maintaining renal perfusion and function. Essentially that requires adequate volume replacement with the addition of a mannitol infusion and low dose dopamine. Attention is then turned to the iliac vessels. The root of the mesentery is dissected off the aorta, and the dissection is carried down the anterior face and onto the right iliac artery. The left iliac artery may be approached in one of two directions. If the retroperitoneum is relatively free of haematoma, then the peritoneum can be lifted from the anterolateral abdominal wall and the vessel exposed as it runs along the psoas muscle. This approach is particularly useful in gaining access to the iliac bifurcation. For more proximal exposure, it is necessary to lift the sigmoid mesentery and mobilize the common iliac artery. In all the approaches care must be taken not to damage the ureter as it crosses the iliac bifurcation or the common iliac veins lying behind the iliac arteries. The lower limit of the dissection will be governed by the lower extent of the aneurysm. If the lesion does not extend beyond the aortic bifurcation, then there may be little need to mobilize distal to the common iliac vessels, provided common iliac artery control can be achieved with safety. It is important to repair all existing aneurysms, even though they may involve the common, internal or external iliac arteries. In addition, stenotic lesions of the iliac artery may need to be bypassed. In our experience the repair involves a bifurcation graft going to the common iliac bifurcation in over 80% of cases.

The aneurysm can now be opened, the clot and thrombus removed and sent for culture and sensitivity. Patent lumbar vessels are stitch-tied with non-absorbable sutures. The appropriate sized graft must now be selected. In general, a size 18 mm is about right for an average-sized man. Minimizing blood loss is important, and for this reason a woven dacron graft or collagen-impregnated graft should be used, but any graft that has a low porosity is satisfactory. The upper end is sutured with a continuous 3/0 Prolene suture. A clamp is placed on the graft just distal to the upper anastomosis, and the upper clamp is removed. Bleeding points should be oversewn at this stage when a good circumferential view of the anastomosis is available, but a small ooze will usually stop with gentle packing. If the graft is to be a straight one, then the distal anastomosis will be very close to the aortic bifurcation. It is important to avoid stenosing the origin of the iliac vessels. If there is any doubt regarding the patency of the iliac origins, then it is preferable to perform a bi-iliac procedure. In this case the lower anastomoses are constructed end-to-end. The common iliac vessels are transected in an oblique fashion to avoid stenosis, and the anastomosis is carried out with a continuous 4/0 Prolene suture.

Once the graft is in place and haemostasis achieved, the aneurysm sac is sutured over the graft. Care is taken to separate the fourth part of the duodenum from the upper anastomosis. The old sac is most commonly used, but occasionally a free omental graft is useful if complete coverage of the graft is not achieved with the old sac. Following the removal of the clamps, the blood pressure may fall precipitously, so release should be gradual by finger control of the graft, the amount of blood flow being determined by the blood pressure response. Volume replacement may be necessary to prevent hypotension and the table is changed to a foot-up position temporarily.

Unusual problems

Control of haemorrhage is the most crucial aspect of surgery for ruptured aneurysm. Haemorrhage is generally responsible for the common causes of death following aneurysm repair: these include renal failure, stroke, myocardial ischaemia, coagulopathies and refractory hypotension. The blood loss is usually arterial, but venous blood loss can indeed be large and unremitting.

The commonest site of major venous blood loss follows damage to the iliac veins, usually incurred during dissection of the iliac arteries. Care must be exercised when dissecting in this region. Often it is unnecessary to dissect all the way around the iliac arteries; one can apply the clamp with the vein still adherent to the arterial wall, though this can result in damage to the vein. Achieving distal control by an extraperitoneal approach to the external and internal iliac arteries can avoid damage to the common iliac veins, and in general the distal vessels are free of haematoma, allowing full visualization of the vessels. This is our preferred approach. Common iliac and vena cava bleeding at the aortic bifurcation can be difficult to control. Such bleeding is usually due to fibrous adhesion between the veins and the aorta. Transection of the aortic or iliac arteries may be necessary to gain adequate visualization to repair the venous damage.

Aortocaval fistula may present either alone or coexistent with frank rupture of an aortic aneurysm. Miani et al (1984) reviewed 226 ruptured aortic aneurysms and found caval ruptures in 5.7%. Clinical features include heart failure, venous congestion, tachycardia and a loud machinery bruit. Priapism has been a feature (Thompson & Bergan 1987). If there is prior warning of a likely fistula, precautions should be taken to prevent pulmonary embolism from dislodgement of intramural thrombi. The best management is to close the fistula from within the aneurysm and not attempt to separate the IVC from the aorta.

Division of the left renal vein is still a somewhat controversial manouvre in gaining better access to the neck of the aneurysm. By ligating and dividing the left suprarenal and gonadal veins, the left renal vein can be mobilized to enhance exposure without the need to divide it. Szilagyi et al (1969) reported the use of temporary transection but suggested that the vein be anastomosed after the repair was completed. Since then there have been a number of reports concerning the ligation of the renal vein (Rastad et al 1984, Solheim et al 1985, Adar et al 1985). Adar and colleagues compared two groups of patients, one of which had had the vein ligated, the other not, and found no difference between the two in terms of renal outcome. Solheim's group found no untoward sequelae in 11 patients. Rastad et al, however, found that complications were common in six patients who had had their vein ligated.

Venous anomalies can similarly be responsible for major venous bleeding. Brener et al (1974) reported and reviewed the literature of venous anomalies in aortic surgery. The four anomalies most commonly encountered are: duplication of the IVC (2.2–3.0%), retroaortic left renal vein (1.8–2.4%), circumaortic renal collar (1.5–8.7%) and transposition of the IVC (0.2–0.5%). These figures are derived from anatomical dissections and include minor anomalies that would not be of importance in a surgical setting. Brener points out that in patients with a duplication, the left IVC may go unnoticed due to its small size, and it may be ligated. The retroaortic vein drains in a more caudal direction to join the IVC. If it is not recognized it will be damaged during mobilization of the neck. In Brener's series, 40% of these veins were injured during surgery. The circumaortic collar poses a particular threat, because having identified the anterior portion of the renal vein, the posterior one may not be noticed. The posterior limb runs in a similar direction to the retroaortic vein, i.e. caudal. If it is damaged, then to gain access may require transection of the neck of the aneurysm.

The transposed IVC is easily recognized at operation. The major problem is coping with the obstruction to the aortic neck caused by the vein crossing from left to right at the level of the right renal vein. Often the IVC can be retracted either up or down, but occasionally transection is required. Transection must be performed below the level of the renal veins. Connelly et al (1980) collected six cases and reviewed the literature on horseshoe kidney. The incidence of this anomaly in the general population is approximately 0.25% (Perlmutter et al 1979). In routine operations for aortic aneurysms this problem will be noted on the preoperative CT scan, but in emergency procedures it will be an intraoperative finding. On finding a horseshoe kidney the arterial supply must be established. Connelly's review found that 60% of the patients had an anomaly of at least one renal artery. Only 20% of patients have two renal arteries (Pappin 1972). Preservation of the renal arterial supply is achieved by excision of a Carrel patch and implantation into the graft. Often the upper arteries are sufficiently high to leave in situ. The ureters usually cross the symphysis anteriorly and lie more medially than usual, but they may be retracted to allow access to the aneurysm. Divison of the symphysis is straightforward and generally free of complications.

Primary rupture of the aneurysm into the duodenum can occur, albeit rarely. The aneurysm becomes adherent to the fourth part of the duodenum and ruptures into the mucosa without penetration into the lumen (Thompson et al 1987). Infection then results in frank rupture into the lumen resulting in major haemorrhage. Almost all these patients have a herald bleed, which may be either haematemesis or melaena. Pain is not a feature. Although infection is a part of the pathology, repair may be performed in the usual fashion. The duodenum can be repaired by either simple closure or Roux-en-Y, depending on the size of the defect. The aortic surgery can then be performed in the usual way. Extra care must be taken to separate the duodenum from the anastomosis line. Results with this form of management are most acceptable, as Sweeney & Gadacz (1984) have demonstrated. If there is gross infection, then an extra-anatomic bypass is indicated.

Complications

One-third of all complications following rupture of aortic aneurysms are related to acute renal failure. This condition is followed by respiratory or cardiac problems, which are responsible for another one-third of problems. Other complications include haemorrhage, ischaemic colitis, spinal ischaemia, distal emboli and abnormal clotting function (Garrett & Ilabaca 1982, Lambert et al 1986). Although relating to elective procedures, Bush (1983) emphasized some precautions to decrease the incidence of renal failure following aneurysm repair. The main factor in preventing renal failure is the maintenance of adequate extracellular volume (Crawford et al 1981, Shires et al 1961). An important adjunct is the maintenance of a satisfactory blood pressure and encouragement of renal function using mannitol and an infusion of low dose dopamine.

Postoperative bleeding is less common with the inclusion method of aneurysm repair. The sac causes a degree of tamponade, limiting the bleeding. In Lambert's series, only one out of 66 deaths was caused by postoperative bleed. Crawford (1983) recommends the use of angiography to identify the site of haemorrhage. He suggests that a negative investigation is often reassuring, and there have been a number of unexpected positive findings. There were no false negative examinations.

The exact incidence of ischaemic colitis following aortic surgery is unknown but may be around 6%. This figure is based on macroscopic changes at colonoscopy. Taking into account the incidence of clinical colitis, the figure is probably closer to 1.5–5%, but it has been quoted as high as 15%. The mortality rate of clinically evident ischaemic colitis is around 80% and therefore constitutes a major problem secondary to aortic surgery. As well as the florid case of ischaemic colitis, there are likely to be unknown numbers of patients suffering from subclinical ischaemia. Clinical symptoms of ischaemic colitis include diarrhoea, tenderness and distension, but they are notoriously inaccurate. Symptoms of subclinical ischaemic colitis include general malaise, slow recovery from major surgery and late stricture formation. The general malaise is probably related to the increased permeability of the bowel wall to micro-organisms and the subsequent bacteraemia. Crawford (1983) has drawn attention to the patient who has undergone a previous right hemicolectomy and has therefore lost the marginal artery on which his colon will survive. At the end of the operation the colon must be carefully inspected, and if there is any doubt regarding its viability then the inferior mesenteric artery must be implanted into the graft.

Spinal cord ischaemia occurs in approximately 0.25% of cases (Szilagyi 1983) and is ten times more common in patients with ruptured aneurysms than in those with non-ruptured aneurysms, yielding an incidence of around 2% in the ruptured group. The arterial supply to the lumbar chord is variable but is largely derived from the radicular branches, which originate from the ascending cervical, intercostal, and lumbar arteries. The cord between T10 and L4 is supplied by two radicular branches, the main one being the arteria radicularis magna of Adamkiewicz. The origin of this artery can vary. The usual point of origin is from a lumbar vessel between T11 and L1, but it may be as low as L2 or L3. As long as it derives from the higher of the alternatives, then even a high intra-abdominal clamping of the aorta will not cause problems, but if the origin is low,

then normal clamping can cause ischaemia. Szilagyi suggests that an additional cause is the stasis that follows hypotension, especially if it is associated with hypercoagulability. The prognosis in this group is somewhat better, either partial or complete recovery being possible (Joseph et al 1988).

Distal emboli will cause lower limb ischaemia, and care must be exercised to prevent this complication. The two main sites of origin of emboli are the aorta itself and the common iliac arteries. For this reason clamping of the external iliac arteries should be achieved as soon as possible after control of the proximal aorta is achieved. In elective or expanding aneurysms these vessels are clamped before the neck of the aneurysm is controlled and the body of the aneurysm is handled. This technique was verified in a study by Starr et al (1979), who found an embolization rate of 0.23%. Ruptured aneurysms can be treated in the traditional way by clamping the neck first, but with the proviso that minimal handling of the sac occurs before the distal clamps are applied in an attempt to decrease the incidence of distal emboli. Once the graft has been completed, a meticulous routine of flushing and irrigation should be used to ensure that there is no risk of distal embolization. If there is any doubt regarding thrombosis distal to the clamp, then a Fogarty catheter must be passed and thrombus or embolus withdrawn.

Depending on the amount of blood lost during repair of the aneurysm, there is a risk of consumption coagulopathy (Hicks et al 1975, Gardner et al 1978). Although Wakefield et al (1982) could not demonstrate such a correlation, Lambert et al (1986) noted an increased probability of survival in those who had had preoperative fresh frozen plasma. It has also been noted that aneurysms per se can cause disseminated intervascular coagulopathy even without rupture (Thompson et al 1986, Mulcare et al 1974, 1976). The associated bleeding disorders seen in patients with rupture has led to the common practice of not using systemic heparin in the emergency situation. When rupture occurs in patients on Warfarin anticoagulant therapy, the infusion of cryosupernate or fresh frozen plasma will correct the tendency to bleed.

Results of rupture

There has been a noticeable fall in the morbidity and mortality rates following elective aortic aneurysm repair, but this has not been as evident in patients undergoing emergency repair. Most series report a mortality rate of between 40 and 60% (Hoffman et al 1982). Crawford (1983) reported a rate of 25%, while Lambert et al (1986) claimed a survival rate of 25%. In general the need to travel to major centres has selected a more favourable group in these reports. Prolonged hypotension, angina and myocardial infarction preoperatively are indicators of poor outcome, while maintenance of blood pressure above 110 mm Hg and normal renal function are good prognostic indicators. Intraoperatively, those factors associated with a poor prognosis included prolonged operation time, prolonged hypotension, large estimated blood loss and large blood transfusion. Postoperatively any form of organ failure is associated with a raised mortality: renal 53%, respiratory 59%, cardiac 60%, and 75% for ischaemic colitis (Wakefield et al 1982).

Visceral artery aneurysms

Although aneurysms of visceral arteries are uncommon, they are responsible for occasional emergency procedures. These aneurysms arise from foregut vessels, the most common being the splenic artery, which accounts for 56% of all splanchnic aneurysms (Whitehouse et al 1982). The next most common are hepatic artery aneurysms, followed by mesenteric, coeliac, and gastroduodenal aneurysms (Williams et al 1987).

Splenic artery aneurysms

Splenic artery aneurysms were first described in 1770 by Beaussier (1770). Their incidence in the general population is ill defined. In unselected series of autopsies, the incidence was 0.098–0.16% (Moore et al 1970, Sheps et al 1958). Stanley & Fry (1974) looked at angiograms and found an incidence of 0.78%, which in patients with cirrhotic portal hypertension rose to 7.1%. In patients over the age of 60, the incidence of splenic artery aneurysm is 10.4% (Bedford & Lodge 1960); in fact they occur mainly in the seventh decade, but there is also a peak in the third decade (Stanley et al 1970). The earlier peak is related to splenic artery aneurysms occurring during pregnancy. The close relationship between pregnancy and splenic artery aneurysm has been confirmed by most studies (Stanley & Fry 1974, Trastek et al 1985, Moore & Lewis 1961). Indeed in Stanley's study (1974) of 60 cases, 80% were women: once arteritis, portal hypertension, splenomegaly and arterial fibrodysplasia had been ruled out, 40% of the women in the study had completed at least six pregnancies.

Splenic artery aneurysms occur at bifurcations, most commonly in the distal third on the main trunk (Fry 1983, Trastek et al 1985, Williams et al 1987). They tend to be saccular and measure less than 20 mm in diameter (Fry 1983, Stanley & Fry 1974), but they range in size from 6 to 300 mm (Trastek et al 1985). The aetiology of these aneurysms is diverse, including fibromuscular disease, portal hypertension, focal arteritis (including mycotic endarteritis and secondary to pancreatitis), multiple pregnancy, atherosclerosis and trauma. Early reports of splenic artery aneurysms suggested that they were dangerous, with a rupture rate of 46% (Owens & Coffey 1953). More recent studies suggest that these aneurysms are more benign. The rupture rate in Stanley & Fry's series (1974) was 5.3%, and in that reported by Trastek et al (1982) was 3%.

Symptomatology of splenic artery aneurysms is rather nonspecific. More than 80% of patients are asymptomatic (Whitehouse et al 1982). Of those patients who do have symptoms, the most common complaint is left upper quadrant discomfort. In the study by Trastek et al (1982), 17% had symptoms, invariably abdominal pain. In the same study 4% had symptoms and signs of rupture, but only half the ruptures were of a splenic aneurysm, the remainder were ruptures of a coexisting aneurysm. Other presentations of splenic artery aneurysms include a bruit, palpable mass and indentation of the stomach on barium meal (Whitehouse et al 1982, Williams et al 1987, Trastek et al 1985). All these features are rare. Rupture of a splenic artery aneurysm is mainly characterized by signs of acute blood loss, usually intraperitoneally. Often it ruptures at first into the lesser sac, allowing for tamponade and therefore time for surgical intervention. As the pressure builds up, there will be secondary rupture into the peritoneal cavity. This phenomenon is often referred to as 'double rupture' and may occur minutes or days later (Jorgensen 1985, Stanley et al 1970, Trastek et al 1982, Vries et al 1982).

Occasionally aneurysms of the splenic artery can rupture into adjacent organs. The symptomatology will be complex and depend on the organ involved, which is most commonly the pancreas. Pancreatitis may be responsible for a number of ruptured splenic artery aneurysms. Twenty cases of upper gastrointestinal bleeding secondary to a ruptured splenic artery aneurysm have been reported. 'Haemosuccus pancreaticus' describes the syndrome of bleeding into the pancreatic duct with blood loss through the ampulla of Vater. Pseudoaneurysm of the splenic artery can follow severe pancreatitis. Bleeding from this source is a rapidly lethal complication of pancreatitis (Stabile et al 1983).

Undoubtedly the most important group of patients with splenic artery aneurysms are pregnant women. They are both the largest subgroup of patients with the condition (Stanley & Fry 1974), and the most likely to rupture. While the chance of rupture in the whole group is less than 2%, for pregnant women the figure is closer to 80% (Stanley et al 1970, Fry 1983). In pregnant women who do go on to rupture, the mortality rate for mothers is 70%, and for the fetus it is almost 100% (O'Grady et al 1977).

There are three indications for elective surgery: aneurysms larger than 20 mm diameter (where the mortality rate associated with rupture is approximately 25%: Fry 1983), women of childbearing age, and pregnancy. Pregnant women should therefore be advised to undergo resection during the third trimester. The exact operative procedure will depend on the position of the aneurysm, but an attempt should be made to preserve the spleen whenever possible. Splenectomy will be necessary if the aneurysm is close to or within the spleen itself. The complications of splenectomy have to be considered, and the necessary postoperative precautions taken. If the aneurysm is located beyond the pancreas but outside the spleen, the aneurysm may be excised and the splenic artery tied off. The spleen will be able to survive on the abundant blood supply from the short gastric vessels. Those aneurysms that lie in close proximity to the pancreas may simply be ligated and left in situ. All branches must be ligated, including those that run posteriorly to supply the pancreas itself.

Hepatic artery aneurysms

Although hepatic artery aneurysms are rarely seen, they are the second most common visceral aneurysm and constitute about 20% of all such aneurysms (Curran & Taylor 1986). Unlike splenic artery aneurysms, they have a high probability of rupture (Stanley et al 1970). The major aetiological factor is atheroma, which accounts for about 32%; then degeneration of the media (24%); trauma (including surgical injury) accounts for 22%. Other causes included mycotic lesions, but these are far less common than they used to be (Rutherford 1977, Guida & Moore 1966).

All ages are at risk, but the mean age is around 38 years. Men are affected twice as often as women (Erskine 1973). Hepatic aneurysm can be classified into intra- and extrahepatic. In a review of the world literature of 148 aneurysms, 117 were extrahepatic, 25 intrahepatic and six were both intra- and extrahepatic (Guida & Moore 1966). The hepatic artery proper and the right hepatic artery are affected equally; the cystic, left hepatic, and gastroduodenal arteries are rarely involved.

Clinical presentation of a ruptured aneurysm depends on the exact site of the rupture. Intraperitoneal rupture is common, occurring in about 50% of patients (Harlafris & Akin 1977). Alternatively rupture occurs into an adjacent organ (Williams et al 1987) such as bile duct, portal vein, duodenum or liver. Right upper quadrant pain is common; it may be sudden and occasionally radiates to the back. Guarding and rebound are usually associated with signs of acute blood loss. Haemobilia occurs in about 62% of patients and jaundice in over 50% (Croom et al 1976). The triad of abdominal pain, haemobilia and obstructive jaundice is present in only one-third of patients (Kibbler et al 1985).

Diagnosis is often difficult, but it may be inappropriate to waste time with investigations if the patient is bleeding heavily. There may be an opportunity to consider simple investigations such as a plain abdominal radiograph, which may demonstrate a calcified rim in the right upper quadrant. Free rupture of a hepatic aneurysm into the peritoneal cavity calls for immediate surgery; there is no place for delay or for other investigations. In the evaluation of haemobilia or upper gastrointestinal bleeding when the patient is stable, CT scanning, ultrasound scanning and angiography do have a place. Ultrasound and CT scans will show the relationship of the aneurysm to the bile ducts and the portal vein, and also whether it is intra- or extrahepatic.

Elective resection of hepatic aneurysms is strongly advised because their high rate of rupture. This advice especially relates to extrahepatic aneurysms. The major difference between elective and emergency surgery for this lesion is the preparation. Depending on the position of the aneurysm, surgery may involve simple ligation, cable graft, excision, embolization or a partial hepatectomy. A full preoperative investigation will help define the very variable hepatic blood supply. Patients undergoing emergency surgery do not enjoy these benefits. Preoperative placement of a balloon catheter by the radiologist may be helpful in controlling the proximal hepatic artery, the balloon catheter being withdrawn once the vessel is adequately clamped.

Rupture of an extrahepatic aneurysm requires immediate surgery. If the aneurysm is located on the common hepatic artery proximal to the gastroduodenal artery, the arterial supply to the liver should be maintained by the collaterals from the superior mesenteric artery, and the aneurysm can be ligated. Excision of the aneurysm may be attempted if no vital structures are involved. Mycotic aneurysms may necessitate an aggressive approach to debridement.

More distal aneurysms, in which the collateral circulation is thought to be inadequate, will require a cable graft. The saphenous vein is considered the most suitable. It is flexible, and the

diameter is appropriate for the hepatic artery. If there is doubt about the adequacy of the blood supply to the liver, then a trial of occlusion can be carried out, assessing the viability of the liver after 10–15 min. Collateral flow can also be assessed by observing the backflow from the distal cut end of the hepatic artery. Continuity can be restored by anastomosis of the distal hepatic artery to any major artery in the area, such as the superior mesenteric or splenic artery.

Percutaneous embolization of these aneurysms has recently been described in patients who are undergoing angiography as part of the investigation of upper gastrointestinal bleeding. In general, it is not indicated for extrahepatic lesions because of the importance of maintaining hepatic blood supply.

Superior mesenteric artery aneurysms

These aneurysms are very much rarer than either splenic or hepatic aneurysms. About 100 cases have been reported in the literature (Hans et al 1977). The most common aetiology today is atherosclerosis, although in the past infection was the main cause (Jorgensen 1985). Williams et al (1987) suggest otherwise, pointing out that a large proportion of these aneurysms are found in either intravenous drug addicts or patients with subacute bacterial endocarditis (Yellin 1977). According to Wright et al (1982), two-thirds of these aneurysms are mycotic. It is therefore necessary to rule out bacterial endocarditis as a cause of a specific lesion. Trauma and arterial dysplasia can also be responsible for this type of aneurysm (Graham et al 1980). The exact incidence of rupture is not known, but it is believed to be about 50% if left untreated (Hans et al 1977). The mortality following rupture has been reported by Stanley et al (1970) as 20%.

Occasionally these patients present before rupture with abdominal pain and possibly an abdominal mass. In the presence of subacute bacterial endocarditis, these symptoms should alert one to the possibility of a visceral aneurysm (Jorgensen 1985). Another mode of presentation is intestinal ischaemia. This may be due to either embolization of the contents of the aneurysm, or sudden thrombosis of the aneurysm, causing occlusion. Both these events occur more frequently in the non-mycotic aneurysms (Stanley et al 1970).

As with most emergency procedures, it is important that the approach to a ruptured superior mesenteric aneurysm is through a vertical incision, because control may require clamping the aorta at the diaphragmatic hiatus. Good exposure of the origin of the SMA requires mobilization of the duodenojejunal junction and elevation of the pancreas. An extraperitoneal approach is possible by reflecting the left colon and the duodenum to the right. These approaches will allow access to the origin of the vessel.

Following the first successful treatment of an SMA aneurysm by DeBakey and Cooley in 1949 (1953), it was noted that restoration of continuity was often unnecessary. Small-bowel viability is not usually threatened. The reason is not clear but may be related to the gradual narrowing of the lumen by the aneurysm and the subsequent development of collateral arterial supply (Williams et al 1987). Thus the most common procedure is aneurysmectomy. If there is any doubt regarding the small bowel viability, then some form of arterial continuity will be necessary. Often an end-to-end anastomosis is possible following excision of the aneurysm. Other alternatives include a saphenous vein graft. The use of an insert prosthesis should be discouraged because of the high incidence of mycotic aneurysm.

Olcott & Ehrenfeld (1977) have suggested endoaneurysmorrhaphy for mycotic and false aneurysms of visceral vessels. This procedure involves control of both the afferent and efferent vessels, opening the aneurysm and the main artery, debridement of the sac, then closure of the vessel without excision of any of the vessel wall. The postoperative management must include a prolonged course of the relevant antibiotic to prevent reformation of the aneurysm.

Gastroduodenal artery aneurysms

These are rare. Indeed in 1985 Taheri & Mueller collected all reports of gastroduodenal aneurysms and found 22 cases. Of these patients 87% were male, and the average age was 49 years. The commonest means of diagnosis was by angiogram, although CT scan has been suggested as an effective means of diagnosis. Neither endoscopic nor barium studies have been shown to be useful in detecting these aneurysms (Williams et al 1987). The commonest aetiological factor is pancreatitis, which is responsible for over 50% of cases (Ekhauser et al 1980). Other causes include atheroma and trauma (Stanley et al 1970). These aneurysms present with abdominal pain or occasionally with jaundice, but in Stanley's series 50% presented with rupture into the retroperitoneum or gastrointestinal tract.

Treatment of these aneurysms includes simple ligation and intra-arterial embolization (Thakkar et al 1983). In either case the mortality rate is high. Williams et al favour the use of transcatheter embolization as it avoids a difficult operation and the results are acceptable. It should be pointed out that it does have complications, including aneurysm rupture and organ necrosis (Taheri & Mueller 1985). Ekhauser et al (1980) reported a mortality of 47% in patients suffering from pancreatitis.

Miscellaneous foregut artery aneurysms

Aneurysms of the coeliac, gastric and gastroepiploic arteries have been reported (Stanley et al 1970). They are rare, and little is known about their natural history. The assumption has been that they will grow in size and eventually rupture. The symptoms these aneurysms cause depend on the adjacent structures, but more commonly patients remain symptom free until they rupture or are discovered incidentally. These aneurysms are more common in middle-aged men (Deterling 1971). The aetiology is arteriosclerosis, although Stanley et al (1970) suggest that some may be congenital. Most cases have already ruptured on presentation (Stanley et al 1970). Two-thirds cause massive upper gastrointestinal bleeding (Isaacson & Delancy 1978).

Treatment generally involves simple ligation of

the vessel, but occasionally it requires resection of an adjacent organ. In patients with an aneurysm of the coeliac artery, an attempt should be made to restore the hepatic branch. Liver necrosis will not necessarily follow ligation (Appleby 1953), and one can clamp the vessel to assess the likelihood of serious ischaemia before performing graft surgery.

REFERENCES

Adar R, Rabbi I, Bass A et al 1985 Left renal vein division in abdominal aortic aneurysm operations. Effect on renal function. Archives of Surgery 120: 1033–1036

Appleby L H 1953 The celiac axis in the expansion of the operations for gastric carcinoma. Cancer 6: 704–707

Beaussier M 1770 Sur un anévrisme de l'artère splénique dont les parois se sont ossifiées. Journal de Medecine, Chirurgie, Pharmacie (Paris) 32: 157

Bedford P D, Lodge B 1960 Aneurysm of the splenic artery. Gut 1: 312–320

Brener B J, Darling R C, Frederick P L, Linton R R 1974 Major venous anomalies complicating abdominal aortic surgery. Archives of Surgery 108: 159–165

Bush H L 1983 Renal failure following abdominal aortic reconstruction. Surgery 93: 107–109

Connelly T L, McKinnon W, Smith R B, Perdue G D 1980 Abdominal aortic surgery and horseshoe kidney. Report of six cases and a review. Archives of Surgery 115: 1459–63

Cooperman M, Deal K F, Wooley C F, Evans W E 1977 Spontaneous aorta-caval fistula with paradoxical pulmonary embolism. American Journal of Surgery 134: 647–649

Crawford E S 1983 Symposium: Prevention of complications of abdominal aortic reconstruction. Introduction. Surgery 93: 91–96

Crawford E S, Saleh S A, Babb J W, Glaeser D H, Vaccaro P S, Silvers A 1981 Infrarenal abdominal aortic aneurysm: Factors influencing survival after operation performed over a 25 year period. Annals of Surgery 193: 699–709

Cronenwett J L, Murphy T F, Zelenock G B et al 1985 Actuarial analysis of variables associated with rupture of small abdominal aortic aneurysms. Surgery 98: 472–483

Croom R D, Frantz P T, Thomas C G, Hothem A O 1976 Aneurysms of the hepatic artery. Southern Medical Journal 69: 1013–1017

Curran F T, Taylor S A 1986 Hepatic artery aneurysm. Postgraduate Medical Journal 62: 957–959

Dale W A, Bernstein E F 1976 Management of the small aneurysm. In: Varco R L, Delaney J P (eds) Controversy in surgery. WB Saunders, Philadelphia, pp 261–265

Darling R C 1970 Rupture arteriosclerotic abdominal aortic aneurysms. American Journal of Surgery 119: 397–416

Darling R C, Messina C R, Brewster D C, Otinger L W 1977 Autopsy study of unoperated abdominal aortic aneurysms: The case for early resection. Circulation 56: 161–164

DeBakey M E, Cooley D A 1953 Successful resection of mycotic aneurysm of the SMA: Case report and review of the literature. American Journal of Surgery 19: 202–212

Deterling R A 1971 Aneurysm of the visceral arteries. Journal of Cardiovascular Surgery 12: 309–322

Ekhauser F E, Stanley J C, Zelenock G B et al 1980 Gastroduodenal and pancreaticoduodenal artery aneurysms: A complication of pancreatitis causing spontaneous GI bleed. Surgery 88: 335–344

Erskine J M 1973 Hepatic artery aneurysm. Vascular Surgery 7: 106–125

Foster J H, Gobbel W G, Scott H W 1969 Comparative study of elective resection and expectant treatment of abdominal aortic aneurysm. Surgery Gynecology and Obstetrics 129: 1–9

Fry W J 1983 Splanchnic Artery Aneurysms In: Najarian J S, Delaney J P (eds) Advances in vascular surgery. Year Book Medical Publications, Chicago, pp 311–315

Gardner R J, Gardner N L, Tarnay T H, Warden H E, James E C, Watne A L 1978 The surgical experience and a one to sixteen year follow up of 277 abdominal aortic aneurysms. American Journal of Surgery 135: 226–239

Garrett H E, Ilabaca P A 1982 The ruptured abdominal aortic aneurysm. In: Bergen J J, Yao J S T (eds) Aneurysm: Diagnosis and Treatment. Grune & Stratton, New York

Graeber G M, Bredenberg C E, Gregg R O, Parker F B, Webb W R 1978 Diagnosis and management of spontaneous aortoenteric fistulas. American Journal of Surgery 136: 269–272

Graham J M, McCollum C H, DeBakey M E 1980 Aneurysms of the splanchnic arteries. American Journal of Surgery 140: 797–801

Guida P M, Moore S W 1966 Aneurysm of the hepatic artery. Report of five cases with a brief review of the previously reported cases. Surgery 60: 299–310

Hans S S, Gordon M, Lee P T 1977 Saccular atherosclerotic aneurysm of the superior mesenteric artery. Archives of Surgery 112: 854

Harlafris N N, Akin J G 1977 Hemobillia from ruptured hepatic artery aneurysm. American Journal of Surgery 133: 229–232

Hicks G L, Eastland M W, DeWeese J A, May A G, Rob C G 1975 Survival improvement following aortic aneurysm resection. Annals of Surgery 181: 863–869

Hoffman M, Avellone J C, Plecha F R et al 1982 Operation for ruptured abdominal aortic aneurysm: a community wide experience. Surgery 5: 597–602

Isaacson R, Delancy H 1978 Intragastric rupture of a left gastric artery aneurysm. Journal of the Medical Association of Georgia 67: 648–647

Johnson J M, Wood M 1978 Arteriovenous fistula secondary to rupture of atherosclerotic abdominal aortic aneurysm. Report of five cases. American Journal of Surgery 136: 171–175

Jorgenson B A 1985 Visceral artery aneurysms. Danish Medical Bulletin 32: 237–242

Joseph M G, Langsfeld M, Lusby R J 1988 Infrarenal aortic aneurysms — An unusual cause of paraparesis. ANZ Journal of Surgery 59: 743–4

Khaw H, Soltiurai V S, Craighead C C, Baston R C 1986 Ruptured abdominal aortic aneurysm presenting as a symptomatic inguinal mass; report of 6 cases. Journal of Vascular Surgery 4: 384–389

Kibbler C C, Cohen D L, Cruickshank J K, Kushwaha S S, Morgan M Y, Dick R D 1985 Use of CAT scanning in the diagnosis and management of hepatic artery aneurysm. Gut 26: 752–756

Lambert M E, Baguley P, Charlesworth D 1986 Ruptured abdominal aortic aneurysms. Journal of Cardiovascular Surgery 27: 256–261

Louras J C, Welch J P 1984 Masking of ruptured abdominal aortic aneurysm by incarcerated inguinal hernia. Archives of Surgery 119: 331–332

Merchant R F, Cafferata H T, DePalma R G 1981 Pitfalls in the diagnosis of abdominal aortic aneurysm. American Journal of Surgery 142: 756–758

Mercurias-Taylor L A, Kurer M H 1986 Haematuria and abdominal aortic aneurysm. Journal of Cardiovascular Surgery 27: 565–567

Miani S, Mingazzini P, Piglionica R, Biasi G M, Ruberti U 1984 Influence of the rupture site of abdominal aortic aneurysm with regard to post operative survival rates. Journal of Cardiovascular Surgery 25: 515–519

Mohr L, Smith L 1975 Arteriovenous fistula from ruptured abdominal aortic aneurysm. Archives of Surgery 110: 806–812

Moore M D, Lewis R J 1961 Splenic artery aneurysm. Annals of Surgery 153: 1033–1045

Moore S W, Guida P M, Schumaker H W 1970 Splenic artery aneurysm. Bulletin dela Société Internationale de Chirurgie (Bruxelles) 29: 210–218

Mulcare R J, Royster T S, Wiess H J et al 1974 Disseminated intravascular coagulation as a complication of abdominal aortic aneurysm repair. Annals of Surgery 180: 343–349

Mulcare R J, Royster T S, Phillips L L 1976 Intravascular coagulation in surgical procedures on the abdominal aorta. Surgery Gynecology and Obstetrics 143: 730–734

O'Grady J P, Day E J, Toole A L, Paust J C 1977 Splenic artery aneurysm rupture in pregnancy. A review and case report. Obstetrics and Gynecology 50: 627–630

Olcott C, Ehrenfeld W K 1977 Endoaneurysmorrhaphy for visceral artery aneurysms. American Journal of Surgery 133: 636–639

Owens J C, Coffey R J 1953 Aneurysm of the splenic artery, including a report of 6 additional cases. International Abstracts of Surgery (Chicago) 97: 313–335

Pappin E 1972 Abdominal aortic aneurysm and horseshoe kidney. British Journal of Surgery 59: 513–517

Perlmutter A D, Retik A B, Bauer S B 1979 Anomalies of the upper urinary tract. In: Harrison H J, Gutes R F, Permutter A D (eds) Urology, 4th edn. WB Saunders & Co. Philadelphia, pp 1330–1335

Rastad J, Almgren B, Bowald S et al 1984 Renal complications to left renal vein ligation in abdominal aortic surgery. Journal of Cardiovascular Surgery 25: 432–436

Rosenthal D, Clark M D, Stanton P E, Lamis P A 1986 "Chronic contained" ruptured abdominal aortic aneurysm: Is it real? Journal of Cardiovascular Surgery 27: 723–724

Rutherford R B 1977 Infrarenal aortic aneurysms. In: Rutherford R B (ed) Vascular surgery, 2nd ed. WB Saunders, Philadelphia, pp 755–771

Senapati A, Hurst P A E, Thomas M L, Browse N L, Burnard K G 1986 Differentiation of ruptured aortic aneurysm from acute expansion by computerised tomography. Journal of Cardiovascular Surgery 27: 719–722

Sheps S G, Spittel J A, Fairbairn J F, Edwards J E 1958 Aneurysms of the splenic artery with special reference to bland aneurysms. Proceedings of the Staff Meetings of the Mayo Clinic 33: 381–390

Shires T, Williams J, Brown F 1961 Acute changes in extracellular fluids associated with major surgical procedures. Annals of Surgery 154: 803–810

Solheim K, Krag L E, Nerdrum H J 1985 Ligation of the left renal vein. Acta Chirurgica Scandinavica 151: 603–606

Stabile B E, Wilson S E, Debas H T 1983 Reduced mortality from bleeding pseudocysts and pseudoaneurysms caused by pancreatitis. Archives of Surgery 118: 45–51

Stanley J C, Fry W J 1974 Pathogenesis and clinical significance of splenic artery aneurysms. Surgery 76: 898–909

Stanley J C, Thompson N W, Fry W J 1970 Splanchnic artery aneurysms. Archives of Surgery 101: 689–697

Starr D S, Lawrie G M, Morris G C 1979 Prevention of distal embolism during arterial reconstruction. American Journal of Surgery 764–769

Swanson R J, Littooy F N, Hunt T K, Stoney R J 1980 Laparotomy as a precipitating factor in the rupture of intra-abdominal aneurysms. Archives of Surgery 115: 299–304

Sweeney M S, Gadacz T R 1984 Primary aorto-duodenal fistula: Manifestation, diagnosis and treatment. Surgery 96: 492–497

Syme J 1831 Editorial. Medical and Surgical Journal (Edinburgh) 36: 104

Szilagyi D E 1983 Spinal chord ischaemia in surgical procedures with temporary clamping of the abdominal aorta. Surgery 93: 110–111

Szilagyi D E, Smith R F, DeRusso F J, Elliott J P, Sherrin F W 1966 Contribution of abdominal aortic aneurysmectomy to prolongation of life. Annals of Surgery 164: 678–699

Szilagyi D E, Smith R F, Elliott J P 1969 Temporary transection of the left renal vein: A technical aid in aortic surgery. Surgery 65: 32–40

Taheri S A, Mueller G 1985 Surgical approach and review of the literature on gastroduodenal aneurysm: a case report. Angiology 36: 895–898

Thakkar R V, Gajjar B, Wilkins R A, Levi A J 1983 Embolization of gastroduodenal artery aneurysm caused by chronic pancreatitis. Gut 24: 1094–1098

Thompson J E, Bergan J J 1987 The ruptured abdominal aortic aneurysm. In: Bergan J J, Yao J S T (eds) Vascular surgical emergencies. Grune & Stratton, New York, pp 285–297

Thompson J E, Hollier L H, Patman R D, Persson A V 1975 Surgical treatment of abdominal aortic aneurysm: Factors affecting mortality and morbidity — a 20 year experience. Annals of Surgery 181: 654–661

Thompson R W, Adams D H, Cohen J R, Mannick J A, Whittemore A D 1986 Disseminated intravascular coagulation caused by abdominal aortic aneurysm. Journal of Vascular Surgery 4: 184–186

Trastek V F, Pairolero P C, Joyce J W, Hollier L H, Bernatz P E 1982 Splenic artery aneurysms. Surgery 91: 694–699

Trastek V F, Pairolero P C, Bernatz P E 1985 Splenic artery aneurysm. World Journal of Medicine 9: 378–383

Vries J E de, Schattenkerk M E, Malt R A 1982 Complications of splenic artery aneurysm other than intraperitoneal rupture. Surgery 91: 200–204

Wakefield T W, Whitehouse W M, Wu S et al 1982

Abdominal aortic aneurysm rupture: Statistical analysis of factors affecting outcome of surgical treatment. Surgery 5: 586–595

Whitehouse W M, Graham L M, Stanley J C 1982 Aneurysms of the celiac, hepatic, and splenic arteries. In: Bergan J J, Yao J S T (eds) Aneurysms — diagnosis and treatment. Grune & Stratton, New York, pp 405–415

Williams R A, Milliken J C, Wilson S E 1987 Splanchnic artery aneurysms. In: Wilson S E, Veith F J, Hobson R W et al (eds) Vascular surgery. Principles and practice. McGraw-Hill, New York, pp 504–512

Wright C B, Schoepfle W J, Kurtock S B, Corry R J et al 1982 Gastrointestinal bleeding and mycotic superior mesenteric aneurysm. Surgery 92: 40–44

Yellin A E 1977 Rupture mycotic aneurysm: A complication of parenteral drug use. Archives of Surgery 112: 981–986

Index